C. Esposito · G. Esposito (Eds.)

Pediatric Surgical Diseases
A Radiologic Surgical Case Study Approach

C. Esposito · G. Esposito (Eds.)

C.T. Albanese · M. Fujioka · G. MacKinlay · N. Rollins
F. Schier (Ass. Eds.)

Pediatric Surgical Diseases

A Radiologic Surgical Case Study Approach

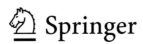 Springer

Ciro Esposito, MD, PhD
Associate Professor of Pediatric Surgery
Department of Pediatrics
Chair of Pediatric Surgery
Federico II University of Naples
School of Medicine
Via S. Pansini 5
80131 Naples
Italy

Giovanni Esposito, MD, PhD
Emeritus Professor of Pediatric Surgery
Federico II University of Naples
School of Medicine
Via S. Pansini 5
80131 Naples
Italy

ISBN 978-3-540-71515-3   e-ISBN 978-3-540-71516-0

DOI 10.1007/978-3-540-71516-0

Library of Congress Control Number: 2008939686

© 2009 Springer-Verlag Berlin Heidelberg

Cover design: Frido Steinen-Broo, eStudio Calamar, Spain

Printed on acid-free paper

9 8 7 6 5 4 3 2 1

springer.com

To my mentors, Ettore Ruggieri, Giuseppe Zannini and François
D'Allaines, who showed me the way to be a part of the medical world.
With gratitude,
Giovanni Esposito

To my father, the best pediatric surgeon I have ever known,
and the man who instilled in me the thrill, challenge and satisfaction
of lifelong learning.
I thank him for his continuous teaching, and for transferring to me
his love for the children we care for every day.
With gratitude,
Ciro Esposito

Preface

The idea to write this book was born about 3 years ago when we were changing the seat at the Unit of Pediatric Surgery of the University of Naples "Federico II."

We realized that during the 30-year activity of our unit we had collected a large number of rare and interesting cases of pediatric surgical diseases.

The difficulties met in the diagnosis of many of these cases gave us the idea to publish some of the most important ones, each with a collection of images accompanied by text providing a practical guide to reach the final diagnosis.

Since our idea was welcomed by numerous colleagues and friends, we proposed to Springer to publish this book.

All the authors who accepted to participate in our project (pediatricians, pediatric surgeons, pediatric and adult radiologists) are considered leading world experts in the diagnosis and treatment of pediatric surgical dis-

eases, and we are extremely grateful to them for their contribution and for devoting their time to producing such outstanding reviews.

Thus, with their precious help, we have created an educational text, focusing on more than 200 case reports of pediatric surgical diseases, which will certainly be very useful to all professionals working in pediatrics who need to prepare themselves when approaching a variety of diagnostic and therapeutic problems in conditions affecting infants and children.

We would like to thank in particular our associate editors, Craig T. Albanese, Masayuki Fujioka, Gordon MacKinlay, Nancy Rollins, and Felix Schier, whose great competence and extensive experience in this field helped us in writing, collecting, and organizing this material.

Ciro Esposito, Giovanni Esposito
Editors

Contents

Associated Editors

Craig T. Albanese, Prof.
Chief of Pediatric Surgery
Department of Surgery
Stanford University Medical Center
Division of Pediatric Surgery
Lucile Packard Children's Hospital
780 Welch Road, Suite 206
Stanford, CA 94305-5733
USA

Masayuki Fujioka, Prof.
Stroke Center
Neurology and Neurosurgery
Helios General Hospital Aue
Dresden University of Technology
Gartenstr. 6
08280 Aue
Germany
and
Kansai Medical University
2-3-1 Shinmachi
Hirakata City
573-1191 Osaka
Japan

Gordon MacKinlay, Prof.
Department of Pediatric Surgery
University of Edinburgh
Scotland
UK
and
Royal Hospital for Sick Children
9 Sciennes Road
Edinburgh
Scotland
UK

Nancy Rollins, Prof.
Department of Pediatric Radiology
Children's Medical Center Dallas
University of Texas
Southwestern Medical Center Dallas
and Holder of the Charles Cameron Sprague Chair
in Medical Science
1935 Motor Street
Dallas, TX 75235
USA

Felix Schier, Prof.
Department of Pediatric Surgery
University Medical Center Mainz
Langenbeckstr. 1
551101 Mainz
Germany

List of Contributors

Yves Aigrain, Prof.
Department of Pediatric Surgery and Urology
Hôpital Necker Enfants Malades
149 rue de Sèvres
75015 Paris
France

Craig T. Albanese, Prof.
Chief of Pediatric Surgery
Department of Surgery
Stanford University Medical Center
Division of Pediatric Surgery
Lucile Packard Children's Hospital
780 Welch Road, Suite 206
Stanford, CA 94305-5733
USA

Francesca Alicchio, Dr.
Chair of Pediatric Surgery
University of Naples "Federico II"
Via Pansini 5
80131 Naples
Italy

Michele Ametrano, Dr.
Department of Pediatrics
University of Naples "Federico II"
Via Pansini 5
80131 Naples
Italy

Brice Antao
Department of Paediatric Surgery
Leeds Teaching Hospitals NHS Trust
Beckett Street
Leeds LS9 7TF
UK

Giuseppe Amici, Prof.
Chair of Pediatric Surgery
University of Ancona
Via Corridoni 11
60123 Ancona
Italy

Giuseppe Ascione, Dr.
Chair of Pediatric Surgery
University of Naples "Federico II"
Via Pansini 5
80131 Naples
Italy

Richard A. Barth, Prof.
Chair of Radiology, Department of Radiology
Lucile Packard Children's Hospital at Stanford
Stanford University School of Medicine
725 Welch Road
Stanford, CA 94305-5654
USA

François Becmeur, Prof.
Service de Chirurgie Infantile
Hôpital de Hautepierre
67091 Strasbourg Cedex
France

Sophie Branchereau, Dr.
Service de Chirurgie Pediatrique
Hôpital de Bicêtre
78 Rue de General Leclerc
94275 Le Kremlin Bicêtre Cedex
France

Hervé Brisse, Dr.
Department of Radiology
Curie Institute
26 rue d'Ulm
75248 Paris Cedex 05
France

Luigi Califano, Prof.
Department of Maxillofacial Surgery
University of Naples "Federico II"
Via Pansini 5
80131 Naples
Italy

Antonella Centonze, Dr.
Pediatric Surgery Unit
Pugliese Hospital
Via Pio X 111
88100 Catanzaro
Italy

Christophe Chardot, Prof.
University of Geneva Children's Hospital
Paediatric Surgery Unit
Rue Willi Donzè 6
CH 1205 Geneve
Switzerland

Aurelie Chiappinelli, Dr.
Chair of Pediatric Surgery
University of Naples „Federico II"
Via Pansini 5
80131 Naples
Italy

Priscilla Chiu, Dr.
Staff Surgeon, Scientist-Track Investigator
Division of General Surgery
University of Toronto
The Hospital for Sick Children
555 University Avenue
Toronto
Ontario M5G 1X8
Canada

Fabrizio Cigala, Prof.
Department of Orthopedics and Traumatology
School of Medicine
University of Naples "Federico II"
Via Pansini 5
80131 Naples
Italy

Bruno Cigliano, Dr.
Chair of Pediatric Surgery
University of Naples "Federico II"
Via Pansini 5
80131 Naples
Italy

Alba Cruccetti, Dr.
Pediatric Surgery Unit
Salesi Children's Hospital
Via Corridoni 11
60123 Ancona
Italy

Anne Dariel, Dr.
Pediatric Surgery Department
Hopital Mère-Enfant
7 Quai Moncousu
44000 Nantes
France

Carolina De Fazio, Dr.
Gabriele D'Annunzio University
School of Medicine
Via Vestini 150
66100 Chieti
Italy

Luis de la Torre, Prof.
Hospital Angeles Puebla
Unidad de Pediatria
Av. Kepler no. 2143
Col. Unidad Territorial Atlixcayotl
Puebla CP 72810
Mexico

Concetta De Luca, Dr.
Chair of Pediatric Surgery
University of Naples "Federico II"
Via Pansini 5
80131 Naples
Italy

Ugo de Luca, Dr.
Pediatric Surgery Unit
Santobono Children's Hospital
Via Mario Fiore 15
80129 Naples
Italy

Marianna De Marco, Dr.
Chair of Pediatric Surgery
University of Naples "Federico II"
Via Pansini 5
80131 Naples
Italy

Vincenzo Di Benedetto, Prof.
Department of Pediatric Surgery
University of Catania
95100 Catania
Italy

Hana Dolezalova, Dr.
Chair of Pediatric Radiology
University of Naples "Federico II"
Via Pansini 5
80131 Naples
Italy

Sanjeev Dutta, Prof.
Division of Pediatric Surgery
Department of Surgery
Lucile Packard Children's Hospital
Stanford Medical Center
Stanford, CA 94305-5733
USA

Alaa El-Ghoneimi, Prof.
Department of Pediatric Surgery and Urology
Hôpital Robert Debré
48 Boulevard Sérurier
75935 Paris Cedex 19
France

Ciro Esposito, Prof.
Associate Professor of Pediatric Surgery
Department of Pediatrics
Chair of Pediatric Surgery
Federico II University of Naples
School of Medicine
Via S. Pansini 5
80131 Naples
Italy

Giovanni Esposito, Prof.
Emeritus Professor of Pediatric Surgery
Chair of Pediatric Surgery
Federico II University of Naples
School of Medicine
Via S. Pansini 5
80131 Naples
Italy

Paola Esposito, Dr.
Ss. Annunziata Hospital
Via dei Vestini 150
66100 Chieti
Italy

Vincenzo Farina, Prof.
Department of Pediatrics
University of Naples "Federico II"
Via Pansini 5
80131 Naples
Italy

Amedeo Fiorillo, Prof. Dr.
University of Naples Federico II
Department of Pediatrics
Via S. Pansini 5
80131 Naples
Italy

Donald Frush, Prof.
Duke Medical Center
Department of Radiology
1905 McGovern-Davison Children's Health Center
Box 3808 DUMC
Durham, NC 27710
USA

Masayuki Fujioka, Prof.
Stroke Center
Neurology and Neurosurgery
Helios General Hospital Aue
Dresden University of Technology
Gartenstr. 6
08280 Aue
Germany
and
Kansai Medical University
2-3-1 Shinmachi
Hirakata City
573-1191 Osaka
Japan

Frédéric Gauthier, Prof.
Service de Chirurgie Pediatrique
Hôpital de Bicêtre
78 Rue de General Leclerc
94275 Le Kremlin Bicêtre Cedex
France

Valerio Gentilino, Dr.
Department of Pediatric Surgery
Gaslini Children Hospital
University of Genoa
Largo Giannina Gaslini 5
16100 Genoa
Italy

Emanuela Giordano, Dr.
Chair of Pediatric Surgery
University of Naples "Federico II"
Via Pansini 5
80131 Naples
Italy

Chiara Grimaldi, Dr.
Service de Chirurgie Pediatrique
Hôpital de Bicêtre
78 Rue de General Leclerc
94275 Le Kremlin Bicêtre
France

Sylviane Hanquinet, Prof.
University of Geneva Children's Hospital
Paediatric Radiology Unit
Rue Willi Donzé 6
CH 1205 Genève
Switzerland

Yves Heloury, Prof.
Department of Pediatric Surgery
Hopital Mère-Enfant
7 Quai Moncousu
44000 Nantes
France

Salvatore Iacobelli, Dr.
Chair of Pediatric Surgery
University of Naples "Federico II"
Via Pansini 5
80131 Naples
Italy

Vincenzo Jasonni, Prof.
Department of Pediatric Surgery
Gaslini Children Hospital
University of Genoa
Largo Giannina Gaslini 5
16100 Genoa
Italy

Nadia Khan, Dr.
Department of Neurosurgery
University of Zurich
Frauenklinikstrasse 10
8091 Zurich
Switzerland

Korgun Koral, Prof.
Department of Radiology
University of Texas Southwestern Medical
Center at Dallas and Children's Medical Center
1935 Motor Street
Dallas, TX 75235
USA

Jacob C. Langer, Prof.
Department of Surgery
University of Toronto
The Hospital for Sick Children
555 University Avenue
Toronto
Ontario M5G 1X8
Canada

Marc-David Leclair, Dr.
Pediatric Surgery Department
Hopital Mère-Enfant
7 Quai Moncousu
44000 Nantes
France

Selvaggia Lenta, Dr.
Department of Pediatrics
University of Naples "Federico II"
Via Pansini 5
80131 Naples
Italy

Mario Lima, Prof.
Chair of Pediatric Surgery
University of Bologna
Department of Pediatric Surgery
Policlinico S. Orsola
Via Massarenti 11
40138 Bologna
Italy

Francesco Longo, Dr.
Department of Maxillofacial and ENT Surgery
National Cancer Institute of Naples
"Fondazione Pascale"
Via Semmola
80131 Naples
Italy

François I. Luks, Prof.
Division of Pediatric Surgery
Alpert Medical School of Brown University
Hasbro Children's Hospital
2, Dudley Street, Suite 180
Providence, RI 02905
USA

Marcelo Martinez-Ferro, Prof.
Professor of Surgery and Pediatrics
Deparment of Surgery
"Fundacion Hospitalaria" Private Children's Hospital
Cramer 4601, 3rd Floor
C1429AKK
Buenos Aires
Argentina

Gordon A. MacKinlay, Prof.
The University of Edinburgh
The Royal Hospital for Sick Children
Sciennes Road
Edinburgh EH9 1LF
Scotland
UK

Luigi Mansi, Prof.
Department of Radiology
University of Naples "SUN"
Via Pansini 5
80131 Naples
Italy

Antonio Marte, Prof.
Associate Professor of Pediatric Surgery
Second University of Naples
Via Pansini 5
80131 Naples
Italy

Luciano Mastroianni, Dr.
Pediatric Surgery Unit
Salesi Children Hospital
Via Corridoni 11
60123 Ancona
Italy

Girolamo Mattioli, Prof.
Department of Pediatric Surgery
Gaslini Children Hospital
University of Genoa
Largo Giannina Gaslini 5
16100 Genoa
Italy

Mongi Mekki, Prof.
Service de Chirurgie Pédiatrique
University of Monastir
CHU Monastir 5000
Tunisia

Carl Muroi, Dr.
Department of Neurosurgery
University of Zurich
Frauenklinikstrasse 10
8091 Zurich
Switzerland

Azad Najmaldin, Prof.
Department of Paediatric Surgery
Leeds Teaching Hospital NHS Trust
St. James's University Hospital
Beckett Street
Leeds LS9 7TF
UK

Deepika Nehra, Dr.
Division of Pediatric Surgery
Department of Surgery
Lucile Packard Children's Hospital
Stanford Medical Center
Stanford, CA 94305-5733
USA

Abdellatif Nouri, Prof.
Service de Chirurgie Pédiatrique
University of Monastir
CHU Monastir 5000
Tunisia

Francesco Onorati, Dr.
Cardiac Surgery Unit
Policlinico di Germaneto
Università Magna Grecia
Via Europa
Germaneto
88100 Catanzaro
Italy

Daniel Orbach, Dr.
Department of Pediatric Oncology
Curie Institute
26 rue d'Ulm
75248 Paris Cedex 05
France

Alfonso Papparella, Prof.
Second University of Naples
Pediatric Surgery, Department of Pediatrics
Via Pansini 5
80131 Naples
Italy

Pio Parmeggiani, Prof.
Professor of Pediatric Surgery and Chief
Second University of Naples
Pediatric Surgery, Department of Pediatrics
Via Pansini 5
80131 Naples
Italy

Annalisa Passariello, Dr.
Department of Pediatrics
Federico II University of Naples
Via S. Pansini 5
80129 Naples
Italy

Flavio Perricone, Dr.
Chair of Pediatric Surgery
University of Naples "Federico II"
Via Pansini 5
80131 Naples
Italy

Pascale Philippe-Chomette, Dr.
Department of Pediatric Surgery and Urology
Hôpital Robert Debré
48 Boulevard Sérurier
75935 Paris Cedex 19
France

Alessio Pini Prato, Dr.
Department of Pediatric Surgery
Gaslini Children Hospital
Largo Giannina Gaslini 5
16100 Genoa
Italy

Guillaume Podevin, Dr.
Pediatric Surgery Department
Hopital Mère-Enfant
7 Quai Moncousu
44000 Nantes
France

Pier Francesco Rambaldi, Dr.
Department of Radiology and Nuclear Medicine
Second University of Naples
Piazza Miraglia 3
80138 Naples
Italy

Attilio Renzulli, Prof.
Cardiac Surgery Unit
Policlinico di Germaneto
Università Magna Grecia
Via Europa
Germaneto
88100 Catanzaro
Italy

Samuel Rice-Townsend, Dr.
Division of Pediatric Surgery
Department of Surgery
Lucile Packard Children's Hospital
Stanford Medical Center
Stanford, CA 94305-5733
USA

Corrado Rispoli, Dr.
General Surgery Unit
Ascalesi Hospital
80143 Naples
Italy

Nancy Rollins, Prof.
Department of Pediatric Radiology
Children's Medical Center Dallas
University of Texas
Southwestern Medical Center Dallas
and Holder of the Charles Cameron Sprague Chair
in Medical Science
1935 Motor Street
Dallas, TX 75235
USA

Mercedes Romano, Dr.
Second University of Naples
Pediatric Surgery, Department of Pediatrics
Via Pansini 5
80131 Naples
Italy

Carmelo Romeo, Prof.
Department of Pediatric Surgery
University of Messina
Viale Gazzi Padiglione NI
98124 Messina
Italy

Giovanni Ruggeri, Dr.
Chair of Pediatric Surgery
University of Bologna
Policlinico S. Orsola
Via Massarenti 11
40138 Bologna
Italy

Maria Domenica Sabatino, Dr.
Chair of Pediatric Surgery
Second University of Naples
Via Pansini 5
80131 Naples
Italy

Francesco Sadile, Prof.
Department of Orthopedics and Traumatology
School of Medicine
University of Naples "Federico II"
Via Pansini 5
80131 Naples
Italy

Sabine Sarnacki, Prof.
Department of Pediatric Surgery and U 793
Hôpital Necker Enfants Malades
149 rue de Sèvres
75015 Paris
France

Antonio Savanelli, Dr.
Chair of Pediatric Surgery
University of Naples "Federico II"
Via Pansini 5
80131 Naples
Italy

Cristina Savanelli, Dr.
Department of Endocrinology
University of Naples "Federico II"
Via Pansini 5
80129 Naples
Italy

Felix Schier, Prof.
Department of Pediatric Surgery
University Medical Center Mainz
Langenbeckstr. 1
551101 Mainz
Germany

Jürgen Schleef, Dr.
Department of Paediatric Surgery
IRCCS Burlo Garofolo
Via dell´Istria 65/1
34100 Trieste
Italy

Françoise Schmitt, Dr.
Department of Pediatric Surgery
44000 Nantes
France

Reinhard Schumacher, Prof.
Department of Pediatric Radiology
University Medical Center Mainz
Langenbeckstr. 1
551101 Mainz
Germany

Luigi Scippa, Dr.
Department of Pediatrics
University of Naples "Federico II"
Via Pansini 5
80131 Naples
Italy

Alessandro Settimi, Prof.
Chair of Pediatric Surgery
University of Naples "Federico II"
Via Pansini 5
80131 Naples
Italy

Carla Settimi, Dr.
Department of Pediatrics
University of Naples "Federico II"
Via Pansini 5
80129 Naples
Italy

Giacomo Sica, Dr.
Cardiac Surgery Unit
Policlinico di Germaneto
Università Magna Grecia
Via Europa
Germaneto
88100 Catanzaro
Italy

Etienne Suply, Dr.
Department of Pediatric Surgery
44000 Nantes
France

Gianluca Terrin, Dr.
Department of Pediatrics
University of Naples "Federico II"
Via Pansini 5
80131 Naples
Italy

Claudia Tiano, Dr.
Department of Pediatrics
University of Naples "Federico II"
Via Pansini 5
80131 Naples
Italy

Juan A. Tovar, Prof. Dr.
Departamento de Cirugía Pediátrica
Hospital Universitario La Paz
P. Castellana 261
28046 Madrid
Spain

Antonino Tramontano, Dr.
Pediatric Surgery Unit
Santobono Children Hospital
Via Mario Fiore 15
80129 Naples
Italy

Jean Stephane Valla, Prof.
Department of Pediatric Surgery and Urology
Fondation Hôpital Lenval
Avenue de Californie 55
06200 Nice
France

Gianfranco Vallone, Dr.
Department of Radiology
University of Naples "Federico II"
Via Pansini 5
80131 Naples
Italy

Isabelle Vidal, Dr.
Pediatric Surgery Department
Hôpital Mère-Enfant
7 Quai Moncousu
44000 Nantes
France

Salam Yazbeck, Prof.
Department of Pediatric Surgery
San Justine Children Hospital
Montreal
Canada

Yasuhiro Yonekawa, Prof. emeritus
Dept. of Neurosurgery
University of Zurich
Haldenbachstrasse 12
8091 Zurich
Switzerland

Abbreviations

AP	Anteroposterior		**GI**	Gastrointestinal
ALT	Alanine aminotransferase		**HCG**	Human chorionic gonadotropin
AST	Aspartate aminotransferase		**ICU**	Intensive care unit
CE	Contrast enhanced		**IV**	Intravenous
CRP	C-reactive protein		**IVU**	Intravenous urogram
CT	Computed tomography		**MCDK**	Multicystic dysplastic kidney
DMSA	Dimercaptosuccinic acid		**MIBG**	Metaiodobenzylguanidine
ECG	Electrocardiogram		**MR**	Magnetic resonance
ERCP	Endoscopic retrograde cholangiopancreatography		**NMR**	Nuclear magnetic resonance
			NPO	Nil per os
EXIT	Ex utero intrapartum treatment		**PET**	Positron emission tomography
FDG	[(18)F]-fluorodeoxyglucose		**SIOP**	International Society of Pediatric Oncology
FLAIR	Fluid attenuated inversion recovery			
FNAB	Fine-needle aspiration biopsy		**STIR**	Short tau inversion recovery
Gd	Gadolinium		**US**	Ultrasonography
Gd-DTPA	Gadolinium-diethylenetriamine pentaacetic acid		**UTI**	Urinary tract infection
			VATS	Video-assisted thoracoscopic surgery
GER	Gastroesophageal reflux		**VCE**	Video capsule endoscopy
			VUR	Vesicoureteral reflux

Introduction

We think that a quick introduction is necessary to explain how this book is organized and how it should be read.

The book is divided into eight sections, six of them focusing on different parts of the human body and two sections dedicated to emergency, trauma, and tumors.

The book is easy to read and includes more than 200 case reports of different pathological conditions. Each radiological surgical case comprises no more than two printed pages.

The question page (Q) is a right-hand page; the answer page (A) is found overleaf.

The Q page contains radiological images (radiography, CT, MRI, scintigraphy, ultrasonography etc.), focusing on a specific case. Accompanying the figures is the clinical history of the patient along with some questions on the interpretation of the images for the diagnosis and management of the case presented.

The A page contains the interpretation of the images shown on the Q page, and possibly other figures of diagnostic procedures performed in the same case in order to obtain a clear diagnosis. The A page also includes information about the particular condition affecting the patient and the management of the case shown, including therapy and follow-up. Most case reports end with a short "Suggested Reading" list.

1

Head and Neck

Introduction

The patient of pediatric neurosurgery ranges from the preterm infant to the adolescent. The diseases addressed in pediatric neurosurgery include congenital disorders such as hydrocephalus, spina bifida, and craniosynostosis, particular types of tumors of the central nervous system, cerebrovascular diseases including vascular malformations and moyamoya disease, intractable epilepsy, and traumatic brain injury or acquired disorders. Pediatric neurosurgery requires team work that involves pediatric specialists from various fields including pediatric anesthesia, neurology, neuro-oncology, plastic surgery, psychology, and neuroradiology.

In this section, 13 pediatric cases of head or neck diseases are presented. These include brain tumors and cerebrovascular diseases. The imaging studies performed for the diagnosis of these pathological conditions are computed tomography, magnetic resonance imaging, cerebral angiography, and single photon emission computed tomography. The brain tumors discussed in this section are craniopharyngioma, ganglioglioma, medulloblastoma, choroid plexus papilloma, pilocytic astrocytoma, dysembryoplastic neuroepithelial tumor, anaplastic astrocytoma, and atypical meningioma. Cerebral arterial aneurysm, moyamoya disease, and moyamoya syndrome are also presented.

All patients underwent neurosurgical operations and had a good recovery after the surgery. We hope the readers will enjoy learning the characteristics of diagnostic imaging in these surgical cases.

Q 1

Nancy Rollins

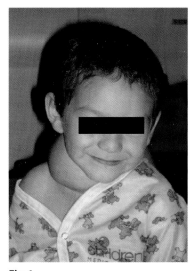

Fig. 1

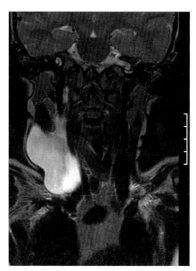

Fig. 2

A 4-year-old boy presented with a soft, slowly enlarging,
right cervical soft-tissue mass (Fig. 1).
- What is the differential diagnosis?
- What is the best imaging strategy?
- What does the MR image show (Fig. 2)?
- Should the lesion be biopsied or resected?
- Is there a nonsurgical alternative for treatment?

A 1

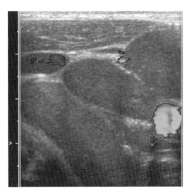
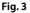

Fig. 3

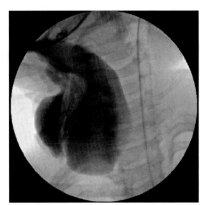

Fig. 4

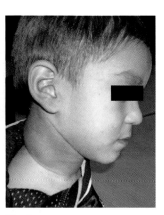

Fig. 5

The differential diagnosis includes a low-flow vascular malformation, neuroblastoma or nerve-sheath tumor, or possibly a rhabdomyosarcoma. Contrast-enhanced MR imaging is used to define the internal architecture of the lesion, e.g., solid vs. cystic, slow flow vs. high flow, and the extent of the lesion proximity to vital structures such as the carotid sheath. Lymphatic malformations are usually low signal on T1 images; however, the signal intensity on the T1 images may be similar to or higher than that of regional muscle if bleeding has occurred into the lymphatic malformation or if the fluid has a high protein content. The presence of fluid-fluid levels is almost pathognomonic of a lymphatic malformation. On T2 images and STIR sequences (Fig. 2), the fluid shows very bright signal although blood products may decrease in signal intensity. Ultrasonography may show a cyst(s) with absence of echoes or medium levels of echoes in high proteinaceous or hemorrhagic fluid (Fig. 3). The MR image shows a large, fluid-filled, unilocular cyst extending from the skull base to the supraclavicular region anterior to the sternocleidomastoid muscle. The imaging findings are classic for a macrocystic lymphatic malformation and biopsy is not indicated. The lesion is best treated with sclerotherapy.

Lymphatic malformations are composed of dysplastic vesicles or pouches filled with lymphatic fluid. The pouches of fluid may be large (macrocystic) or microcystic. Lymphatic malformations are often admixed with a venous malformation, e. g., venolymphatic malformations. Macrocystic lymphatic malformations and mixed venolymphatic malformations are amenable to sclerotherapy, whereas microcystic lesions and microcystic components of lymphatic malformations are usually not. Sclerotherapy is usually performed under fluoroscopic guidance, although ultrasonography is useful in puncturing nonpalpable lesions. The cyst should be emptied of fluid as much as possible. Contrast medium is injected to document correct intralesional positioning of the needle and lack of extravasation of contrast and of the sclerosing agent (Fig. 4). Effective sclerosing agents include OK-432, absolute alcohol, and doxycycline. OK 432 (picibinal) is a lyophilized mixture of a low-virulence strain of *Streptococcus pyogenes* mixed with benzypenicillin. Intralesional hemorrhage may complicate sclerotherapy, which is seen as an abrupt increase in the size of the lymphatic malformation and change from a soft spongy lesion to a tense slightly painful one. Intralesional hemorrhage does not, as a rule, require drainage since the hemorrhage will slowly resolve. Figure 5 shows the patient 2 weeks after sclerotherapy.

Q 2

Nancy Rollins

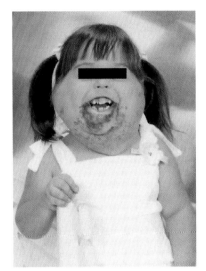

Fig. 1

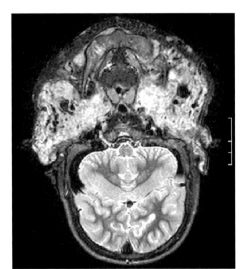

Fig. 2

A 3-year-old girl presented with a large disfiguring facial mass that failed to involute with high-dose pulsed
steroids and alpha interferon. Figure 1 shows the patient
at presentation. Figure 2 is a cross-sectional image of the
face.

- What is the differential diagnosis?
- Should this lesion be biopsied?
- What are the options for medical management?
- What does the MR imaging show?

A 2

MR imaging (Fig. 2) shows a large nonlipomatous mass which enhances and which has extensive involvement of the parotid glands and muscles of mastication as well as the infratemporal fossa. Branches of the external carotid arteries are dilated as are the internal jugular veins indicating a high-flow lesion.

The patient underwent sequential arterial embolizations using particles and coils with considerable decrease in the size of the lesion. Figure 3 shows the patient 1 year later. There is residual facial deformity due to residual fibro-adipose tissue that will be corrected surgically. Laser therapy will be used to treat the remaining cutaneous component.

Hemangiomas usually appear within 2 weeks after birth as a small red blemish or bump, which grows rapidly. The lesion may spontaneously regress, usually between 12–18 months of age. Complete regression results in the lesion being inapparent by age 3–5 years of age, with no or only minor residual scaring. In other patients, involution may take longer; 50% will involute by age 5, 70% by age 7, and 90% by the age of 9. Lesions which regress slowly are often associated with scaring, atrophoderma, stria, and cutaneous discoloration. Hemangiomas that require early aggressive treatment include those that are cosmetically deforming, growing rapidly, or obstructing vision, hearing, breathing, eating or, any other body function.

Systemic corticosteroids 2–3 mg/kg, given for 4-8 weeks comprise the first-line therapy for complicated hemangiomas; regression rates of up to 90% have been reported. Intralesional corticosteroid injections may be used for lesions that are smaller than 3 cm in diameter and well-defined and for lesions that show ulceration. Three to five intralesional injections are usually given at 6-week intervals; each dose should not exceed 3 mg/kg.

Hemangioma not responsive to corticosteroid therapy may be treated with both alpha and the 2a form of alpha interferon. However, treatment with interferon is associated with the development of irreversible spastic diplegia in about 20% of children. Vincristine is now recommended for hemangiomas with airway, eyelid, and orbital involvement, disseminated neonatal hemangiomatosis of the skin, liver, kidney, and cardiac failure. A weekly dosage of 1 mg/m(2) is injected intravenously. The dose is tapered depending on the clinical response. The reported range of injections is 5–25 with a length of treatment of 1.5–8 months. Dramatic response may be

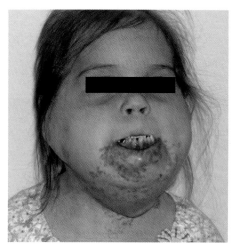

Fig. 4

observed within 1 month of treatment, although a slow protracted response may also occur.

Superficial hemangiomas may be treated with pulsed dye laser, but deeper lesions are not treatable with this modality as the depth of laser penetration is only 1–2 mm. For large multicompartmental facial lesions, arterial embolization is usually effective at accelerating the regression of the hemangiomas. The procedure involves superselective catherization of branches of the external carotid arteries and occlusion of arteries supplying the hemangiomas using particulate material and small endovascular coils. The internal carotid arteries should also be studied to assess what, if any, contributions to the hemangiomas arise from the internal carotid arteries and to exclude carotid stenosis in patients with PHACE syndrome (posterior fossa brain malformations, hemangiomas, arterial anomalies, coarctation of the aorta and cardiac defects, and eye abnormalities).

Sequential embolizations are needed to devascularize the lesions because arterial collaterals form rapidly. Potential complications of embolization include inadvertent embolization of the central retinal artery causing blindness as well as stroke and damage to the femoral arteries resulting in leg length discrepancy. If surgical removal or reconstruction is needed, preoperative superselective embolization is recommended to minimize intraoperative blood loss.

Q 3

François Luks

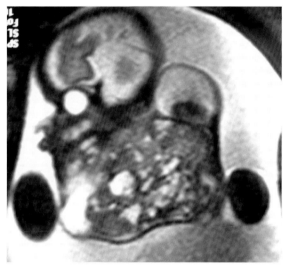

Fig. 1

On routine prenatal ultrasound at 22 weeks, a complex cystic mass was found in the cervical region of an otherwise normal-appearing fetus.

On subsequent examinations at 24 and 26 weeks, the mass was seen to increase dramatically in size. At 26 weeks, moderate polyhydramnios was noted. The remainder of the examination was normal.

MR imaging was performed to better characterize the mass (Fig. 1). At that time, the total size of the mass was larger than the fetal head. Again, polyhydramnios was noted.

- What is the most likely diagnosis, and what is the differential diagnosis?
- How should the expecting couple be counseled?
- Is intervention before birth indicated?
- How should the pregnancy be further monitored, and what might prompt early intervention? Should time, place, and/or mode of delivery be altered?
- Is neonatal intervention required? If so, how soon after delivery?
- What is the prognosis for a fetus with this condition?

A 3

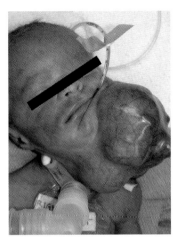

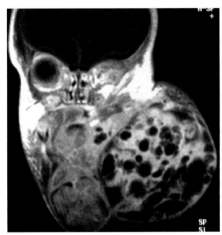

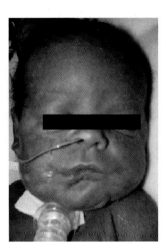

Fig. 2   **Fig. 3**   **Fig. 4**

The size of the lesion and its complex, cystic/solid and heterogeneous appearance are typical of a cervical teratoma. If predominantly cystic, the only other possible diagnosis would be a cystic hygroma.

Head and neck teratomas are far less frequent than pelvic and sacrococcygeal ones, and are less likely than sacrococcygeal teratomas to cause significant vascular steal, fetal hydrops, or mirror syndrome (concomitant maternal preeclampsia). However, the size and location of this lesion are likely to cause some degree of respiratory obstruction at birth. The presence of polyhydramnios suggests that fetal swallowing is impaired, causing further concern about neonatal respiratory distress.

In the past, the mortality rate of large cervical teratomas exceeded 50% because of airway obstruction at birth. In addition, the presence of polyhydramnios increases the risk of premature rupture of membranes and preterm delivery.

Because of the rapid growth of the lesion, several multidisciplinary meetings were held to plan an EXIT procedure: ex-utero, intrapartum treatment of the upper airway obstruction. This approach requires a planned and controlled C-section whereby uterine contractions are suppressed, preventing separation of the placenta. Only the head and neck of the fetus are delivered, leaving the umbilical cord in utero. Thus, an airway can be obtained while the infant remains on placental support.

Once the airway is secured, the cord can be clamped and the infant delivered. This approach requires a very high level of control and collaboration between maternal-fetal medicine specialists (perinatologists), maternal anesthesiologists, pediatric surgical specialists, and neonatologists. Obtaining an airway can range from simple orotracheal intubation to rigid bronchoscopy as a temporary airway and tracheostomy or even (partial) resection of the obstructing mass. EXIT procedures of up to 60–90 min have been described, although the average duration of this procedure is about 20 min.

Because of the polyhydramnios and the risk of preterm labor, it is important to choose the time of delivery by EXIT carefully: in the present case, the mother experienced some contractions at 29 weeks, and an EXIT was performed at 32 weeks. Several days before the planned procedure, glucocorticoids were administered to the mother to accelerate lung maturation.

At delivery, the diagnosis of cervical teratoma was confirmed (Fig. 2). Intubation proved impossible, and a tracheostomy was performed.

MR imaging was performed in the ensuing days (Fig. 3), and semi-elective resection of the entire mass was performed at 8 days of life. Despite the massive distortion of normal structures, these lesions are not invasive, and symmetry is usually restored postoperatively (Fig. 4).

Q 4

Giovanni Esposito and Ciro Esposito

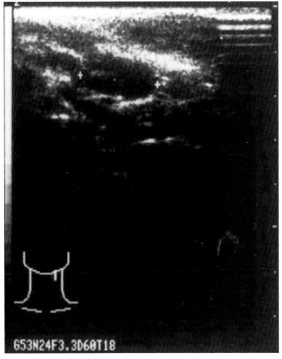

Fig. 1

A 4-year-old child without previous medical problems, apart from an episode of bilateral parotitis at the age of 3 months, was admitted to hospital after the mother noticed a swelling on the child's left cheek. After objective examination a painless mass was found with indistinct margins in the left parotid region. An ultrasound study (Fig. 1) and other examinations were performed, indicating the need for surgical intervention.

- What does the ultrasound demonstrate?
- What other examinations were performed?
- What was the suspected diagnosis?
- What was the surgical treatment?
- What was the definitive diagnosis?
- What was the follow-up?

A 4

The ultrasound shows a small hypoechogenic lesion in the left parotid region.

A fine-needle aspiration biopsy (FNAB) was carried out, which demonstrated the presence of adipocytes mixed with acinic cells at histologic examination.

The diagnosis was a lipoma of the parotid gland. The surgical treatment comprised superficial parotidectomy with conservation of the facial nerve. On the basis of a histologic examination of the removed specimen (Fig. 2), demonstrating the presence of mature adipocytes with abnormal mature and multilobular adipose tissue combined with inflammatory cells (Fig. 3), the definitive diagnosis was that of parotid lipomatosis.

The postoperative course was uneventful and the child was discharged from hospital 6 days after the operation. At the 5-year follow-up, the child had recovered completely.

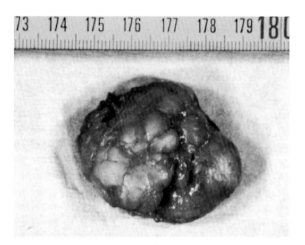

Fig. 2

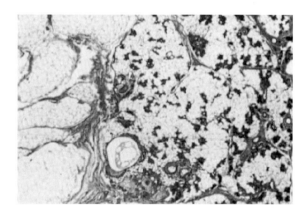

Fig. 3

Suggested Reading

1. Al-Arfaj AA, Arora RK, El Hassan AY, Al-Metwalli RR. Lipomatosis of the parotid gland in children. Saudi Med J 2003 Aug; 24(8):898–900

2. Holland AJ, Baron-Hay GS, Brennan BA. Parotid lipomatosis. J Pediatr Surg 1996 Oct; 31(10):1422–3

3. Sinha DD, Joshi M, Sharma C, Chaturvedi V. Infantile congenital parotid lipomatosis: a rare case report. J Pediatr Surg 2005 Sep; 40(9):e15–6

4. Som PM, Scherl MP, Rao VM, Biller HF. Rare presentations of ordinary lipomas of the head and neck: a review. AJNR Am J Neuroradiol 1986 Jul–Aug; 7(4):657–64

5. Walts AE, Perzik SL. Lipomatous lesions of the parotid area. Arch Otolaryngol 1976 Apr; 102(4):230–2

Q 5

Luigi Califano and Francesco Longo

A 13-year-old girl presented with a history of parotid swelling from 15 months, which was not related to eating. During this period she did not experience fever or pain.

When the girl presented to our department, she had already undergone many cycles of antibiotic therapy, without any result. The results of blood examinations were normal.

The surgeon asked for a CT scan with iodine medium.

- What does Fig. 1 show?
- Why did the surgeon perform this examination?
- Are there further examinations to be performed in this case?
- What pathological condition is affecting this girl?
- What is the best way to manage this condition?

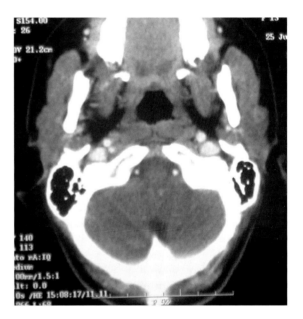

Fig. 1

A 5

This girl was affected by a parotid acinic cell neoplasm. The history and clinical examination already pointed to a parotid tumor. A CT scan with iodine medium allows one to gain more information about the precise location of the neoplasm and to define its borders and its relationships with closer structures.

Figure 1 shows a roundish, inhomogeneous lesion of 10-mm diameter, without peripheral anomalies compatible with pleomorphic adenoma or noninfiltrating neoplasms, localized in the superficial part of the parotid gland. There was no involvement of the neck lymph nodes.

For a preoperative diagnosis to be made, it is necessary to perform fine-needle aspiration biopsy (FNAB), which has very good accuracy with very little discomfort for the patient. Obtaining an almost-certain diagnosis allows one to plan the intervention with better accuracy and to prepare the patient for the surgical procedure. The FNAB in this case showed a solid proliferation of acinic cells arranged in solid blocks, suggesting an acinic cell tumor.

The patient underwent total parotidectomy under general anesthesia. A face lift approach was used on this young patient to minimize the effect of scars (Fig. 2). Moreover, in an attempt to avoid the risk of Frey syndrome, a temporalis fascia flap was used to cover the nerve and to reduce the gap left by the parotid gland excision (Figs. 3–4). No sign of facial nerve damage was evident after intervention. Histological examination of the surgical specimen confirmed the preoperative diagnosis of acinic cell tumor.

The patient was followed up every 3 months with ultrasonography and twice a year with CT in the first year, and then with ultrasonography twice a year and CT once a year. Four years after the intervention, the patient was free of disease.

Suggested Reading

1. Mathew S, Ali SZ. Parotid fine-needle aspiration: a cytologic study of pediatric lesions. Diagn Cytopathol 1997; 17:8–13
2. Orvidas LJ, Kasperbauer JL, Lewis JE, Olsen KD, Lesnick TG. Pediatric parotid masses. Arch Otolaryngol Head Neck Surg 2000; 126:177–84

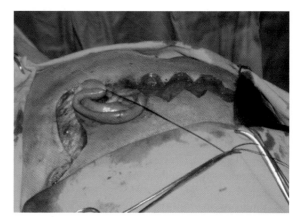

Fig. 2

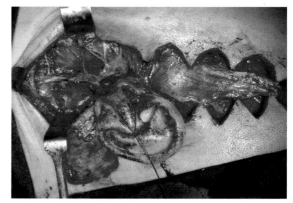

Fig. 3

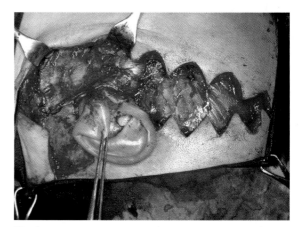

Fig. 4

Q 6

Luigi Califano, Paola Esposito, and Francesco Longo

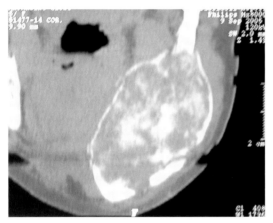

Fig. 1

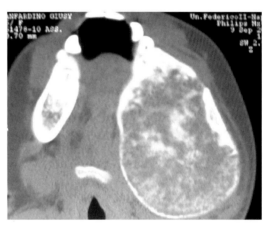

Fig. 2

A 3-year-old girl presented with mandibular swelling that had appeared 6 months earlier.

The girl had growth hormone deficit and psychomotor retardation, facial dysmorphism (telecantus), and an arachnoid cyst in the adenohypophyseal region. The child had the clinical picture of an atypical facial-cardiocutaneous syndrome.

After the girl's mother noted swelling of the mandible, a pediatrician performed CT (Figs. 1, 2) and referred the child to a maxillofacial surgeon.

- What do Figs. 1 and 2 show?
- What other diagnostic examinations can be performed?
- What is the diagnosis?
- What is the appropriate treatment?
- What is the prognosis for this young patient?

A 6

This child is affected by fibrous dysplasia of the mandible, a condition in which normal medullary bone is gradually replaced by abnormal fibrous connective proliferation. This disease is localized in the head in less than 10% of cases and produces monostotic or polyostotic lesions, isolated or in association with McCune-Albright syndrome.

This disease most commonly presents as an asymptomatic, slow enlargement of the involved bone. The monostotic form is the most common (80%) and more frequently affects the ribs, long bones, pelvis, jaws, and skull. Maxillary lesions occur more frequently than mandibular ones.

Fibrous dysplasia characteristically occurs during the first and second decade of life and becomes stable after puberty.

In the classic presentation, as shown in Figs. 1 and 2, the radiographic appearance is described as homogeneous radio-opacity with numerous trabeculae of woven bone imparting a ground glass appearance. Lesions of fibrous dysplasia may also present as unilocular or multilocular radiolucencies. There are no alterations in laboratory values.

A three-dimensional CT scan can be very useful in showing the complete extension of the disease and in planning preoperatively the margins of surgical intervention.

Typical histological features are represented by proliferation of fibrous connective tissue with trabeculae of immature bone tissue. A histological differential diagnosis with osteoma, fibroma, or Paget's disease can be difficult to make without the correct interpretation of clinical and radiological findings.

Once a jaw lesion is diagnosed, the extent of skeletal involvement should be investigated, with plain radiographs, total-body CT, or scintigraphy. In our case, there was only one lesion.

Because of the stabilization of growth after puberty, the treatment consists only of biopsy for confirmation of the diagnosis and periodic follow-up for small lesions and bone recontouring via a transoral approach to treat

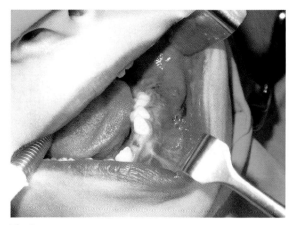

Fig. 3

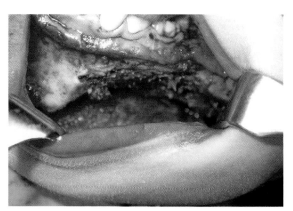

Fig. 4

functional or cosmetic disability (Figs. 3, 4). En bloc resection is unnecessary considering the lesion's slow-growing and non-neoplastic nature.

The incidence of malignant transformation is very rare, less than 1%, and is related to cases in which patients were treated with radiotherapy, which should always be avoided considering the benign nature and limited growth of the lesion.

Q 7

Luigi Califano and Francesco Longo

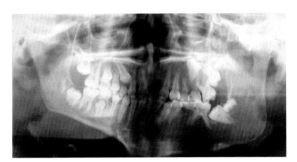

Fig. 1

An 11-year-old girl presented with a history of facial asymmetry that had started 18 months previously with dental crowding.

The patient was in general good health and had menarche when she was 10 years old. She did not complain of any pain or discomfort.

When the girl presented to our department, she had a deviation of the chin and a cross-bite and had already started orthodontic treatment without any result.

The surgeon asked for a panoramic plain radiograph followed by CT with three-dimensional reconstruction.

- What do Figs. 1–3 show?
- Should further examinations be performed in this case? If so, why?
- What condition is affecting this girl?
- What is the best way to manage this pathological condition?

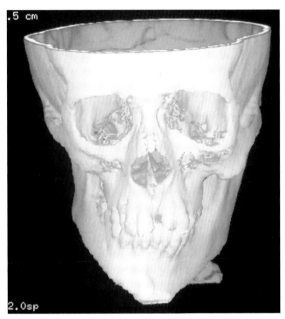

Fig. 2

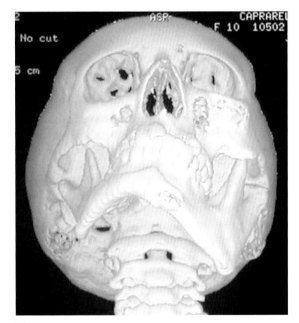

Fig. 3

A 7

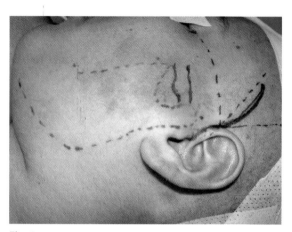

Fig. 4

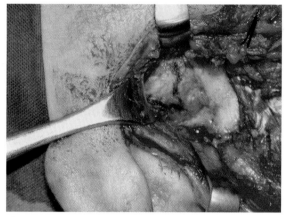

Fig. 5

This girl was affected by hemimandibular hyperplasia. Hemimandibular hyperplasia is a developing anomaly of the mandible which appears at puberty and often continues in the following years. Its features are asymmetry of the lower third of the face, deviation of the mandible to the opposite side of the affected hemimandible, and secondary growth anomaly of the maxilla.

A panoramic plain radiograph (Fig. 1) shows an elongation and enlargement of one side of the mandible, i.e., enlargement of the condyle, condylar neck and ascending and horizontal rami; the head of the condyle can be normal in cases of slow growth or enlarged in cases of rapid evolution. A cephalometric study shows variable dental compensation in the sagittal and vertical planes. CT with three-dimensional reconstruction (Figs. 2, 3) clearly shows the hemimandibular enlargement.

To manage correctly these patients, it is very important to collect all clinical data. In fact, a history of rapid changes suggests an active growth, while a history showing an old presentation and slow changes indicates inactivity or reduced activity of the condylar process. Bone scans are very useful for confirming an active growth, but there is a high risk of false-positive findings.

In cases of active growth, as in our case, condylectomy is the treatment of choice. The patient needs close follow-up and orthodontic treatment to prepare for a two-jaw surgery if the maxilla is also affected.

Our patient underwent condylectomy via a rhitidectomy approach to minimize scars and avoid any risk of facial nerve damage (Fig. 4). An intraoperative view of the condyle is presented in Fig. 5.

The patient was followed up for 3 years, with progressive improvement of the occlusion and facial symmetry.

Suggested Reading

1. Chen YR, Bendor-Samuel RL, Huang CS. Hemimandibular hyperplasia. Plast Reconstr Surg 1996; 97:730–7
2. Ferguson JW. Definitive surgical correction of the deformity resulting from hemimandibular hyperplasia. J Craniomaxillofac Surg 2005; 33:150–7
3. Marchetti C, Cocchi R, Gentile L, Bianchi A. Hemimandibular hyperplasia: treatment strategies. J Craniofac Surg 2000; 11:46–53

Q 8

Luigi Califano and Francesco Longo

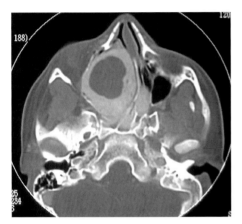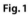

Fig. 1

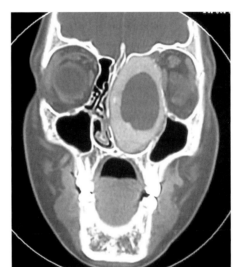

Fig. 2

A 14-year-old boy presented with facial asymmetry, nasal obstruction, and exophthalmus that had started 1 year previously.

The patient was in general good health. He did not complain of any pain, but reported diplopia.

To evaluate the airway status, the surgeon asked for a CT scan.

- What do Figs. 1 and 2 show?
- What is the diagnosis?
- What treatment plan should be followed?

A 8

The patient had juvenile aggressive ossifying fibroma. Juvenile aggressive ossifying fibroma occurs in young patients generally before the age of 15 years. The most common sites of occurrence include the maxilla, frontal bones, ethmoid bones, and paranasal sinus.

At clinical presentation, facial asymmetry, nasal obstruction, and exophthalmus with visual disturbances are generally present. The tumor presents a progressive and often rapid enlargement with thinning and erosion of adjacent bone.

The CT studies show an expansile, destructive, radiopaque, or hyperintense nonhomogeneous lesion (Figs. 1, 2).

The approach to juvenile aggressive ossifying fibroma is surgical. Depending on the size, location, and extension of the tumor, the goal of treatment should be complete excision, which in many cases requires an aggressive surgical procedure. En bloc resection should be evaluated in cases of large or recurrent lesions and can cause significant deformities especially in the case of orbital or cranial involvement.

Close follow-up is mandatory, since the reported recurrence rate for this tumor is between 30% and 60%; however, no case of metastasis has been reported.

Our patient underwent submental intubation to avoid the presence of an anesthesia tube in the operative field. The lesion was reached and removed via a bipartite Le Fort 1 fracture (Fig. 3). The fracture lines were fixed with biodegradable plates to avoid any alteration of the residual growth of the maxilla (Fig. 4).

The patient was followed-up for 3 years with clinical examinations and CT every 4 months, and at the time of writing was free of disease (Fig. 5).

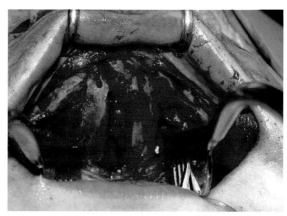

Fig. 3

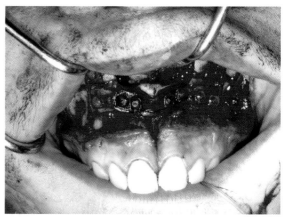

Fig. 4

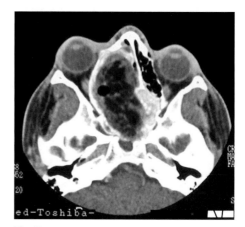

Fig. 5

Suggested Reading

1. Bertrand B, Eloy P, Cornelis JP, Gosseye S, Clotuche J, Gilliard C. Juvenile aggressive cemento-ossifying fibroma: case report and review of the literature. Laryngoscope 1993; 103:1385–90
2. Brannon RB, Fowler CB. Benign fibro-osseous lesions: a review of current concepts. Adv Anat Pathol 2001; 8:126–43
3. Marvel JB, Marsh MA, Catlin FI. Ossifying fibroma of the mid–face and paranasal sinuses: diagnostic and therapeutic considerations. Otolaryngol Head Neck Surg 1991; 104:803–8

Q 9

Craig T. Albanese

A routine screening ultrasound at 20 weeks' gestation was performed (Fig. 1) revealing a large mass (*arrows*) protruding from the fetal oral cavity (*open arrow*). The exact origin could not be delineated by this examination. There were calcifications (*arrowhead*) in the mass.

MR imaging (Fig. 2) was performed, which confirmed the diagnosis of an oral cavity-based mass (*arrow*). There was polyhydramnios (*asterisk*) secondary to the obstructing mass in the oral cavity.

- What is the diagnosis?

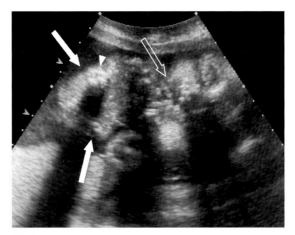

Fig. 1

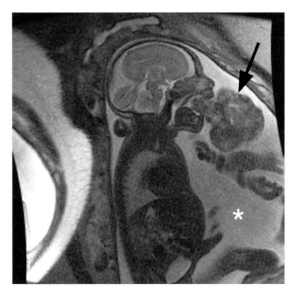

Fig. 2

A 9

This large mass with calcifications is most consistent with an oral teratoma (epignathus).

Because of the risk of airway compromise, the fetus was delivered using the EXIT (ex utero intrapartum treatment) strategy. During the procedure, the uterus is opened and the mass is removed while the fetus is still connected to the placenta. After resecting the mass (Fig. 2) that was emanating from the area of the hard palate, orotracheal intubation was performed, the umbilical cord cut, and the baby delivered. The child recovered uneventfully.

Suggested Reading

1. Abendstein B, Auer A, Pumpel R, Mark E, Desch B, Tscharf J. Epignathus: prenatal diagnosis by sonography and magnetic resonance imaging Ultraschall Med 1999 Oct; 20(5):207–11

2. Chattopadhyay A, Patra R, Vijaykumar. Oral tumors in newborn. Indian J Pediatr 2003 Jul; 70(7):587–8

3. Ozeren S, Yuksel A, Altinok T, Yazgan A, Bilgic R. Prenatal ultrasound diagnosis of a large epignathus. J Obstet Gynaecol 1999 Nov; 19(6):660–1

Q 10

Masayuki Fujioka, Carl Muroi, Nadia Khan, and Yasuhiro Yonekawa

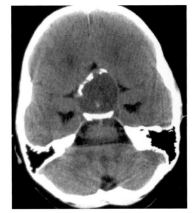

Fig. 1

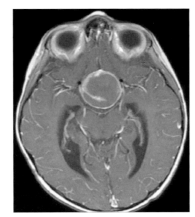

Fig. 2

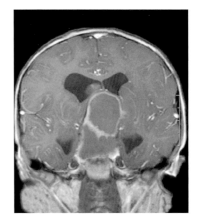

Fig. 3

A 6-year-old girl suffered from headaches, poor appetite, general fatigue, and projectile vomiting for 3 days.

According to her father, the girl had recently been saying that it was dark even during the day. The presence of increased intracranial pressure and visual disturbance was suspected.

On admission to hospital, the bilateral light reflex (direct and indirect) was weak. CT scanning of the head was performed (Fig. 1).

She had decreased skin turgor suggestive of dehydration associated with polyuria (low specific gravity). Her blood glucose level was normal and the plasma natrium level was moderately increased. She also presented with growth failure and short statue.

- What does Fig. 1 show?
- What pathophysiology should be suspected?
- What does the MR imaging study (Gd-T1-weighted) of the head show (Figs. 2–4)?

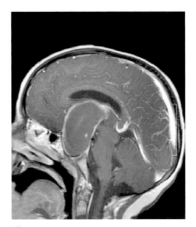

Fig. 4

- What diagnosis can be considered?
- What treatment should be performed?

A 10

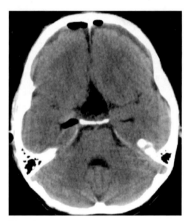

Fig. 5

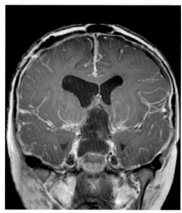

Fig. 6

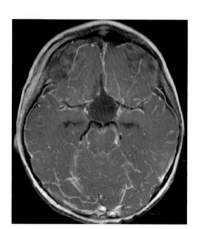

Fig. 7

The CT scan (Fig. 1) and T1-weighted MR images with administration of gadolinium-diethylenetriamine pentaacetic acid (Gd-DTPA; Figs. 2–4) reveal a cystic tumor extending from the sella turcica through the suprasellar cistern to the third ventricle. The CT scan shows calcification in some portions of the cyst wall. The tumor cyst wall is enhanced on the Gd-T1-weighted MR image. The MR images show dilatation of the bilateral lateral ventricle due to the obstruction of the foramen of Monro (obstructive hydrocephalus).

The differential diagnosis for brain tumor in this region includes craniopharyngioma, germ cell tumor, pituitary adenoma, glioma, and meningioma.

The simultaneous presence of dehydration and excessive urination of low specific gravity suggests diabetes insipidus. In addition, the patient had growth failure suggestive of pituitary dwarfism. The endocrinological study showed hypopituitarism with decreased blood levels of growth hormone, insulin-like growth factor-1 (somatomedin-C), and thyroid-stimulating hormone.

Craniopharyngioma is the most probable diagnosis for a suprasellar cystic tumor with partially calcified wall, leading to hypopituitarism in this 6-year-old girl. The tumor occupying the third ventricle was totally removed, without additional deficits, via an interhemispheric transrostrum corporis callosi and lamina terminals approach with the patient in the supine position.

The postoperative CT scan and MR images (Figs. 5–7) demonstrate the total removal of the tumor. The histological diagnosis is adamantinomatous craniopharyngioma. The characteristic features include peripheral palisading of nuclei, loose arrangements of squamous cells, and nodules of keratin and calcification.

In general, the features of craniopharyngioma on CT images include cyst formation with calcification and enhancement effects of the cyst wall and solid portion. The signal behavior of craniopharyngioma on T1-weighted images varies according to its cystic contents (hypo-, iso-, and hyper-intensity). The increased intensity on T1-weighted images seems to result partly from the high concentration of liquid cholesterol. On T2-weighted images, craniopharyngiomas are commonly hyperintense. The solid portions are heterogeneously enhanced and the cyst wall is strongly enhanced on Gd-T1-weighted images.

Postoperative hormonal replacement therapy was initiated with administration of adrenal corticosteroid, thyroid hormone, and antidiuretic hormone. After 6 months, the patient had improved visual acuity (right 0.2 and left 0.6) and no apparent recurrence of craniopharyngioma.

Q 11

Giovanni Esposito, Aurelie Chiappinelli, Gianfranco Vallone, and Ciro Esposito

An infant weighing 3,350 g, born at term after a normal pregnancy and delivery, had a mass in the submandibular left region, the size of a walnut, in front of the sternocleidomastoid muscle. On US the mass appeared to be a characteristic lymphangioma, and therefore it was decided not to treat the lesion but to follow its evolution.

Because the mass increased in size, hospitalization was decided when the child was 3 months old.

On admission, the child was in good condition, without any local or general anomalies except for the presence of the mass.

The left submandibular region was deformed by an irregular ovoidal swelling with a maximum diameter of 8 cm, showing partly cystic and partly solid consistency.

Laboratory test results were normal.

After another US study, an intervention was decided on (Fig. 1).

- What does Fig. 1 show?
- What was the diagnosis?
- What was found during the intervention and what was performed?
- What was the definitive diagnosis?
- What was the follow-up?

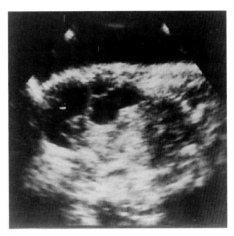

Fig. 1

A 11

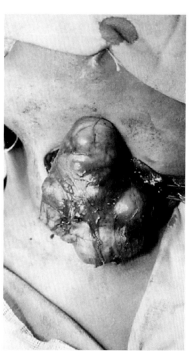

Fig. 2

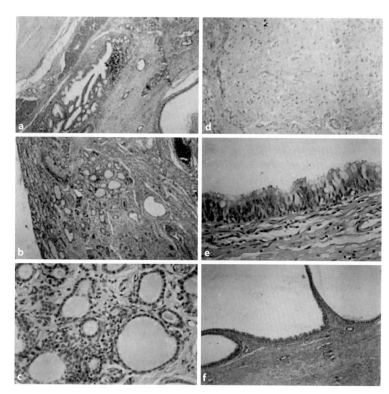

Fig. 3

The US shows a mass with a complex structure characterized by multiple eccentric fluid areas around a central solid irregular area.

The diagnosis was cervical teratoma.

At surgery, the multicystic mass was reached via a transversal cut along its maximum diameter. The mass was excised with some difficulties because it extended to the back of the trachea reaching the paravertebral space. The mass, measuring 6×4×2.5 cm, showed multiple small cysts around a central solid area (Fig. 2).

On the basis of the histologic examination, which showed embryogenic tissues including mainly mature thyroid tissue, the definitive diagnosis was that of thyroid teratoma (Fig. 3).

The postoperative course was uneventful, and at follow-up after 2 years the boy was in good condition without any relapse.

Q 12

Ugo De Luca

A 9-year-old boy had an asymptomatic, midline anterior cervical mass initially interpreted by his parents as the Adam's apple (Figs. 1, 2). The mass was mobile during swallowing, firm, and it had well-defined margins. The growth had been slow and no infections occurred.

The patient underwent ultrasonography (Fig. 3), which revealed a hypoechoic cystic mass very close to the hyoid bone.

- What is the diagnosis?
- What is the differential diagnosis?
- What is the treatment?
- What complications can be expected?

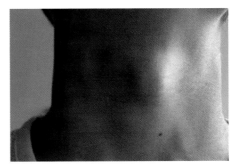

Fig. 1

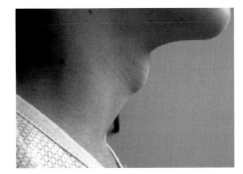

Fig. 2

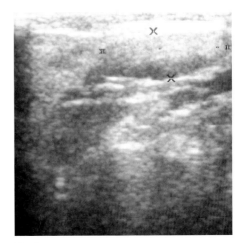

Fig. 3

A 12

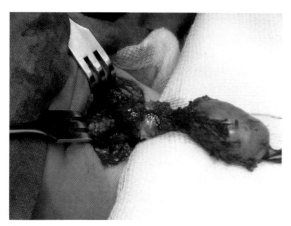

Fig. 4

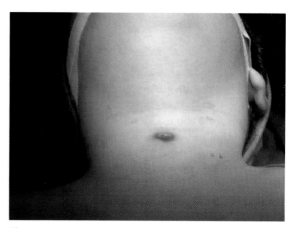

Fig. 5

The midline cervical mass was a large thyroglossal duct cyst (TDC). It did not become infected and slowly increased in volume.

The differential diagnosis must include lymph node hyperplasia and dermoid cyst.

The treatment of choice for TDC is surgery via the Sistrunk procedure. Once the surgeon has isolated the cyst through a transverse cervical incision, the hyoid bone body (1–2 cm) must be resected together with the cyst, and the dissection should be continued until the foramen cecum at the base of the tongue (Fig. 4).

Accurate hemostasis must be achieved and closure in layers realized. No drainage is necessary and the child can be discharged on the same day of surgery.

Complications of unoperated TDC are recurrent infections, fistulization (Figs. 5, 6) to the skin with consequent retracting scar, and possible, although rare, cancerization.

Complications of operated cases are postoperative infection and recurrence of the cyst, which is very high if the Sistrunk procedure is not radical; the recurrence rate is 4% in complete Sistrunk operations and rises to 20% if several cyst infections precede the radical operation.

Moreover, attention must be paid to the distal portion (toward the pyramidal lobe of the thyroid gland) of the thyroglossal duct, if present; if this is ignored, it could be responsible for relapse.

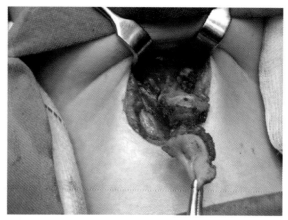

Fig. 6

Suggested Reading

1. C. Boglino, A. Inserra, A. Silvano et al. La chirurgia del dotto tireoglosso in età pediatrica. Minerva Chir 1993; 48:393–402

2. Bratu, J.M. Laberge. Day Surgery for thyroglossal duct cyst excision : a safe alternative. Pediatr Surg Int 2004; 20:675–678

3. J. Maddalozzo, T.K. Venkatesan, P. Gupta. Complications associated with the Sistrunk Procedure. Laryngoscope 2001; 111: 119–123

Q 13

Nancy Rollins

A 13-month-old girl presented with a slow-growing, soft, purplish mass involving the left buccal surface and lip (Fig. 1). The lesion was seen at birth as a small bluish region. The parents were told the lesion represented a small hemangioma which would involute with time.

- What is the differential diagnosis?
- What is the best imaging strategy?
- Should the lesion be biopsied or resected?
- Is there a nonsurgical alternative for treatment?

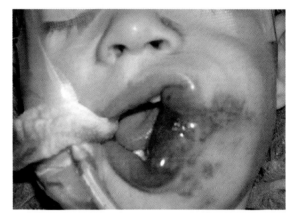

Fig. 1

A 13

The purplish lesion is a venous malformation. The patient underwent MR imaging using gadolinium-DTPA. An axial short tau inversion recovery (STIR) sequence (Fig. 2) and a post-contrast T1 spin echo (Fig. 3) sequence through the lesion were performed. The lesion is well-circumscribed, nonlipomatous, with moderately intense enhancement and no dilated feeding arteries. The lesion represents a congenital venous malformation. The patient underwent sclerotherapy with absolute alcohol repeated four times 4–6 weeks apart (Figs. 4, 5). Figure 6 shows the final result. Residual cutaneous discoloration was treated with laser.

The venous malformation should not be confused with a hemangioma. Attempts at surgical resection would be disfiguring and unlikely to affect a complete cure. Biopsy is contraindicated. The patient was therefore referred for sclerotherapy. Prior to sclerotherapy, cross-sectional imaging is mandatory and is best performed with MR imaging. MR with contrast is needed to define the composition of the lesion; i.e., venous, lymphatic, or mixed, as well as to assess the extent of the lesion and the proximity to neurovascular structures. Lesions that have a sharp abrupt transition from the surrounding tissue respond better to sclerotherapy than do lesions with ill-defined margins that cross tissue and fascial planes. Sclerotherapy is the injection of aqueous or oleic solutions into abnormally dilated vascular or lymphatic channels inducing damage to the endothelial lining and resulting in thrombosis, fibrosis, stenosis, and local scarring. Residual cosmetic deformity due to formation of scar tissue within the venous malformation is treated with surgery. Blood loss is minimized by the sclerotherapy and complete resection of the lesion is more readily accomplished. For deeper venous malformations that present with pain or functional impairment in the absence of cosmetic deformity, subsequent surgery is not usually needed. Large multi-compartmental venous malformations of the face and extremities often have phleboliths, calcified blood clots that are diagnostic of venous malformations and which are not seen in hemangiomas. These large lesions are usually not curable and treatment in the form of sequential sclerotherapy is designed to decrease pain and promote full functionality. Venous malformations usually demonstrate significant growth with the onset of puberty, especially in female subjects.

There are multiple agents used for sclerotherapy including bleomycin, sodium tetradecyl, ethibloc (etha-

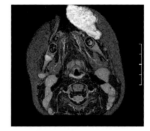
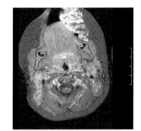

Fig. 2   **Fig. 3**

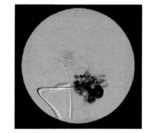
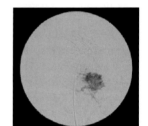

Fig. 4   **Fig. 5**

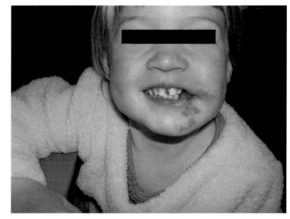

Fig. 6

nolamine oleate), absolute alcohol, and doxycycline. Bleomycin is a chemotherapeutic agent known to cause pulmonary fibrosis and should be avoided for nonmalignant disease in children. Absolute alcohol denudes the endothelial cells upon direct contact with the vessel wall. Permanent damage to the vessel wall results in complete obliteration of the vessel lumen, which prevents recanalization. Sclerosing agents are usually mixed with nonionic contrast and the installation of the sclerosant should be performed under fluoroscopic guidance to limit complications resulting from extravasation of the sclerosing agent into the regional soft tissue or draining veins.

Complications of sclerotherapy using absolute alcohol include skin necrosis, neuropathy, muscle atrophy, and cardiovascular collapse. Absolute alcohol is particularly dangerous, and installation of absolute alcohol into venous structures should be performed with careful monitoring of the patient's vital signs by the anesthesiologist. No more than 1.0 cc/kg ethanol should be given during sclerotherapy. Reported complications include respiratory depression, cardiac arrhythmias, seizures, rhabdomyolysis, hypoglycemia, and death. The treated site undergoes marked often very painful swelling.

Doxycycline is a tetracycline derivative commonly used for malignant pleural effusions via direct intrapleural injection. Animal studies have shown that doxycycline can induce a marked decrement in neural function when applied to the subepineural layers of the sciatic nerve in the rat, and phrenic nerve paralysis after intrapleural installation of doxycycline has been reported. Caution should be used therefore when a facial venous malformation involves the distribution of the facial nerve.

Suggested Reading

1. Berenguer B, Burrows PE, Zurakowski D, Mulliken JB. Sclerotherapy of craniofacial venous malformations: complications and results. Plast Reconstr Surg 1999; 104:1–11
2. Esterly NB. Cutaneous hemangiomas, vascular stains and malformations, and associated syndromes. Curr Probl Pediatr 1996; 26(1):3–39
3. Goyal M, Causer PA, Armstrong D. Venous Vascular Malformations in Pediatric Patients: Comparison of Results of Alcohol Sclerotherapy with Proposed MR Imaging Classification. Radiology 2002 223:639–644
4. Mason KP et al. Serum Ethanol Levels in Children and Adults after Ethanol Embolization or Sclerotherapy for Vascular Anomalies. Radiology 2000; 217:127–132

2

Thorax

Introduction

Pediatric surgical pathology in the chest can occur in the heart, the lung, the mediastinum, or the chest wall. Mechanisms of disease can range from congenital anomalies, infectious or inflammatory conditions, trauma, neoplasia, or disorders of organ function. This section addresses a wide variety of thoracic problems encountered by the pediatric surgeon, and gives examples of how these problems can be diagnosed and managed effectively.

The diagnosis of thoracic surgical problems starts with a careful history and physical examination. For many pulmonary, tracheal, and mediastinal problems, attention to the subtleties of breathing patterns, stridor, chest wall movement and symmetry, and auscultation will permit the surgeon to narrow down the diagnostic alternatives before any imaging is done. Similarly, it is on the basis of the clinical evaluation of the patient that the clinician will be able to prioritize interventions. The "ABCs" (rapid evaluation of *a*irway, *b*reathing, and *c*irculation) are more important in thoracic diseases than in any other part of the body.

There are several levels of imaging commonly used for the evaluation of thoracic disease. Chest radiography is one of the oldest and most commonly used modalities, and will often reveal everything the surgeon needs to know. In many cases the chest radiograph may be more sensitive than physical examination for identifying lung pathology, air or fluid in the pleural space, and mediastinal masses. More recently, the use of computerized tomography has provided additional information and sensitivity over plain chest radiography, but at the expense of significantly higher radiation dose, which must be kept in mind when using this modality. Ultrasound has had limited utility in the chest, because the air in the lungs interferes with the sound waves. However, for evaluation of the heart, blood flow in vessels, and pleural fluid collections, ultrasound offers excellent imaging without radiation. Magnetic resonance imaging also has the advantage of providing excellent images without radiation, but it has been underutilized in the chest. This is an area for future development.

More invasive diagnostic modalities include bronchoscopy, with or without bronchoalveolar lavage, image-guided needle and core biopsies, and video-assisted thoracoscopic surgery, which of course is increasingly being used for therapeutic purposes as well.

Finally, the widespread use of prenatal diagnostic techniques, ranging from the maternal alpha-fetal protein test to sophisticated ultrasound, has resulted in identification of many thoracic anomalies before birth. This has provided the opportunity for counseling, altering the location or mode of delivery, and in some cases performing fetal interventions for life-threatening conditions.

Q 14

Jürgen Schleef

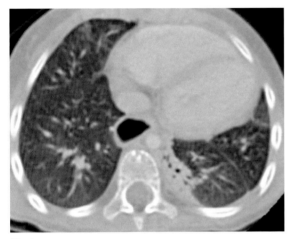

Fig. 1

A 4-year-old girl had a history of recurrent pulmonary infections from the age of 20 months, which were usually treated with antibiotics.

The mother informed the pediatrician that the girl had a prenatal diagnosis of a small lung malformation, but that a plain radiograph of the chest at the age of 1 year was normal. No further investigations were performed.

The girl was brought to our hospital again with fever and a cough. The white blood cell count was pathologic at 22,000; the CRP value was 8.2.

The doctor in the emergency department decided, on the basis of the history provided by the mother, to ask for a CT scan.

- What does Fig. 1 show?
- Why did the surgeon in the emergency department decide to perform a CT scan?
- What condition is affecting this child?
- How should this condition be treated?

A 14

Figure 1 shows a CT scan of the thorax. In the inferior part, a pulmonary malformation (congenital cystic adenomatoid malformation; CCAM) is visible. The radiologist described this malformation and ruled out extrapulmonary sequestration, since no separate blood supply from the inferior aorta could be identified.

The history of the child is typical of a connatal condition (pulmonary malformation). In most of these cases, a chest radiograph is not indicated to rule out a postnatal persisting malformation. A CT scan (or MR imaging) is mandatory in every case.

CCAM is a condition that is frequently found at prenatal ultrasound examination. If this pathological condition is not treated, persistent pulmonary infections resistant to antibiotic treatment are very frequent. In rare cases, an associated malignancy has been described in the literature.

The therapy is usually surgical. In extrapulmonary sequestration, an embolization of the supplying vessel is proposed by some authors as an alternative treatment.

In this case an atypical resection of the malformation was performed by thoracoscopy. Figure 2 shows the thoracoscopic view, while Fig. 3 shows the postoperative CT scan.

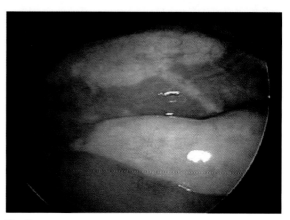

Fig. 2

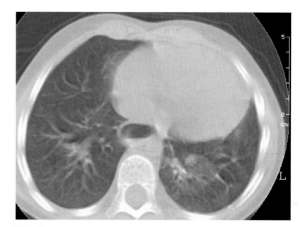

Fig. 3

Suggested Reading

1. Davenport M, Warne SA, Cacciaguerra S, Patel S, Greenough A, Nicolaides K. Current outcome of antenatally diagnosed cystic lung disease. J Pediatr Surg 2004; 39(4):549–56

2. Gornall AS, Budd JL, Draper ES, Konje JC, Kurinczuk JJ. Congenital cystic adenomatoid malformation: accuracy of prenatal diagnosis, prevalence and outcome in a general population. Prenat Diagn 2003; 15; 23(12):997–1002

3. Illanes S, Hunter A, Evans M, Cusick E, Soothill P. Prenatal diagnosis of echogenic lung: evolution and outcome. Ultrasound Obstet Gynecol 2005; 26(2):145–9

4. Pai S, Eng HL, Lee SY, Hsiao CC, Huang WT, Huang SC Rhabdomyosarcoma arising within congenital cystic adenomatoid malformation. Pediatr Blood Cancer 2005; 45(6): 841–5

5. Shanmugam G, MacArthur K, Pollock JC. Congenital lung malformations–antenatal and postnatal evaluation and management. Eur J Cardiothorac Surg 2005; 27(1):45–52

Q 15

Jürgen Schleef

An 11-year-old girl was brought to our hospital with a chest wall deformity. The mother reported that the girl was growing normally, but the deformity, which had been present since birth, was getting worse and the pectus had become "deeper" in the last year.

The girl was very shy, avoided sport activities, and told the surgeon that she sometimes felt short of breath.

The surgeon decided, on the basis of the history supplied by the mother, to ask for a CT scan of the thorax, an electrocardiogram (ECG), echocardiography, and a pulmonary function test.

- What does Fig. 1 show?
- Why did the surgeon ask for these examinations?
- What pathological condition is affecting this child?
- How should this condition be treated?

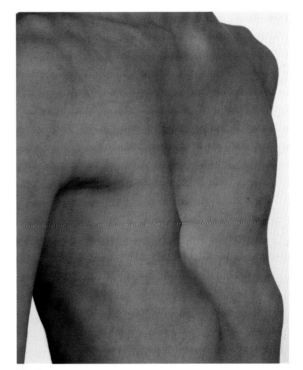

Fig. 1

A 15

Figure 1 is a picture of the chest of an 11-year-old girl. The deformity is a typical pectus excavatum. Note the retraction of the sternum.

Figure 2 is a CT slice of the thorax as requested by the surgeon. It shows the typical configuration of a pectus excavatum with a left side shift of the heart. The anterior thoracic wall is retracted.

The surgeon asked for the examination to rule out further associated diseases. In most cases, the heart or the lungs are not affected.

The treatment of this condition can be surgical. Different techniques are described in the literature. The most popular technique is a thoracoscopic-assisted approach with retrosternal bar implantation, as described by Donald Nuss. Figure 3 shows the clinical result 2 years after surgery on this patient.

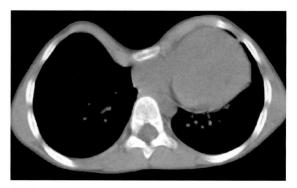

Fig. 2

Suggested Reading

1. Croitoru DP, Kelly RE Jr, Goretsky MJ, Gustin T, Keever R, Nuss D. The minimally invasive Nuss technique for recurrent or failed pectus excavatum repair in 50 patients. J Pediatr Surg 2005; 40(1):181–6; discussion 186–7
2. Goretsky MJ, Kelly RE Jr, Croitoru D, Nuss D. Chest wall anomalies: pectus excavatum and pectus carinatum. Adolesc Med Clin 2004; 15(3):455–71
3. Krasopoulos G, Dusmet M, Ladas G, Goldstraw P. Nuss procedure improves the quality of life in young male adults with pectus excavatum deformity. Eur J Cardiothorac Surg 2006 Jan; 29(1):1–5. Epub 2005 Dec 5. PMID: 16337131 [PubMed – indexed for MEDLINE]
4. Lawson ML, Mellins RB, Tabangin M, Kelly RE Jr, Croitoru DP, Goretsky MJ, Nuss D. Impact of pectus excavatum on pulmonary function before and after repair with the Nuss procedure. J Pediatr Surg 2005; 40(1):174–80

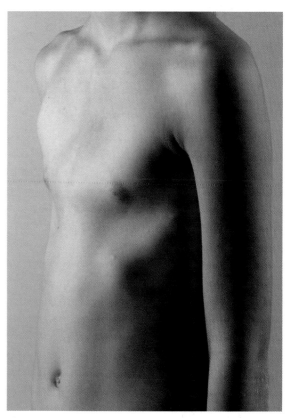

Fig. 3

Q 16

Nancy Rollins and Korgun Koral

A 2-day-old infant presented with respiratory distress.
- What does the chest radiograph show (Fig. 1)?
- What are the CT findings (Figs. 2, 3)?
- What is the differential diagnosis?
- What is the diagnosis?
- What are the types and prognostic implications?
- How is this condition treated?

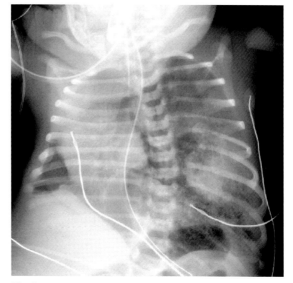

Fig. 1

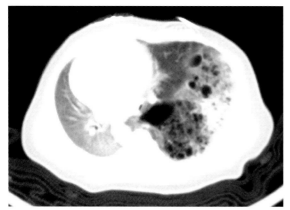

Fig. 2

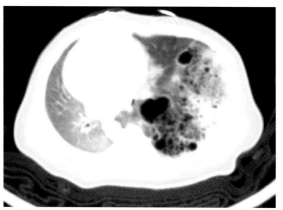

Fig. 3

A 16

There is a rightward shift of the mediastinal structures with expansion of the left hemithorax. A small air cyst can be appreciated in the left lung.

A shift of the mediastinum to the right is seen with a small right lung. There are multiple small cysts in the left lung with areas of solid tissue.

The differential diagnosis includes cystic congenital adenomatoid malformation (CCAM), pulmonary sequestration, congenital diaphragmatic hernia, and cavitary necrosis complicating pneumonia.

The diagnosis is CCAM, type 2. Type 1 consists of one or more large cysts. In type 2, numerous small cysts of uniform size are present. Type 3 appears solid on imaging, but has microcysts. Different types of CCAM do not have different clinical implications.

Treatment is surgical resection.

Suggested Reading

1. Donnelly LF. Pocket Radiologist: Pediatrics. Amirsys Ed. 2002.
2. Kuhn JP, Slovis TL, Haller JO. Caffey's Pediatric Diagnostic Imaging. Elsevier Ed. 2004.

Q 17

Nancy Rollins and Korgun Koral

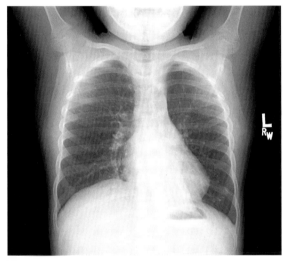

Fig. 1

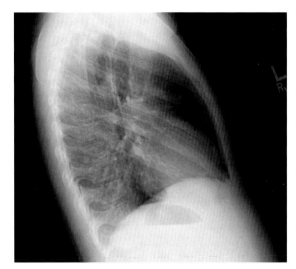

Fig. 2

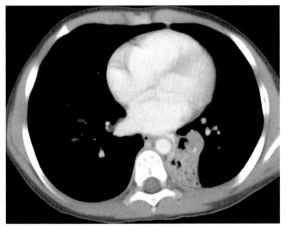

Fig. 3

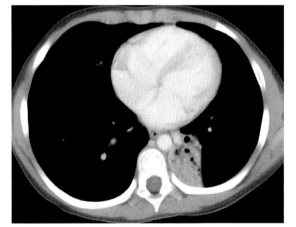

Fig. 4

A 6-year-old boy presented with multiple episodes of left lower lobe pneumonia.

- What are the findings on the posteroanterior and lateral chest radiographs (Figs. 1, 2)?

- What do the CT scans of the chest show (Figs. 3, 4)?
- What is the differential diagnosis?
- What are the types of this abnormality?
- How is it treated?

A 17

There is a well-defined air-space opacity in the posterior segment of the left lower lobe. On the lateral chest radiograph, the lucency of the lungs should increase from the apices to bases; in this case the lung bases are more opaque.

The contrast-enhanced chest CT shows an air-space opacity in the posterior segment of the left lower lobe. The surrounding lung parenchyma appears normal. There is a large vessel within the air-space opacity; however, no direct communication with the descending aorta can be displayed.

Pulmonary sequestration refers to a congenital area of abnormal lung which does not connect to the bronchial tree or pulmonary arteries. It is categorized as extralobar and intralobar. It is not possible to make this distinction on imaging. Extralobar sequestration has its own pleural covering, the intralobar type does not. Pulmonary sequestration usually affects the lower lobe of the left lung. The systemic artery entering into the sequestration is characteristic (different patient; Figs. 5, 6; *arrow*). Sequestration does not contain air, unless infected (Figs. 5, 6; *Ao*, aorta). Treatment is surgical resection.

Suggested Reading

1. Donnelly LF. Pocket Radiologist: Pediatrics. Amirsys Ed. 2002.
2. Siegel MJ, Coley BD. Pediatric Imaging. Lippincott Williams & Wilkins Ed. 2006.

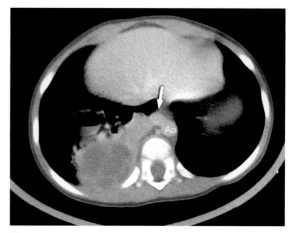

Fig. 5

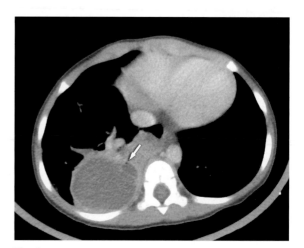

Fig. 6

Q 18

Abdellatif Nouri and Mongi Mekki

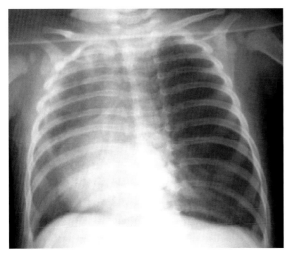

Fig. 1

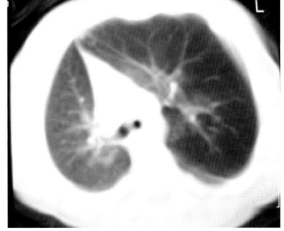

Fig. 2

A 20-day-old full-term male infant at birth presented with respiratory tachypnea with progressive apparition of respiratory distress and cyanosis.

On physical examination, his temperature was 37°C, breath sounds were diminished on the left hemithorax with hyper-resonance on percussion and shift of the mediastinum.

An anteroposterior chest radiograph was obtained (Fig. 1).

• What does Fig. 1 show?
• What are the three diagnoses that can be suggested?

The distress was not severe and a CT scan was performed (Figs. 2, 3).

• What do Figs. 2 and 3 show?
• Which diagnosis do you retain? What are the two differential diagnoses and how do you eliminate them?
• How do you manage this pathological condition?

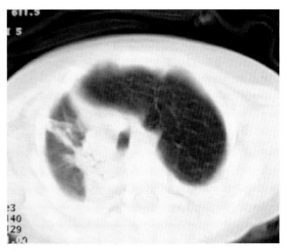

Fig. 3

A 18

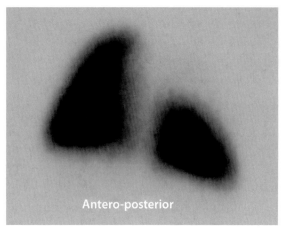

Antero-posterior

Fig. 4

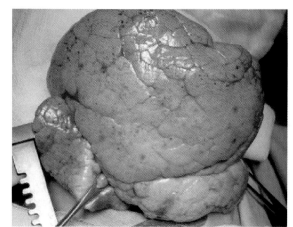

Fig. 5

The chest radiograph (Fig. 1) shows increased translucency of the left hemithorax with herniation of the expanded lung across the midline to the right side. The lower part of the left lung is markedly compressed. The heart and the trachea are displaced to the right and there is a widening of the rib spaces and a depression of the left diaphragm. A chest radiograph is usually sufficient for the diagnosis.

A left pneumothorax can be suspected, but it cannot explain the compression of the lower part of the left lung and there are bronchovascular markings in the hyperlucent chest. The second diagnosis is a huge lung cyst distended by air, but normally it takes an oval shape and is well delimited. The most likely diagnosis is lobar emphysema.

The CT scan (Fig. 2) confirms the emphysema of the left superior lobe with herniation of this hyperinflated lobe to the right side and a mediastinal shift. The right superior lobe is markedly collapsed (Fig. 3).

The most likely diagnosis is congenital lobar emphysema (CLE). The first differential diagnosis is acquired lobar emphysema by mucus plugging, granuloma or lymph node compression of the lobar bronchi. In this case, corticotherapy may induce the patient's recovery. This may explain spontaneous improvement of some lobar emphysema cases. The second differential diagnosis is compensatory emphysema which counterbalances a ventilation defect of the other lobes. If the distress is not severe, pulmonary perfusion scintigraphy can be helpful. The perfusion of the emphysematous lobe is normal in the case of compensatory emphysema and very decreased in the case of CLE. For our patient, pulmonary scintigraphy (Fig. 4) showed the absence of perfusion of the left superior lobe and confirmed CLE.

CLE presenting with distress in neonates requires lobectomy by thoracotomy or thoracoscopy. Figure 5 shows an operative view of the emphysematous superior left lobe.

After a 4-year follow-up, the child was free of symptoms and his chest radiograph was normal because of the compensatory growth of the remaining lung.

Suggested Reading

1. Koontz CS, Olivia V, Gow KW, Wulkan ML. Video assisted thoracoscopic surgical excision of cystic lung disease in children. J Pediatr Surg 2005; 40:835–7
2. Mei-Zahav M, Konen O, Manson D, Langer JC. Is congenital lobar emphysema a surgical disease? J Pediatr Surg 2006; 41:1058–61
3. Ozcelik U, Gocmen A, Kiper N, Dogru D, Dilber E, Yalcin EG. Congenital lobar emphysema: evaluation and long term follow up of thirty cases at a single center. Pediatr Pulmonol 2003; 35:384–91

Q 19

Abdellatif Nouri and Mongi Mekki

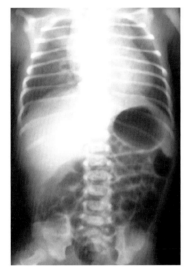

Fig. 1

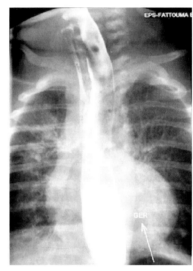

Fig. 3

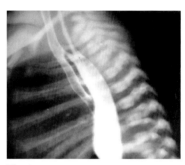

Fig. 4

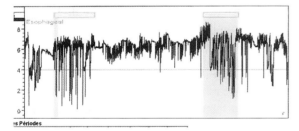

Fig. 2

A 2-month-old boy had a history of recurrent broncho-pulmonary infection, cough, cyanosis, and choking on feeding with alimentary vomiting since birth.

Apart from inspiratory crackles and marked abdominal distension, the physical examination was normal.

A thoracoabdominal radiograph (Fig. 1) was obtained.

- What does Fig. 1 show?

The pediatrician performed a 24-h pH-metry (Fig. 2).
- What does Fig. 2 show?

Medical treatment was prescribed without improvement. A barium meal study was performed (Figs. 3, 4).
- What do Figs. 3 and 4 show?

The medical treatment of this pathological condition was reinforced with the prescription of proton pump inhibitors without improvement of symptomatology.
- What diagnosis should be advocated?
- How do you confirm this diagnosis?
- What is the second exploration that may be helpful for the diagnosis and the treatment?
- How do you prepare this patient for treatment?
- What treatment do you recommend?

A 19

The thoracoabdominal radiograph (Fig. 1) shows a right pneumopathy with bronchial congestion and gaseous distension of the bowel.

The pH-tracing (Fig. 2) shows clusters of numerous episodes of gastroesophageal reflux (GER).

The barium meal study (Fig. 3) shows GER with opacification of the airway by the contrast substance.

The history of cough, cyanosis, and choking on feeding, in addition to the opacification of the airway during the barium meal, allowed the diagnosis of tracheo-esophageal fistula (TEF) to be made.

H-type TEF can be visualized by a tube injection esophagogram performed with the patient in the prone position after the introduction of the tube into the mid-esophagus. Figure 4 shows an H-type TEF above the third thoracic vertebra. Video recording is helpful because the fistula may open transiently. Recently, there has been a great interest in the use of three-dimensional CT for the diagnosis of TEF.

A tracheoscopy is the second helpful exploration for both diagnosis and treatment. It shows the opening of the fistula on the posterior wall of the trachea (Fig. 5) and specifies the distance between the fistula and the carina.

It is important to look for any associated malformations, which are observed in about 50% of cases and correspond to abnormalities of esophageal atresia. The patient's preparation includes medical treatment of GER, respiratory physiotherapy, and replacing oral feeding by nasogastric tube feeding or parenteral nutrition.

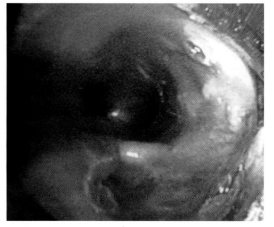

Fig. 5

The treatment of TEF is surgical, although there are some reports of endoscopic techniques consisting in the destruction of the mucosa of the fistula by diathery or laser and its occlusion by injecting glue.

A cervicotomy is the best approach for all fistulae located above the third thoracic vertebra (70%). Below this level, the fistula opening is at the carina and a thoracotomy or a thoracoscopy is needed.

This patient was treated by right cervicotomy. The patient's evolution was uneventful and the GER disappeared after 13 months of medical treatment. At the 3-year follow-up, the child was free of symptoms.

Suggested Reading

1. Allal H, Montes-Tapia F, Andina G, Bigorre M, Lopez M, Galifer RB. Thoracoscopic repair of H-type tracheoesophageal fistula in the newborn: a technical case report. J Pediatr Surg 2004; 39:1568–70
2. Bhatnagar V, Lal R, Sriniwas M, Agarwala S, Mitra DK. Endoscopic treatment of tracheooesophageal fistula using electrocautery and the Nd YAG Laser. J Pediatr Surg 1999; 34:464–7
3. Le SD, Lam WW, Tam PK, Cheng W, Chan FL. H-type tracheooesophageal fistula: appearance of three dimensional computed tomography and virtual bronchoscopy. Pediatr Surg Int 2001; 17:642–3

Q 20

Abdellatif Nouri and Mongi Mekki

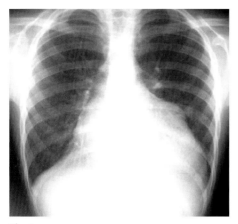

Fig. 1

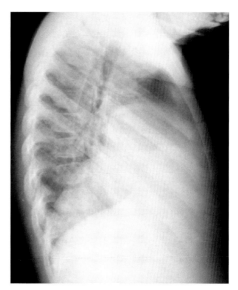

Fig. 2

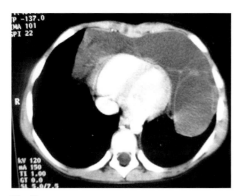

Fig. 3

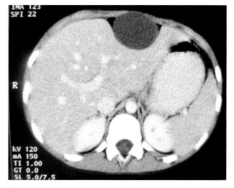

Fig. 4

A 7-year-old girl without a significant previous medical history presented with an epigastric and retrosternal pain, which was noticed 1 month previously, and with recent fever.

The physical examination revealed a temperature of 38°C, polypnea, and a decrease of the breath sounds at the low part of the left hemithorax, which was dull to percussion.

The pediatrician performed the examinations shown in Figs. 1–4.

- What do the recumbent frontal (Fig. 1) and lateral (Fig. 2) chest radiographs show?
- What do the thoracic and abdominal CT scans (Figs. 3, 4) show?
- Which diagnoses can be suggested?
- What is the most helpful exploration for the diagnosis and the surgical approach?
- How do you manage this pathological condition?

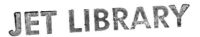

A 20

The frontal and lateral chest radiographs (Figs. 1, 2) show bibasilar densities silhouetting the right and left borders of the heart and the left hemidiaphragm. These densities are anterior to the heart and do not have the typical appearance of pneumonia.

The thoracic CT scan (Fig. 3) shows a multilocular cystic mass casting the anterior and lateral sides of the heart. The septae of the cyst are vascularized and there is no evidence of calcification. This cyst involves the inferior and medium parts of the anterior mediastinum.

The abdominal CT scan (Fig. 4) shows an extension of the cystic mass to the abdomen, probably through a retrosternal defect. This cyst causes a dent on the anterior side of the left liver.

A multilocular cyst of the anterior mediastinum may correspond to a teratoma or a cystic lymphangioma. The absence of calcification, ossification, and fat tissue stands against teratoma.

The ultrasonographic evaluation of intrathoracic cystic lymphangioma has been reported, but mediastinal lesions are better evaluated by CT scan. At present, MR imaging is the most specific exploration that permits one to identify the infiltration by the lymphangioma of the vascular, visceral, and neural structures.

Spontaneous regression of mediastinal lymphangioma has been rarely observed. Rapid enlargement of the lymphangioma, as a result of either hemorrhage or infection, can lead to compression of vital structures with life-threatening risks. Injection of sclerosing agents or radiation therapy has little success and many potential complications. A complete surgical excision of the lymphangioma is the best treatment.

In this case, after the resolution of fever and polypnea by administering antibiotics for 10 days, laparoscopy was performed. A multilocular cyst was discovered, probably corresponding to a multicystic lymphangioma extending to the abdomen through a retrosternal hernia (Fig. 5). Dissection through this defect allowed complete resection of the mediastinal cysts without any complications (Fig. 6). The retrosternal defect was repaired without any drainage. Pathological examination confirmed the diagnosis of cystic lymphangioma.

After a 15-month follow-up, the child was well and free of symptoms. CT scans showed no recurrence.

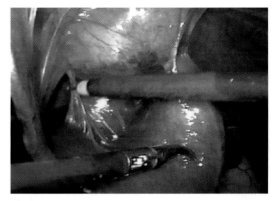

Fig. 5

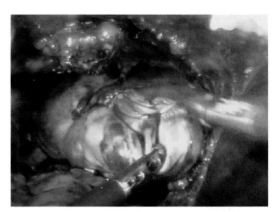

Fig. 6

Suggested Reading

1. Alqahtani A, Nguyen LT, Flageole H, Shaw K, Laberge JM. 25 years' experience with lymphangiomas in children. J Pediatr Surg 1999; 34:1164–8
2. Jeung MY, Gasser B, Gangi A, Bogorin A, Charneau D, Wihlm JM, Dietemann JL, Roy C. Imaging of cystic masses of the mediastinum. Radiographics 2002; 22:S79–93
3. Wu MP, Wu RC, Lee JS, Yao WJ, Kuo PL. Spontaneous resolution of fetal mediastinal cystic hygroma. Int J Gynaecol Obstet 1995; 48:295–8

Q 21

François Luks

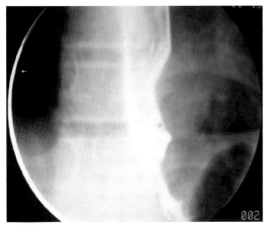

Fig. 1

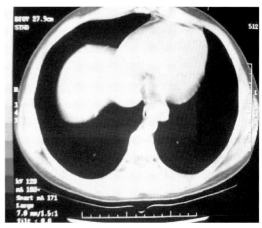

Fig. 2

A 14-year-old girl had been complaining of intermittent epigastric and chest pain for more than 1 year. On further questioning, she reported significant dysphagia with any type of solid food.

She was otherwise healthy, had not lost weight, did not report nausea or vomiting, and had an otherwise normal medical and surgical history.

She was referred to a pediatric gastroenterologist, who ordered an upper gastrointestinal contrast series (Fig. 1).

Following this, CT of the thorax (Fig. 2) and upper endoscopy (Fig. 3) were performed.

She was then referred to a pediatric surgeon, who proposed operative treatment of this condition.

- What does the upper gastrointestinal (GI) series (Fig. 1) show?
- What is the contribution of CT (Fig. 2) and endoscopy (Fig. 3) to the diagnosis?
- What is the optimal treatment for this condition? Which approaches can be offered?
- Is any other test necessary before proceeding with the treatment?

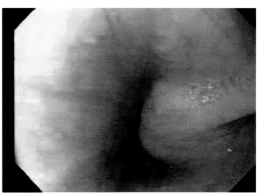

Fig. 3

A 21

Symptoms in this adolescent are vague, and the differential diagnosis list is extensive. Dysphagia, epigastric pain, and chest pain suggest esophageal pathology, but can be manifestations of gastritis and peptic ulcer disease, in addition to gastroesophageal reflux, achalasia, diffuse esophageal spasms, scleroderma, (chronically lodged) esophageal foreign body, or Mallory-Weiss tears, to name only a few.

The upper GI series (Fig. 1) clearly shows a filling defect in the distal third of an otherwise normal appearing esophagus. Not demonstrated in this image, but noted on the full examination, is an absence of gastroesophageal reflux and normal esophageal peristalsis.

An esophageal filling defect may represent an intrinsic esophageal mass, an intramural lesion, or an extrinsic compression. A classical example of extrinsic compression of the esophagus is *dysphagia lusoria* caused by a vascular ring. These filling defects are typically located in the upper esophagus. Tumors of the esophagus are very rare in children; leiomyomas and inflammatory pseudotumors are usually submucosal, while the (extremely rare) leiomyosarcoma may invade superficial layers. Intramural lesions in children are most commonly duplication cysts, whereby the duplication has a separate mucosa and submucosa, but shares a common muscularis with the native esophagus. The endoscopic image (Fig. 3) suggests an intramural or extrinsic process, as the mucosa is pushed in, but is not involved by the process. The CT scan (Fig. 4) is less useful, but demonstrates compression of the esophageal lumen to the right, and a mass effect that appears to be round and cystic.

With a diagnosis of esophageal duplication, resection of the lesion was offered. A left thoracoscopic approach was used, although thoracotomy has traditionally been the approach of choice. In general, a left thoracic approach is preferable for the distal third of the esophagus, whereas the middle esophagus is best approached through the right thorax.

Excision of the duplication cyst was performed after opening the mediastinal pleura (Fig. 5). Dissection of the cyst off the native esophagus was greatly facilitated by concomitant esophageal endoscopy, as the common wall between the two is very thin. Following removal of the cyst, the esophageal muscularis was closed with absorbable sutures.

The patient was discharged 4 days after surgery and has remained symptom-free since then.

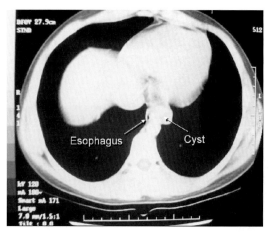

Fig. 4

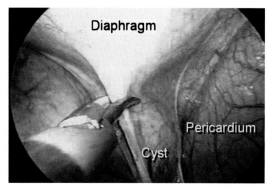

Fig. 5

Suggested Reading

1. Accadia M, Ascione L, De Michele M, et al. Esophageal duplication cyst: a challenging diagnosis of a paracardiac mass. Echocardiography. 2004 Aug; 21(6):551–4

2. Cheynel N, Rat P, Couailler JF, et al. Tubular duplication of the esophagus. Contribution of magnetic resonance imaging in anatomical analysis before surgery. Surg Radiol Anat 2000; 22(5–6):289–91

3. Herbella FA, Tedesco P, Muthusamy R, Patti MG. Thoracoscopic resection of esophageal duplication cysts. Dis Esophagus 2006; 19(2):132–4

4. Joyce AM, Zhang PJ, Kochman ML. Complete endoscopic resection of an esophageal duplication cyst (with video). Gastrointest Endosc 2006 Aug; 64(2):288–9

5. Michel JL, Revillon Y, Montupet P, et al. Thoracoscopic treatment of mediastinal cysts in children. J Pediatr Surg 1998 Dec; 33(12):1745–8

Q 22

François Luks

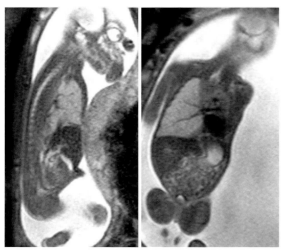

Fig. 1

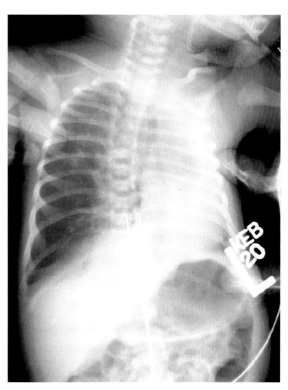

Fig. 2

At 21 weeks of gestation, a fetus was found to have a right-sided chest lesion on routine ultrasonography. The mother was referred for level-2 ultrasonography (detailed examination) and MR imaging of the fetus (Fig. 1).

- What is the differential diagnosis of a chest lesion in a fetus?
- What are the recommendations to the expecting couple?
- Which antenatal interventions, if any, might be considered?
- What is the predicted outcome of a chest lesion in the fetus?

On subsequent ultrasound examinations, at 25, 28, and 32 weeks, the lesion became less obvious, although its size remained stable. The previously noted mediastinal shift (toward the left) gradually resolved.

At birth (38 weeks' gestation), the infant had no respiratory distress and had normal APGAR scores. A chest radiograph within hours of delivery was essentially unremarkable.

At 3 weeks of life, the infant developed increasing dyspnea and tachypnea. A chest radiograph was obtained (Fig. 2). The patient underwent an urgent surgical procedure.

- What does the radiograph in Fig. 2 demonstrate?
- What is the diagnosis, based on this radiograph and an antenatal history of a right-sided chest lesion?

A 22

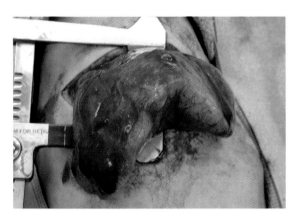

Fig. 3

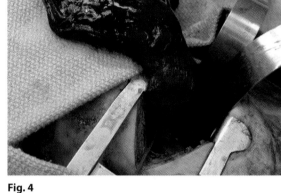

Fig. 4

Fetal chest lesions represent a variety of conditions of seemingly different origins. However, they have more in common than previously realized. The differential diagnosis of a congenital cystic lung lesion is bronchogenic cyst, intralobar and extralobar pulmonary sequestration, and congenital cystic adenomatoid malformation (CCAM). In addition, congenital diaphragmatic hernia may sometimes be mistaken for a primary lesion of the chest.

Congenital lobar emphysema (CLE) is not strictly speaking a cystic lesion of the lung, but is often part of the differential diagnosis. This condition usually occurs in the right middle lobe, presumably as a result of a temporary and/or incomplete occlusion of the right middle lobe bronchus. As a result, fluid trapping distal to the stenosis or obstruction causes dilatation and attenuation of the distal bronchi and an emphysematous appearance of the affected lobe. In the present case, the MR image clearly shows an enlarged right middle lobe, with preservation of the lobar vascular anatomy. This, therefore, is congenital lobar emphysema.

Most congenital cystic lung lesions do not cause fetal distress. If they become very large, they may cause mediastinal shift and hydrops, presumably from impaired systemic venous return. In utero intervention should only be considered in cases of (impending) hydrops. Large,

unilocular cysts can be drained (double pigtail catheter). Solid or complex lesions may require open fetal surgery. However, most lesions, even large ones, will start to regress around 26–28 weeks, and may hardly be detectable at birth. In CLE, spontaneous resolution of the bronchial obstruction and drainage of lung fluid may lead to resolution of the ultrasound findings (as was the case here), but the weakness of the bronchi and bronchioles persists, leading to a risk of air trapping and sudden respiratory distress after birth.

Although the infant was asymptomatic at birth, progressive air trapping in the right middle lobe led to respiratory distress at 3 weeks of life. The repeat chest radiograph (Fig. 2) shows a dramatically overinflated right lung and significant shift of the mediastinum to the left.

This confirmed the diagnosis of CLE, and the patient underwent a right thoracotomy and resection of a severely enlarged and emphysematous right middle lobe (Figs. 3, 4). Figure 3 shows the protrusion through the wound of an extremely hyperinflated right middle lobe. Figure 4 shows the emphysematous and floppy distension of the right middle lobe.

The patient recovered well, was discharged on postoperative day 5, and has been well since then.

Suggested Reading

1. Truitt AK, Carr SR, Cassese J, et al. Perinatal management of congenital cystic lung lesions in the age of minimally invasive surgery. J Pediatr Surg 2006 May; 41(5):893–6

2. Tander B, Yalcin M, Yilmaz B, et al. Congenital lobar emphysema: a clinicopathologic evaluation of 14 cases. Eur J Pediatr Surg 2003 Apr; 13(2):108–11

3. Williams HJ, Johnson KJ. Imaging of congenital cystic lung lesions. Paediatr Respir Rev 2002 Jun; 3(2):120–7

Q 23

Mario Lima and Giovanni Ruggeri

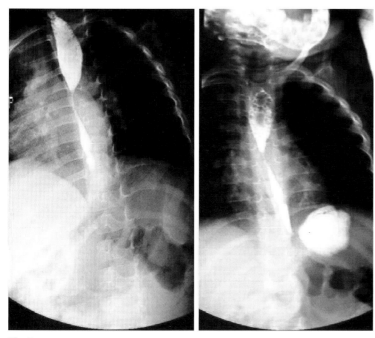

Fig. 1

A malnourished 2 year-old boy, coming from a developing country (Mali, Africa), presented with serious dysphagia. A barium swallow was performed (Fig. 1).

- What does Fig. 1 show?
- What other examinations could be helpful for the diagnosis?
- What is the diagnosis?
- What should be done in similar cases to reach a diagnosis?
- What is the treatment?
- What did the surgeon do in this particular case?
- What is the outcome of the native esophagus?

A 23

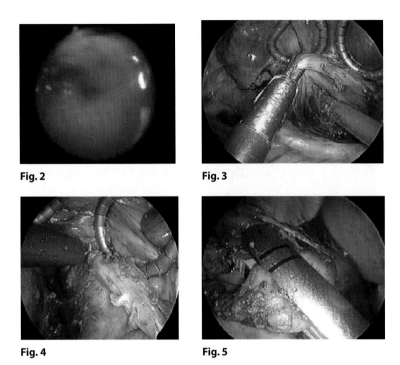

Fig. 2

Fig. 3

Fig. 4

Fig. 5

The young boy had accidentally ingested some household cleaner he had found in a bottle.

The barium swallow shows a dilation of the proximal part of the esophagus and a considerable narrowing of the medial part, making it difficult for the contrast medium to reach the stomach.

The surgeon performed an esophagoscopy (Fig. 2): it shows esophagitis caused by the caustic ingestion, which has caused stenosis of the medial third of the esophagus.

Caustic ingestion is frequent in children under 5 years of age; 90% of cases are a result of alkali burns and 10% are related to acid ingestion. The most common agents involved are potassium hydroxide, sodium hydroxide, and sulfuric acid. Solid granular forms of caustic cleansers are usually irritating and more difficult to swallow than liquid forms, and therefore severe injuries are usually associated with ingestion of liquid agents. With all substances, the volume ingested and the time the mucosa is exposed to the agent determine the extent and depth of the injury.

The management of corrosive injuries is well codified: esophagoscopy is mandatory whenever caustic ingestion is suspected, because it determines whether the esophagus has been injured. It should be performed within the first 24–48 h for diagnosis to be made. With a flexible scope, the entire esophagus may be visualized and the stomach may also be examined. A contrast esophagogram (with water-soluble contrast) should be obtained after 10–14 days; it shows the nature of the esophageal motility, which has predictive value for severe injury and extensive stricture formation. The study can be repeated over time to gain more information.

The goal of treatment is to avoid stricture formation and prevent sepsis. Patients are treated with systemic antibiotics for 7–14 days; prednisone (2–4 mg/kg per day) is often administered for 3–6 weeks. An oral liquid diet followed by soft solids after 2–3 days may be administered. In cases of severe injury, it is best to insert a feeding tube both for enteral nutrition and to maintain access to the esophagus for later bougienage. Concomitant use of acid-secreting inhibitors is widespread but their efficacy has not been proven.

Generally, an aggressive and frequent cycle of dilations allows for recovery of the native esophagus. In our case, this was not possible, and therefore an esophageal replacement was necessary. In our department, we prefer to use the colon.

The esophageal remnant is at high long-term risk for neoplastic degeneration, and so we proceeded with esophagectomy, which was performed thoracoscopically (Figs. 3–5). The child returned to his country and was reported to be doing well.

Q 24

Mario Lima and Giovanni Ruggeri

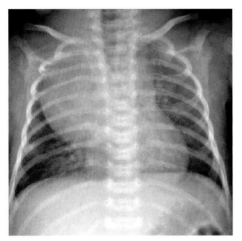

Fig. 1

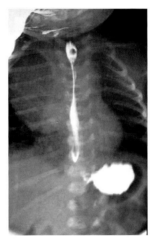

Fig. 2

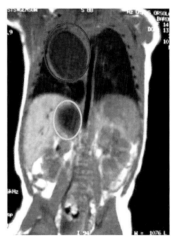

Fig. 3

A 7-day-old newborn was brought to our department with respiratory distress, dysphagia, excessive weight loss, sialorrhea, and frequent regurgitations.

A chest radiograph was acquired (Fig. 1).

- What do you see in Fig. 1?
- Which examination would you perform next? What does it show?
- What is the differential diagnosis?

The surgeon then decided to obtain an esophagogram (see Fig. 2).

- Why did the surgeon order an esophagogram (Fig. 2)? What does it show?
- What did the surgeon do in this case?
- What is the follow-up of this patient?

A 24

The newborn was affected by an esophageal duplication. These duplications are found in the posterior mediastinum and consist of a smooth muscle-walled structure containing mucosal epithelium including gastric heterotopic tissue. The fluid content is ordinarily clear, colorless, and thinly mucoid. Most duplications are 2–4 cm, round, and cystic and can reach huge sizes that may fill the entire thorax.

The chest radiograph shows a large cystic mass, with a clean and regular outline, which occupies a big part of the right hemithorax.

MR imaging was performed. This examination is important so as to also evaluate potential communication with the neural canal. It shows a 4-cm mass in the posterior mediastinum, adjacent to the esophagus, with compressive effect on the right bronchial system (Fig. 3, *red circle*); another 3-cm mass is visible in the right subdiaphragmatic space (*yellow circle*). Both masses have a fluid content. It is not uncommon (10%–15%) for a patient with a mediastinal enteric cyst to have an intraabdominal intestinal duplication.

In the differential diagnosis of mediastinal masses, many pathologies must be considered. They can be divided into two groups: mediastinal cysts and tumors. The former includes thymic, enteric, pericardial, dermoid and bronchogenic cysts and cystic hygromas; the latter includes lymphomas (Hodgkin and non-Hodgkin), neurogenic tumors (ganglioneuroma, neurofibroma, neuroblastoma), thymomas, teratomas, and other rare tumors (hemangiomas, lipomas, rhabdomyosarcomas).

In 20% of the cases the cyst may communicate with the esophagus. This is why the surgeon decided to perform the barium swallow (Fig. 2). In our case there was no communication with the esophagus, which was, instead, compressed, as can be seen by the narrowing in the medial part.

The esophageal duplication was excised thoracoscopically, while the subdiaphragmatic one, which proved to be a jejunal duplication, was removed laparoscopically.

One month after surgery, another barium swallow was performed (see Fig. 4), which showed normal esophageal canalization and gastroesophageal reflux, not related to surgery; for this reason, the young girl undergoes periodic endoscopic checkups.

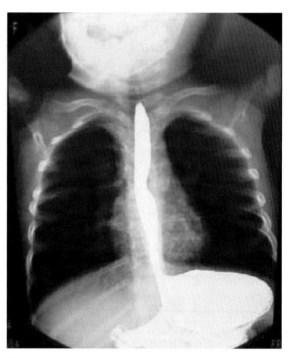

Fig. 4

Suggested Reading

1. Bratu I et al. Foregut duplications: is there an advantage to thoracoscopic resection? J Pediatr Surg 2005; 40:138–41
2. Michel JL et al. Thoracoscopic treatment of mediastinal cysts in children. J Pediatr Surg 1998; 33:1745–8
3. Soares-Oliveira M et al. Intestinal duplications. A survey of 18 cases. An Esp Pediatr 2002; 56:430–3

Q 25

Mario Lima and Giovanni Ruggeri

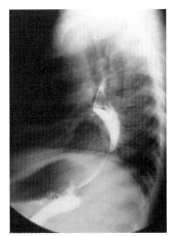

Fig. 1

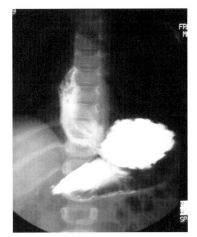

Fig. 2

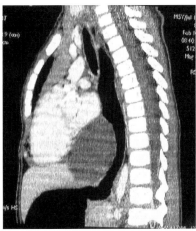

Fig. 3

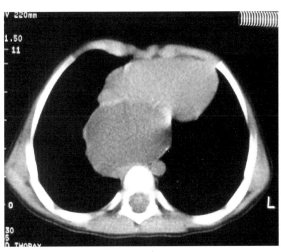

Fig. 4

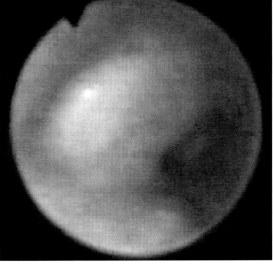

Fig. 5

A 5-year-old boy was brought to our department suffering from progressive dysphagia of recent onset.

A barium swallow was performed (see Figs. 1, 2).

- What do you see in Figs. 1 and 2?

More examinations were performed to reach a diagnosis
(see Figs. 3, 4).

- What do Figs. 3 and 4 show?
- What is the diagnosis?

The surgeon subsequently decided to perform esophagoscopy (see Fig. 5).

- Why did the surgeon decide to perform esophagoscopy? What does it show?
- What did the surgeon do in this case?

A 25

The boy was affected by an esophageal duplication.

The barium swallow (Figs. 1, 2) study shows a posteriorly displaced esophagus, with an ab extrinsic compression in the distal part, along the anterior profile.

MR imaging (Fig. 3) was performed as a first-line examination: it shows a large expansive formation, with round margins, 3 cm in diameter, in the medium mediastinum. Since the differential diagnosis included a bronchogenic cyst, a CT scan was performed (Fig. 4): the lesion is strictly adherent to the esophagus, without a clear cleavage. In some points it seems like the wall of the esophagus and that of the cyst are in continuity but without a real communication between the two. No relationships with the respiratory tree are seen.

The main differential diagnosis is between a bronchogenic cyst and an esophageal duplication, the latter seeming the most likely disease.

If esophageal duplication is suspected, it is useful to know preoperatively whether a communication between the cyst and the esophagus is present; which is why the surgeon decided to perform esophagoscopy (Fig. 5). No communication with the esophagus was seen in this case, but a bulge was visible along the esophageal wall, caused by the compression of the intestinal duplication.

The surgeon decided to excise the lesion thoracoscopically (Fig. 6). Since the duplication was very large, a mini-thoracotomy was necessary (Fig. 7). The fluid content of the cyst was clear, colorless, and thinly mucoid. Some reinforcement stitches were made along the esophageal wall (Fig. 8).

At the time of writing, the boy was well and feeding without any problems.

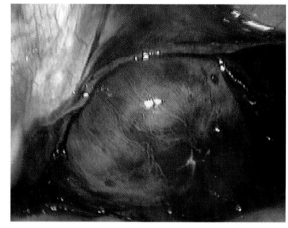

Fig. 6

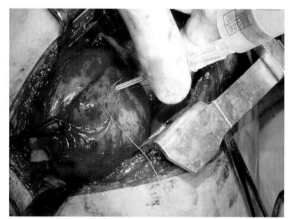

Fig. 7

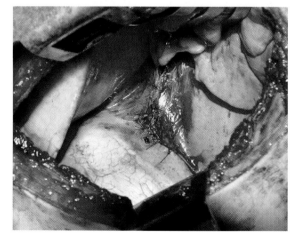

Fig. 8

Suggested Reading

1. Bratu I et al. Foregut duplications: is there an advantage to thoracoscopic resection? J Pediatr Surg 2005; 40:138–41
2. Michel JL et al. Thoracoscopic treatment of mediastinal cysts in children. J Pediatr Surg 1998; 33:1745–8
3. Soares-Oliveira M et al. Intestinal duplications. A survey of 18 cases. An Esp Pediatr 2002; 56:430–3

Q 26

Jacob C. Langer and Priscilla Chiu

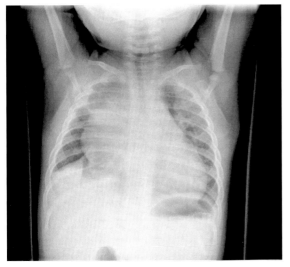

Fig. 1

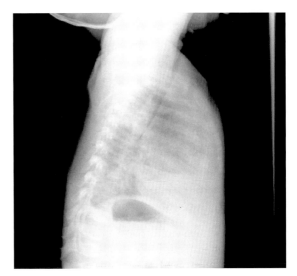

Fig. 2

A 1-year-old boy presented to the local emergency room with cough and fever. His history was otherwise unremarkable and he had no significant birth history.

On clinical examination, the child appeared very well other than having the cough. He had no signs of respiratory distress, displayed no evidence of dyspnea, and his oxygen saturation on room air was normal.

On auscultation, he had diminished air entry to his right chest compared to his left chest. There were no wheezes or crackles. His heart sounds were difficult to auscultate in the right chest.

The child was sent for a chest radiograph, shown in Figs. 1 and 2.

- What are the findings in Figs. 1 and 2?

The surgical team was contacted and a chest CT scan was ordered, shown in Figs. 3 and 4.

- What does the CT scan show?
- What is the differential diagnosis for this lesion based on the features identified on the CT scan?
- What other investigations would you order for this child?
- What is your management plan?
- How would you surgically approach this lesion?

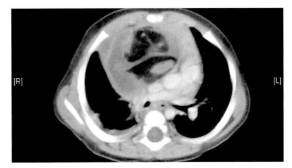

Fig. 3

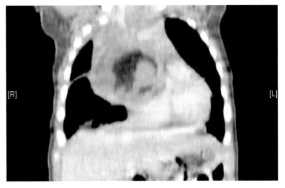

Fig. 4

A 26

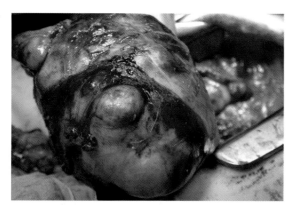

Fig. 5

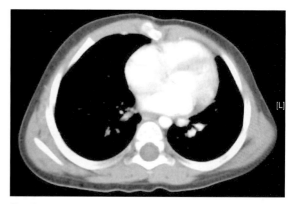

Fig. 6

The chest radiograph clearly shows a large, anterior mediastinal lesion extending into the right chest causing marked left-sided displacement of the heart and atelectasis at the right lung base.

The cough may be secondary to superimposed airway inflammation unrelated to this lesion or the lesion may be compressing the phrenic nerve.

The minimal symptoms may be explained by the gradual increase in the size of the lesion, despite its large size.

Chest radiography is a very effective screening test for chest lesions and should be the first test of choice. However, a chest radiograph may fail to detect a central mediastinal lesion or one that overlaps the cardiac silhouette.

CT can distinguish solid from cystic lesions as well as the relationship to adjacent structures with three-dimensional reconstruction software (Fig. 4).

The boy's CT scan showed a heterogeneous solid mediastinal mass containing fat and calcifications.

The differential diagnosis for an anterior mediastinal mass includes thymic cyst, thymoma, lymphoma, lymphatic malformation, and teratoma. The most likely diagnosis is teratoma based on the CT scan findings.

Teratomas are tumors containing at least two of three germ cell layers. Malignant teratomas include immature teratoma and germ cell tumors that express tumor markers (α-feto-protein, β-human choriogonadotropin) and should be assessed preoperatively with a broad radiological metastatic survey. The adequacy of cardiac function should be assessed preoperatively by echocardiogram. Postoperative surveillance of malignant tumors includes chest radiographs and serum tumor markers.

This patient was negative for serum tumor markers and his echocardiogram showed good function.

The definitive management of anterior mediastinal teratoma is primary resection. After the patient's fever resolved, the tumor was resected through a median sternotomy (Fig. 5). The pathology report indicated a benign, mature teratoma. Postoperative CT showed return of the mediastinal structures to normal position and no recurrence of tumor (Fig. 6).

Suggested Reading

1. Billmire D, Vincouir C, Rescorla F, Rescorla F, Colombani P, Cushing B, Hawkins E, London WB, Giller R, Lauer S. Malignant mediastinal germ cell tumors: an Intergroup study. J Pediatr Surg 2001; 36:18–24

2. Borecky N, Gudinchet F, Laurini R, Duvoisin B, Hohlfeld J, Schnyder P. Imaging of cervico-thoracic lymphangiomas in children. Pediatr Radiol 1995; 25:127–130

3. Bower R, Kiesewetter W. Mediastinal masses in infants and children. Arch Surg 1977; 112:1003–1009

Q 27

Jacob C. Langer and Priscilla Chiu

A 9-year-old boy presented to the local emergency room with left-sided chest pain and shortness of breath. His past medical history was significant for asthma, for which he received inhaled salbutamol treatment. He had not had any recent history of trauma.

On physical examination, his vital signs were stable and his oxygen saturation on room air was 90%. There was a shift of the trachea toward the patient's right side and there was distension of the neck veins.

On auscultation, there was minimal air entry in his left chest. Air entry as well as heart sounds were audible in his right chest.

His initial chest radiograph in the emergency room is shown in Fig. 1.

- What are the significant findings shown in Fig. 1?
- What is your diagnosis?
- What are the immediate management issues for this patient?

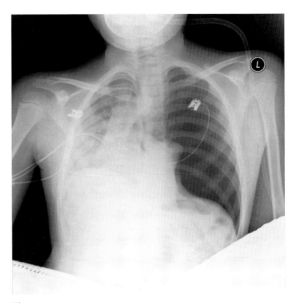

Fig. 1

It was revealed that this was the second episode for this patient and the surgical team was consulted.

A chest CT scan was then ordered.

- What findings are demonstrated in this patient's CT scan, as seen in Fig. 2?
- What are the options for definitive management of this condition?
- What associated disorders increase the risk of developing this condition?

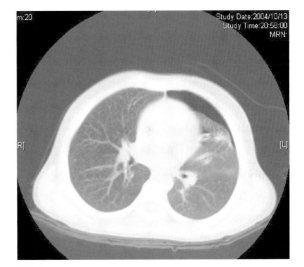

Fig. 2

A 27

This patient had a significant left tension pneumothorax as indicated by the findings of tracheal deviation, distended neck veins, and shortness of breath. The decrease or absence of breath sounds in the left chest distinguishes tension pneumothorax from other causes of acute hemodynamic compromise and respiratory distress.

The differential diagnosis for distended neck veins and shortness of breath includes tension hemothorax, pericardial tamponade, and massive pulmonary embolism.

The immediate management of a tension pneumothorax includes application of supplemental oxygen and needle decompression by placing a large bore needle at the second intercostal space in the mid-clavicular line.

The definitive management is tube thoracostomy. An appropriately sized chest tube (Table 1) is placed in the fifth intercostal space in the anterior axillary line. The tube is connected to an underwater seal chamber with suction applied. In girls, care should be taken to avoid placing the tube through breast tissue as this can lead to abnormal breast development and disfigurement in the future.

In small children, the chest tube should be positioned properly and not curled up in the chest cavity, a situation that can lead to obstruction of the chest tube and re-accumulation of a tension pneumothorax (Fig. 3).

The chest tube should be removed once the pneumothorax is completely evacuated, with no recurrence when the tube is taken off suction, and no further air leaks are detected with maximal inspiratory effort.

Recurrent pneumothoraces in the ipsilateral side suggest underlying pulmonary pathology such as blebs and bullous lung cysts. A second episode of spontaneous pneumothorax warrants further investigation following acute management.

The gold standard for the investigation of recurrent pneumothorax is CT scan to detect underlying cystic lung lesions, typically in the apical segments of the lobes. This imaging should be performed when the pneumothorax has completely resolved, as collapsed lung tissue may mask the presence of small cysts.

The presence of lung cysts combined with patient features such as tall stature and a family history of pneumothorax or vascular disease suggest possible underlying connective tissue disorders such as Marfan's syndrome or Ehlers-Danlos syndrome.

Surgical management of lung blebs or cysts involves thoracoscopic or open apical bullectomy (Fig. 4). Pleurodesis should be used as part of the operation to obliterate the potential space and prevent future pneumothoraces.

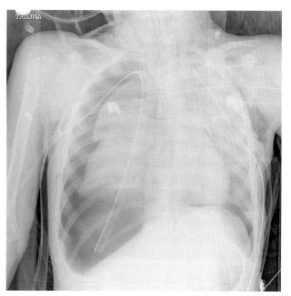

Fig. 3

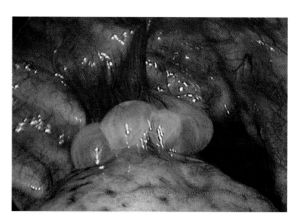

Fig. 4

Table 1 Suggested chest tube size by patient weight

Weight (kg)	Chest tube size (Fr)
3–5	10–12
6–9	12–16
10–11	16–20
12–14	20–22
15–18	22–24
19–22	24–28
23–30	24–32
>30	28–40

Q 28

Jacob C. Langer and Priscilla Chiu

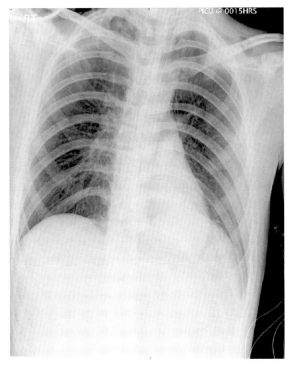

Fig. 1

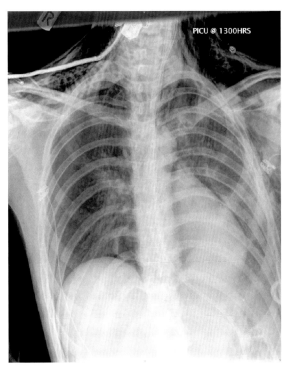

Fig. 2

A 16-year-old boy presented to the local emergency room with a 2-week history of cough, fever, and progressive neurological deficits, requiring emergency intubation for respiratory failure. The intubation was technically difficult and several attempts were made which resulted in esophageal intubation rather than endotracheal intubation.

He was admitted to the intensive care unit. High-dose steroids and antibiotics were started for this patient's pneumonia and acute demyelinating disease. His initial chest radiograph is shown in Fig. 1.

Shortly after intubation, subcutaneous emphysema was noted during the bedside clinical examination. On auscultation, he had fine crackles with air entry to his chest. However, he did not experience any significant deterioration in ventilatory status.

Serial chest radiographs were acquired. Figure 2 shows the chest radiographs of this patient following the development of subcutaneous emphysema.
- What does Fig. 2 show?
- What is the differential diagnosis?
- What other investigations would you order for this patient?

The surgical team was contacted after a significant increase in subcutaneous emphysema.
- What is your management plan?
- What are the complications associated with this condition?

A 28

This patient developed pneumomediastinum and subcutaneous emphysema following traumatic endotracheal intubation and mechanical ventilation.

Most commonly, pneumomediastinum is secondary to pneumothorax with leakage of intrapleural air into the mediastinum. In the absence of associated pneumothorax, pneumomediastinum most commonly results from traumatic injury to the mediastinal aerodigestive tract (i.e., esophagus, trachea, main stem, and proximal bronchi).

Esophageal perforation may be associated with signs such as mediastinitis (fever, pain, respiratory distress) and pleural effusion. In small children, foreign body ingestion with esophageal perforation must be considered in the differential diagnosis.

The treatment of small esophageal perforation is antibiotic administration and drainage of any para-esophageal fluid collections. Large esophageal perforations should be managed by early and aggressive surgical repair, as mediastinitis can lead to fatal sepsis.

Airway injury represents the second most common cause of isolated pneumomediastinum. For this patient, additional factors such as mechanical ventilation, underlying infection, and steroid use may predispose to airway injury.

Treatment of airway perforation may be difficult, especially among the mechanically ventilated patient population. Minimizing airway pressures, treatment with antibiotics for proven infection, and tapering of steroid dosage facilitate spontaneous closure of small airway perforations.

Management of traumatic airway injuries requires early control of the airway with endotracheal intubation beyond the level of injury if possible (e.g., endobronchial intubation). Surgical repair is indicated if the air leak is uncontrolled with endotracheal intubation or fails to resolve with conservative treatment.

Investigations for isolated pneumomediastinum should include an upper gastrointestinal contrast study or esophagoscopy and bronchoscopy to identify the site of injury.

This patient's contrast study (Fig. 3) was normal, but his bronchoscopy revealed a small ulcer at the proximal right mainstem bronchus below the carina, and his CT scan demonstrated impressive pneumomediastinum (Figs. 4). The CT scan also confirmed the absence of any associated pneumothoraces; this is important, since the

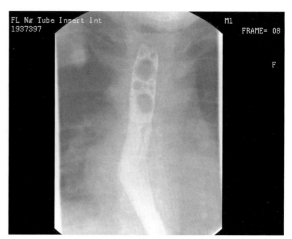

Fig. 3

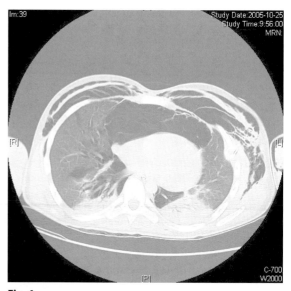

Fig. 4

detection of a pneumothorax on plain film radiographs may be difficult in the setting of extensive subcutaneous emphysema.

Options for surgical repair of airway injuries include primary repair, patch repair using pericardial or pleural autograft, resection and primary anastomosis, and lobectomy (for bronchial injuries). Complications include persistent air leak or bronchopleural fistula, airway granulation tissue, and stenosis.

Q 29

Jacob C. Langer and Priscilla Chiu

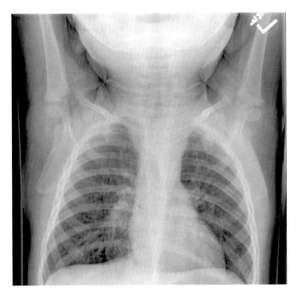

Fig. 1

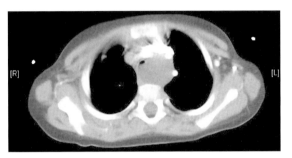

Fig. 2

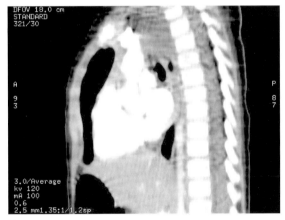

Fig. 3

A 9-month-old boy was taken to the family doctor after his mother noticed progressively noisy breathing. The child was otherwise active and alert.

The patient was afebrile and had no significant past medical history.

The family physician found that the child had significant indrawing with his respirations, but his oxygen saturations were normal on room air and there was air entry bilaterally. There were no crackles on auscultation. The remainder of his physical examination was normal. On further questioning, the patient's mother also reported progressive feeding intolerance with vomiting shortly after feeding.

The child was sent for a chest radiograph, shown in Fig. 1.

- What does Fig. 1 show?

This child came to our attention after chest radiography was performed. The surgeon requested additional examinations, shown in Figs. 2 and 3.

- What do Figs. 2 and 3 show?
- What is the differential diagnosis for this lesion?
- How would you manage this child?

A 29

This child showed signs of respiratory distress suggesting airway obstruction. His chest radiograph showed a mass in the upper mediastinum with deviation and compression of the trachea.

Mediastinal lesions in infants and children are best imaged by CT scan. CT imaging can determine whether the lesion is solid or cystic and the location and extent of the lesion in relation to adjacent structures.

This infant's CT scan of the chest clearly showed a large upper and posterior mediastinal cystic lesion causing compression and rightward deviation of the trachea with near complete obliteration of the esophageal lumen. There was no cystic extension into the spine.

The differential diagnosis includes foregut duplication cyst, mediastinal abscess, and lymphatic malformation. The CT scan showed that the cyst was localized to the mediastinum without septations or evidence of extension into the neck, suggesting it was unlikely to be a cervicomediastinal lymphatic malformation.

Foregut duplication cysts are malformations of foregut development that result in cystic enteric (intestinal) or bronchial remnants within the mediastinum. There may be multiple duplications along the intestinal tract, as duplication cysts can arise in any part of the bowel. Children with foregut duplication cysts may have associated VACTERL anomalies: *v*ertebral, *a*nal, *c*ardiac, *tra*cheo*e*sophageal, *r*enal and *l*imb.

Foregut duplication cysts may be spherical or tubular in shape. The cysts may communicate with the foregut lumen or may be completely separated by the cyst wall. The cysts may harbor ectopic tissues, including gastric mucosa, which may result in acid production, ulcer formation, and bleeding. Occasionally, these cysts can become infected, fistulize to adjacent structures, or rupture.

In contrast, neurenteric cysts are foregut duplications with spinal extension thought to arise from the dorsal

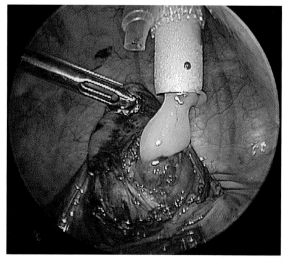

Fig. 4

notochord, representing a different embryological derivation from foregut duplications. Inflammation or cyst enlargement can result in spinal cord compression and paraplegia. The presence of neurological deficits mandates emergency laminectomy to decompress the spinal cord.

Large foregut duplication cysts can cause airway or esophageal obstruction and are sometimes identified prenatally by antenatal ultrasound. The perinatal management of such large cysts may warrant immediate control of the airway at birth.

The definitive management of foregut duplication cysts is surgical resection.

This child underwent thoracoscopic resection of the lesion (Fig. 4). The cyst contained mucus, which was aspirated before the cyst was removed from the chest.

Suggested Reading

1. Azzie G, Beasley S. Diagnosis and treatment of foregut duplications. Semin Pediatr Surg 2003; 12:46–54
2. Bratu I, Laberge JM, Glageole H, Bouchard S. Foregut duplications: is there an advantage to thoracoscopic resection? J Pediatr Surg 2005; 40:138–41
3. Carachi R, Azmy A. Foregut duplications. Pediatr Surg Int 2002; 18:371–4
4. Superina R, Ein S, Humphreys R. Cystic duplications of the esophagus and neurenteric cysts. J Pediatr Surg 1984; 19:527–530

Q 30

Giovanni Esposito and Ciro Esposito

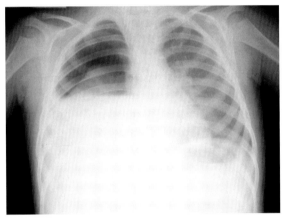

Fig. 1

A 6-year-old boy without any anamnestic findings of disease suffered thoracic trauma after a car accident. He presented with severe respiratory distress and significant dyspnea. On auscultation, hyperphonesis of the right hemithorax was found, and therefore chest radiography was performed (Fig. 1). After this, surgery was carried out.

- What do the thoracic radiographs show?
- Which other procedures should be performed to reach the diagnosis?
- What was the diagnosis?
- What was the treatment?
- What was the follow-up?

A 30

The chest radiographs show a severe right pneumothorax with a collapsed ipsilateral lung.

An explorative puncture was performed at the level of the fifth intercostal space along the mid-axillary line, from which 20 ml of blood came out.

Based on the clinical and radiological features, the diagnosis of hemothorax due to a lung rupture was made.

The treatment consisted in introducing a Petzer tube in the pleural space by minimal incision, connected with an aspiration system (Fig. 2).

During the follow-up, the radiograph of the thorax revealed complete lung expansion; the drainage tube was therefore removed 10 days later and the child was discharged (Fig. 3).

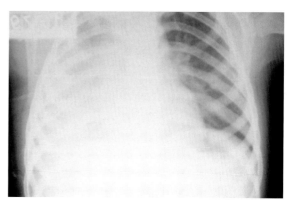

Fig. 2

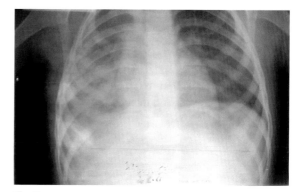

Fig. 3

Suggested Reading

1. Adegboye VO, Ladipo JK, Adebo OA, Brimmo AI. Diaphragmatic injuries. Afr J Med Med Sci 2002 Jun; 31(2): 149–53
2. Karnak I, Senocak ME, Tanyel FC, Buyukpamukcu N. Diaphragmatic injuries in childhood. Surg Today 2001; 31(1): 5–11
3. Shehata SM, Shabaan BS. Diaphragmatic injuries in children after blunt abdominal trauma. J Pediatr Surg 2006 Oct; 41(10):1727–31
4. Soundappan SV, Holland AJ, Cass DT, Farrow GB. Blunt traumatic diaphragmatic injuries in children. Injury 2005 Jan; 36(1):51–4
5. Voeller GR, Reisser JR, Fabian TC, Kudsk K, Mangiante EC. Blunt diaphragm injuries. A five-year experience. Am Surg 1990 Jan; 56(1):28–31

Q 31

Felix Schier

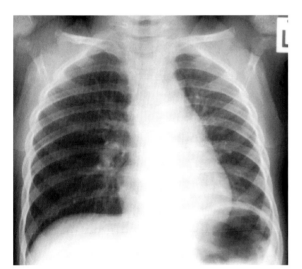

Fig. 1

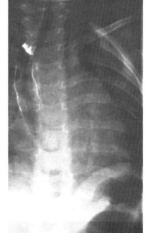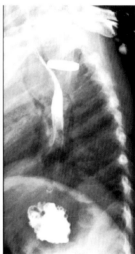

Fig. 2

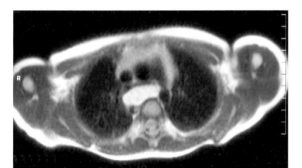

Fig. 3

A 2-year-old boy presented to our department suffering from a recurrent cough. Two episodes of pneumonia had been recorded. There was a slight failure to thrive. All laboratory values were normal. On auscultation there were slightly reduced breath sounds on the right side. The patient underwent imaging, shown in Figs. 1–4.

- What is the most likely diagnosis?

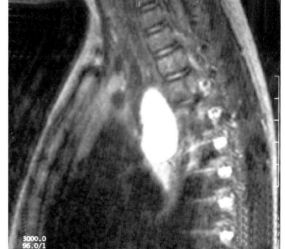

Fig. 4

A 31

The chest radiograph in Fig. 1 shows a moderate mediastinal shift to the left. The right lung is of increased transparency. The right diaphragm is lowered indicating a bronchial valve mechanism.

Figure 2 is an esophagogram. The esophagus is dislocated in a curve to the right and to the back, resulting from a mass at the level of the tracheal bifurcation.

Figures 3 and 4 are axial and sagittal MR images, respectively. A well-delineated high-intensity mass can be identified due to the high protein content of the cyst. The diagnosis is tracheogenic bronchogenic cyst.

Foregut duplications may present in a variety of ways and locations. The histological similarity and anatomic proximity of "bronchogenic cysts" and of intramural "esophageal duplications" support a common origin.

Symptoms vary accordingly. Usually, children with symptomatic bronchogenic cysts suffer from recurrent pneumonia, dysphagia, and failure to thrive.

Surgical excision is curative in these cases, and it is recommended if a symptomatic cystic lung lesion does not respond to medical treatment. The possible complications of bleeding, ulceration, infection, and obstruction of the esophagus or airway should generally lead to resection.

Thoracoscopy is advantageous for isolated intrathoracic bronchogenic cysts. Depending on the location, bronchogenic cysts may also be removed laparoscopically.

Suggested Reading

1. Bratu I, Laberge JM, Flageole H, Bouchard S. Foregut duplications: is there an advantage to thoracoscopic resection? J Pediatr Surg 2005; 40:138–141
2. Koontz CS, Oliva V, Gow KW, Wulkan ML. Video-assisted thoracoscopic surgical excision of cystic lung disease in children. J Pediatr Surg 2005; 40:835–837
3. Nobuhara KK, Gorski YC, LaQuaglia MP, Shamberger RC. Bronchogenic cysts and esophageal duplications: common origins and treatment. J Pediatr Surg 1997; 32:1408–1413
4. Parikh D, Samuel M. Congenital cystic lung lesions: is surgical resection essential? Pediatr Pulmonol 2005; 40:533–537
5. Schier F, Waldschmidt J. Thoracoscopy in children. J Pediatr Surg 1996; 31:1640–1643

Q 32

Brice Antao and Azad Najmaldin

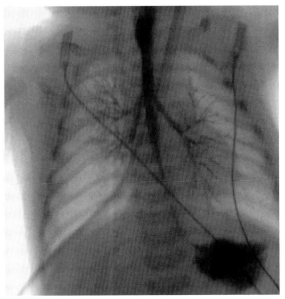

Fig. 1

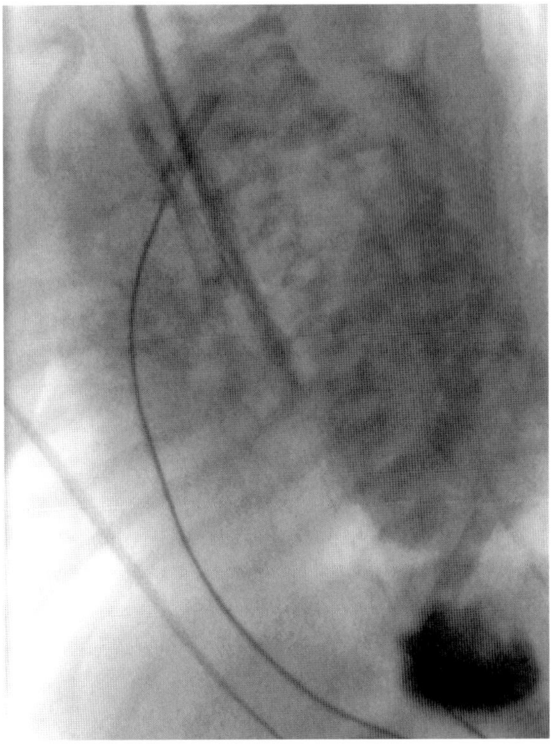

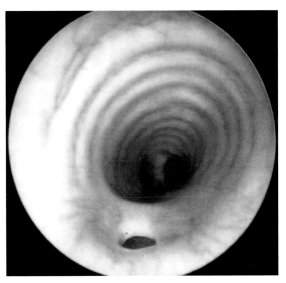

Fig. 2

A male infant was born by normal vaginal delivery at 36 weeks' gestation. He weighed 2,845 g and had good APGAR scores. Soon after birth, he was noted to have increased oral secretions and developed choking, brady-cardia, and apnea with feeds.

- What features are seen in Figs. 1 and 2, suggestive of the diagnosis?
- Why was the examination shown in Fig. 3 performed?
- What other investigations may prove helpful?
- Which is the best approach for treatment of this abnormality?
- What is the outcome of this condition?

Fig. 3

A 32

This neonate had an H-type tracheoesophageal fistula. The classical triad of symptoms of H-type fistula are paroxysm of severe choking and cough precipitated by feeds, abdominal distension due to passage of air from the trachea to the esophagus, and recurrent attacks of pneumonia due to aspiration.

Figures 1 and 2 are anterior and lateral views, respectively, of a tube esophagogram. It clearly demonstrates the fistula. Contrast medium can be seen in the tracheobronchial tree. However, it is important to recognize that contrast medium in the trachea may be a feature of aspiration alone. A routine upper gastrointestinal (GI) contrast study often fails to demonstrate an H-type fistula. A tube esophagogram facilitates contrast medium being injected under high pressure at different levels, and has a better diagnostic yield. It is important to start the tube esophagography high in the cervical esophagus in order to minimize the risk of missing a proximal (high) fistula.

Figure 3 is a bronchoscopic view of the thoracic end of the H-fistula. It usually confirms the diagnosis and allows placement of a catheter through the fistula and precise localization at the time of surgical repair.

Esophagoscopy may also help in identifying an H-type fistula. Although bronchoscopy is a better diagnostic measure than esophagoscopy, usually both procedures are performed in order to diagnose and localize an H-type fistula.

The fistula can be repaired via a cervical or thoracic route. As more than 70% of the H-type fistulas are above the second thoracic vertebra, the majority of surgeons advocate repair via the cervical route. This case was repaired through a cervical incision following a bronchoscopic localization of the fistula. Thoracoscopic repair is an alternative approach.

This child recovered well and was thriving at the 2-year follow-up. Recurrence is a rare complication. On rare occasions more than one H-type fistula may exist and missed during investigations and exploration. Endoscopic evaluation prior to surgery increases the sensitivity of identifying such cases.

Suggested Reading

1. Benjamin B, Pham T. Diagnosis of H-Type tracheoesophageal fistula. J Pediatr Surg 1991; 26:667–671
2. Crabbe DC, Kiely EM, Drake DP, Spitz L. Management of the isolated congenital tracheo-oesophageal fistula. Eur J Pediatr Surg 1996; 6:67–9
3. Ng J, Antao B, Bartram J, Raghavan A, Shawis R. Diagnostic difficulties in the management of H type tracheoesophageal fistula. Acta Radiologica 2006; 8:801–805

Q 33

Craig T. Albanese

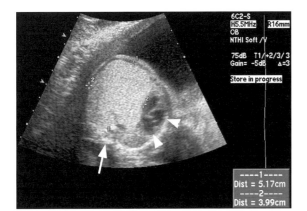

Fig. 1

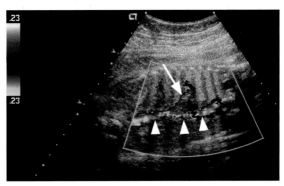

Fig. 2

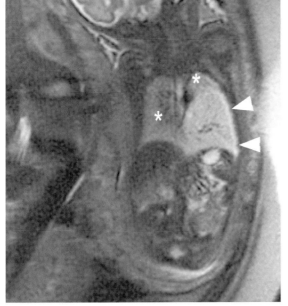

Fig. 3

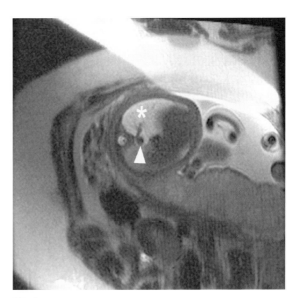

Fig. 4

A large echogenic solid mass (calipers) was noted in the lower left hemithorax of the fetal chest on a 22-week surveillance ultrasound study (Fig. 1). The fetal heart (*arrowheads*) was displaced into the right chest (fetal spine, *arrow*).

Color flow Doppler (Fig. 2) revealed a systemic artery (*arrow*) arising from the aorta (*arrowheads*) feeding this mass. A coronal MR image of the fetus (Fig. 3) showed the bright mass (*arrowheads*) in the left lower

chest. There was normal lung tissue (*asterisks*). A transverse MR image through the lower fetal thorax (Fig. 4) showed the lung mass (*asterisk*) and lower thoracic aorta (*arrowhead*) giving rise to a systemic feeding vessel to the mass.

- What is the anomaly here?
- Which lobes are usually affected?
- Does this mass ever shrink in size prenatally?
- What is the treatment?

A 33

This fetus has a pulmonary sequestration. It can be either extralobar (retains its own pleural investment) or intralobar (within the pleural investment of the adjacent lobes)—this distinction is difficult to make prenatally, unless the sequestered lobe is below the diaphragm (always extralobar in this case). By definition, a sequestration (as opposed to the closely related cystic adenomatoid malformation lesion) has an aberrant blood supply, derived chiefly from the infradiaphragmatic aorta.

Sequestrations are almost always found in the lower lobes. They can diminish in size prenatally but are always noted postnatally on CT scans, even when the plain chest radiograph is normal and the patient is asymptomatic. A newborn chest radiograph (Fig. 5) shows a left lower lobe mass (*arrows*). A chest CT scan (Fig. 6) shows left lower lobe sequestration with systemic arterial feeders (*arrows*) originating from the lower thoracic aorta.

This baby was asymptomatic at birth. The lesion is removed urgently when there are respiratory symptoms. For asymptomatic babies, elective excision is performed since there is a risk of recurrent pulmonary infections and malignant transformation after several decades of life. This child had an intralobar sequestration that was removed thoracoscopically.

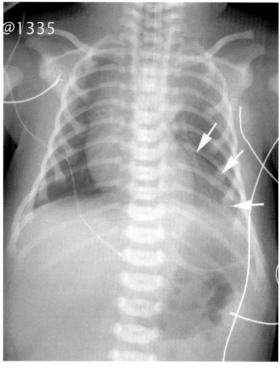

Fig. 5

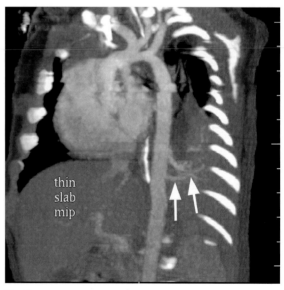

Fig. 6

Suggested Reading

1. de Lagausie P, Bonnard A, Berrebi D, Petit P, Dorgeret S, Guys JM. Video-assisted thoracoscopic surgery for pulmonary sequestration in children. Ann Thorac Surg 2005 Oct; 80(4):1266–9
2. Odaka A, Honda N, Baba K, Tanimizu T, Takahashi S, Ohno Y, Satomi A, Hashimoto D. Pulmonary sequestration. J Pediatr Surg 2006 Dec; 41(12):2096–7
3. Torres LF, Jacob GV, de Noronha L, Seade M, Artigas JL. Congenital pulmonary extralobar intra-abdominal sequestration J Pediatr (Rio J) 1997 Jan-Feb; 73(1):51–3

Q 34

Craig T. Albanese

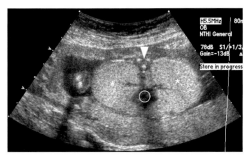

Fig. 1

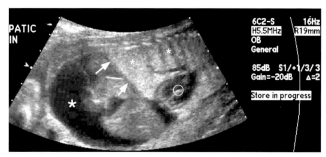

Fig. 2

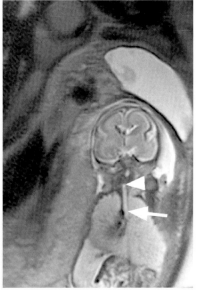

Fig. 3

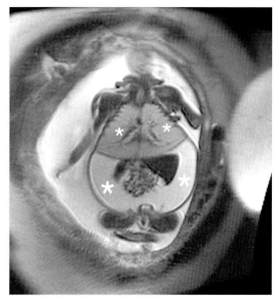

Fig. 4

A pregnant woman was found to have polyhydramnios clinically. Fetal ultrasound (Figs. 1, 2; axial and sagittal views) demonstrated distended pulmonary parenchyma (*small asterisks*), fluid-filled airways, pleural effusion, ascites (large asterisk), and inverted diaphragms (*arrows*). A compressed heart (*circle*) secondary to hyperinflated lungs was seen. Subsequent fetal MR images (Figs. 3, 4) demonstrated a dilated trachea (*arrow*) terminating at the level of the fetal larynx (*arrowhead*), distended lungs (*small asterisks*), fetal ascites (*large asterisks*), and polyhydramnios.

- What is your diagnosis?

A 34

The newborn chest radiograph (Fig. 5) demonstrates hyperinflated lungs and inverted diaphragms.

This neonate has congenital high airway obstruction syndrome (CHAOS). This can be due to any number of complete obstructions at the level of the larynx or trachea. Most commonly, it is due to laryngeal atresia, which is what this patient had.

The baby was delivered using the EXIT strategy and underwent a tracheostomy to secure the airway. A "pigtail" drainage catheter can be noted in the left upper abdomen in Fig. 5, placed to drain the tense ascites.

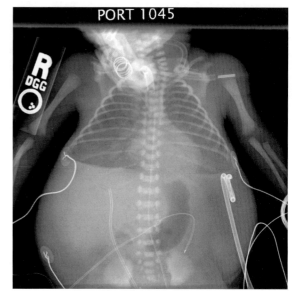

Fig. 5

Suggested Reading

1. Adzick NS. Management of fetal lung lesions. Clin Perinatol 2003 Sep; 30(3):481–92
2. Lim FY, Crombleholme TM, Hedrick HL, Flake AW, Johnson MP, Howell LJ, Adzick NS. Congenital high airway obstruction syndrome: natural history and management. J Pediatr Surg 2003 Jun; 38(6):940–5
3. Marwan A, Crombleholme TM. The EXIT procedure: principles, pitfalls, and progress. Semin Pediatr Surg 2006 May; 15(2):107–15

Q 35

Ciro Esposito and Giovanni Esposito

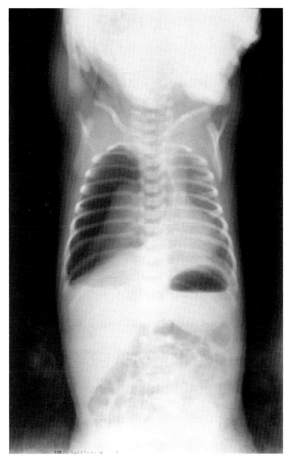

Fig. 1

A newborn requiring vigorous resuscitation because of severe asphyxia at birth presented with respiratory distress a few hours later, which suddenly became worse.

The findings from a plain radiograph (Fig. 1) of the chest suggested urgent treatment.

- What does the radiograph show?
- What was the treatment?
- What was the follow-up?

A 35

The standard radiograph of the chest shows a large pneumothorax on the right site, with a collapse of the lung and a contralateral shift of the mediastinum (Fig. 1).

The pneumothorax was treated by aspiration using a needle, inserted through the second intercostal space along the mid-clavicular line, initially connected with a 10-ml syringe and over the following days to an underwater seal drain without any suction. After 5 days, the lung had expanded and therefore the needle was removed.

After 10 days, the follow-up radiograph of the chest confirmed the complete re-expansion of the lung and the neonate was discharged from hospital (Fig. 2).

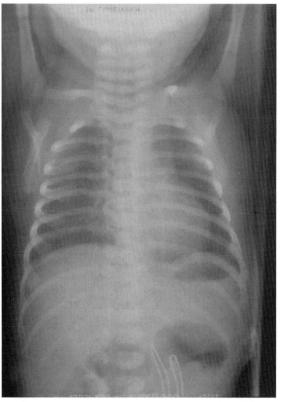

Fig. 2

Suggested Reading

1. Katar S, Devecioglu C, Kervancioglu M, Ulku R. Symptomatic spontaneous pneumothorax in term newborns. Pediatr Surg Int 2006 Sep; 22(9):755–8
2. Kirby C, Trotter C. Pneumothorax in the neonate: assessment and diagnosis. Neonatal Netw 2005 Sep-Oct; 24(5):49–55
3. Margau R, Amaral JG, Chait PG, Cohen J. Percutaneous thoracic drainage in neonates: catheter drainage versus treatment with aspiration alone. Radiology 2006 Oct; 241(1):223–7
4. van den Boom J, Battin M.Chest radiographs after removal of chest drains in neonates: clinical benefit or common practice? Arch Dis Child Fetal Neonatal Ed 2007 Jan; 92(1): F46–8
5. Wenzel V, Russo S, Arntz HR, Bahr J, Baubin MA, Bottiger BW, Dirks B, Dorges V, Eich C, Fischer M, Wolcke B, Schwab S, Voelckel WG, Gervais HW; European Resuscitation Council. The new 2005 resuscitation guidelines of the European Resuscitation Council: comments and supplements. Anaesthesist 2006 Sep; 55(9):958–66, 968–72, 974–9

Q 36

François Becmeur

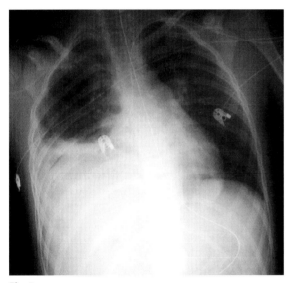

Fig. 1

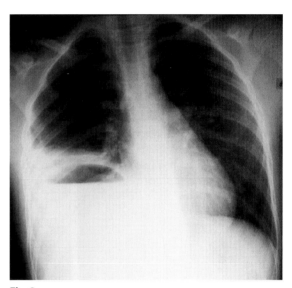

Fig. 2

The majority of the class members of this 9-year-old boy had suffered from gastroenteritis for a few days. This boy presented with vomiting and a fever of about 38°C.

The parents called the doctor on the following evening. After clinical examination, the doctor was able to exclude a diagnosis of appendicitis and suspected gastroenteritis.

Over the next 4 days, the clinical evolution of the boy was variable: he suffered from episodes of septic fever associated with abdominal painful crises.

Five days later, his temperature rose to 40°C. The boy suffered from abdominal pains and especially from severe dyspnea. A clinical examination suggested right pleuritis.

The first radiographic study of the thorax was carried out with the child in bed because he seemed tired (Fig. 1).
- What do you observe in Fig. 1 and which assumptions can you make?

The findings of the first radiograph suggested an infectious pleural pathology. A radiograph of the thorax, with the patient upright, was then obtained (Fig. 2).

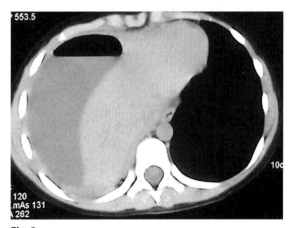

Fig. 3

- What do you observe in Fig. 2 and what is your hypothesis?

A thoracoabdominal CT scan was required (Fig. 3). An interhepatic diaphragmatic abscess is observed with a dense image, probably partially calcified, in the center.
- What is the principal diagnosis and what is your treatment plan?

A 36

Initially, the diagnosis of food poisoning or of gastroenteritis is indeed the most probable diagnosis. A symptomatic treatment (analgesics and antisecretory medication) accompanied by a liquid diet is recommended.

The majority of gastroenteritis cases are of viral origin. The duration of viral gastroenteritis is between 3 and 5 days with a typical chronology of symptoms: vomiting, fever, abdominal pains, and diarrhea. In this patient, the evolution of symptoms over 7 days (from Saturday to Friday), the absence of diarrhea, and the septic fever accompanied by abdominal pains suggest a deep suppuration. No signs of urinary or hepatobiliary involvement were found.

A pleural empyema was initially proposed by the doctors. Pleural empyema generally occurs secondary to an infectious pneumopathy. However, at no time during the week did the patient have respiratory symptoms.

The anteroposterior upright radiograph shows the existence of a fluid–fluid level. The thoracoabdominal scan confirmed the presence of a subdiaphragmatic abscess with a fluid–fluid level testifying to the presence of anaerobic germs. The hyperdense and calcified image within this abscess in the right under the hepatic region suggests the existence of stercoral colitis of appendicular origin. The most probable diagnosis is of a deep abscess with pleural reaction due to subhepatic appendicitis.

Suggested Reading

1. Chandesris MO, Schleinitz N, Gayet S, Bernit E, Crebassa C, Veit V, Harle JR, Kaplanski G. Anaerobic deep abscesses with unusual location: report of 5 cases. Rev Med Interne 2005 Jul; 26(7):534–40
2. Fernandez M, Ortega D, Darras A, Gallardo S, Yarmuch J. Percutaneous drainage of abdominal abscesses Rev Med Chil 1990 Jul; 118(7):772–6
3. Mac Erlean DP, Gibney RG. Radiological management of abdominal abscess. J R Soc Med 1983 Apr; 76(4):256–61
4. Shuler FW, Newman CN, Angood PB, Tucker JG, Lucas GW. Nonoperative management for intra-abdominal abscesses. Am Surg 1996 Mar; 62(3):218–22
5. Useche E, Salazar S, Vetencourt R, Monzon R. Non-surgical drainage of intra-abdominal abscesses. G E N 1991 Jan-Mar; 45(1):9–13

Q 37

François Becmeur

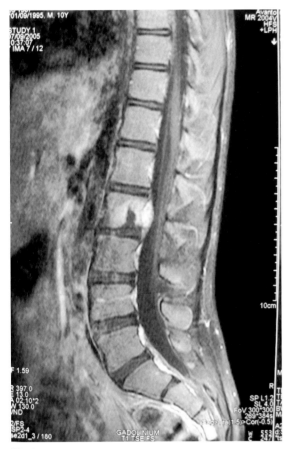

Fig. 1

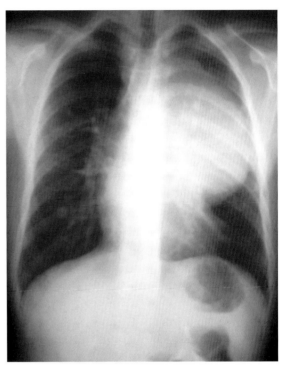

Fig. 2

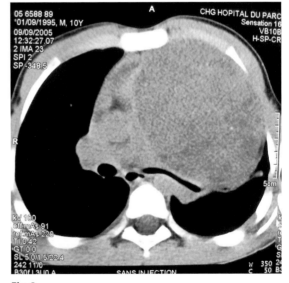

Fig. 3

A 10-year-old boy presented to the emergency department with pain in his left leg that had started 3 weeks earlier without any incident of trauma.

On clinical examination, he was afebrile, there were no hematomas, and the articulations were painless. The pulses were well perceived, and the calf was flexible. A neurological examination revealed pain in the posterior face of the left thigh, extending to the external face of the leg, which involved a limp on walking, without any functional deficit. All osteotendinous reflexes were present except for the left patellar reflex. The cutaneoplantar reflexes were indifferent. A discrete hypoesthesia of the perineum was noted.

A radiological assessment of the rachis was made (Fig. 1).

A reduction in the vesicular murmurs on the left lung was noted during a pulmonary examination. Imaging of the thorax was subsequently performed (Figs. 2, 3).

- Describe Figs. 2, 3.
- What is your diagnosis?

A 37

All the results lead to the diagnosis of a thoracic tumor with metastases. In this age, the most frequent thoracic tumors are lymphomas, neuroblastomas, and germinal tumors.

The diagnosis of germinal tumor was confirmed histologically and chemotherapy was started immediately because of the neurological signs. After a few days, the patient's symptoms improved.

The radiograph of the thorax, in inspiration, highlights an opacity in the upper-left part of the thorax. This is responsible for the deviation of the trachea. A metastasis in the right parenchyma is noted. There is no pleural effusion.

A CT scan of the thorax highlights a very bulky mass in the left mediastinum, measuring 10 cm in diameter, pushing back the mediastinum toward the midline, compressing the left bronchus at the back. This mass is heterogeneous and contains some small calcifications. After injection of contrast medium, a moderate amount of contrast medium is present on the reformatted images, with total vascularization in the form of thread-like vessels.

To assess the germinal tumor, laboratory examinations should measure the levels of alpha-fetoprotein and B-human chorionic gonadotropin, which will be increased. Biopsy of the mass and histological assessment are mandatory.

Suggested Reading

1. Adzick NS. Management of fetal lung lesions. Clin Perinatol 2003 Sep; 30(3):481–92
2. Freud E, Ben-Ari J, Schonfeld T, Blumenfeld A, Steinberg R, Dlugy E, Yaniv I, Katz J, Schwartz M, Zer M. Mediastinal tumors in children: a single institution experience. Clin Pediatr (Phila) 2002 May; 41(4):219–23
3. Gathwala G, Rattan KN. Posterior mediastinal mass: missed diagnosis. Indian J Pediatr 1994 Sep–Oct; 61(5):577–8
4. Glick RD, La Quaglia MP. Lymphomas of the anterior mediastinum. Semin Pediatr Surg 1999 May; 8(2):69–77
5. Tansel T, Onursal E, Dayloglu E, Basaran M, Sungur Z, Qamci E, Yilmazbayhan D, Eker R, Ertugrul T. Childhood mediastinal masses in infants and children. Turk J Pediatr 2006 Jan–Mar; 48(1):8–12

Q 38

Giovanni Esposito and Ciro Esposito

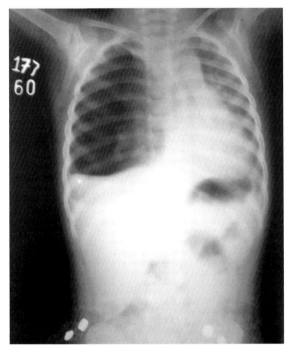

Fig. 1

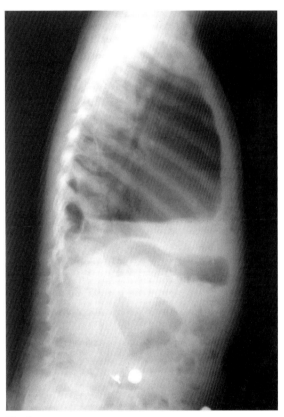

Fig. 2

A 2-year-old child, without a significant previous medical history, was admitted to our hospital because of the sudden onset of a cough and high fever. On objective examination, hypophonesis of the thorax and wet noises were reported. The child was treated with broad-range antibiotics and the symptoms improved remarkably with a reduction of the fever. Two days later, the child presented with respiratory distress along with intense dyspnea and diffuse cyanosis. This time the physical medical report showed no lung sounds in the lung base and a diffused tympanic sound. Radiographs of the thorax (Figs. 1, 2) were acquired.

- What do the radiographs show?
- What was the diagnosis?
- What was the evolution of the disease?
- What was the treatment?
- What was the follow-up?

A 38

The radiographs (Figs. 1, 2) demonstrated the presence of an air–fluid level in the right hemithorax with air in the pleural space and a collapse of the lung with a mediastinal contralateral shift.

The initial diagnosis was tension hydropneumothorax and subsequently after the treatment the diagnosis was tension pyopneumothorax.

The treatment consisted in a minimal pleurotomy of the fifth intercostal space on the axillary midline and introduction of a drainage tube (Petzer probe no. 8) in the pleural space, which allows draining of the pus and air under strong pressure.

The patient was followed up with periodic radiological studies, which demonstrated progressive reduction of the pleural effusion along with progressive expansion of the lung. In fact, as early as the first follow-up 10 days after the water drainage (Fig. 3) there was reduction of the pneumothorax, which completely reverted in successive follow-ups. After 25 days, the water-drainage tube was removed. After 1 month, a radiograph of the thorax showed complete lung expansion with a light pleural air-frame.

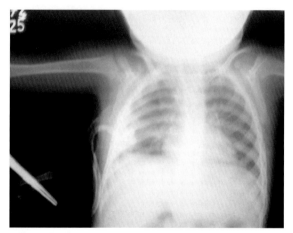

Fig. 3

Suggested Reading

1. Abramzon OM, Kurlaev PP. Prediction of the course of acute purulent diseases of the lung and pleura. Probl Tuberk Bolezn Legk 2006; (7):8–11
2. Chinnan NK, Rathore A, Shabaan AI, Al Samman W. The "forbidden" chest x-ray: tension pyopneumothorax. Am J Emerg Med 2007 Feb; 25(2):200–1
3. Eller P, Theurl I, Koppelstaetter F, Weiss G. Pyopneumothorax due to Streptococcus milleri. Wien Klin Wochenschr 2006 May; 118(7-8):207
4. Hsieh CF, Lin HJ, Foo NP, Lae JC. Tension pyopneumothorax. Resuscitation 2007; 1: 35–38
5. Tsai WK, Chen W, Lee JC, Cheng WE, Chen CH, Hsu WH, Shih CM. Pigtail catheters vs large-bore chest tubes for management of secondary spontaneous pneumothoraces in adults. Am J Emerg Med 2006 Nov; 24(7):795–800

Q 39

Giovanni Esposito and Ciro Esposito

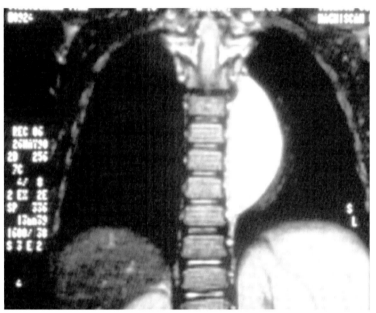

Fig. 1

An 8-year-old child was hospitalized for cryptorchidism treatment, where the incidental radiological finding of thoracic opacity was made. He was transferred to our department, where other examinations were performed that also indicated the need for a thoracic intervention.

- What does Fig. 1 show?
- Which other examinations were performed and what were the results?
- What was the suspected diagnosis?
- What was found during intervention and what was the treatment?
- What was the definitive diagnosis?
- What was the follow-up?

A 39

The radiography study demonstrates the presence of mediastinal opacity on the left side.

MR imaging was subsequently performed along with measurement of urinary vanillylmandelic acid (VMA) and homovanillic acid (HVA) levels.

The MR image (Fig. 1) showed an opacity on the left side of the thoracic spine; the VMA and MVA levels were lower than normal. The suspected diagnosis was of a neurogenic tumor.

At intervention, a mass adherent to the vertebral column was found and was easily excised.

At histologic examination, the tumor proved to be a ganglioneuroblastoma.

The postoperative course was uneventful and the child was discharged on the seventh day after the operation. At the 5-year follow-up, the child was doing well.

Suggested Reading

1. Domanski HA Fine-needle aspiration of ganglioneuroma. Diagn Cytopathol 2005 Jun; 32(6):363–6
2. Geraci AP, de Csepel J, Shlasko E, Wallace SA. Ganglioneuroblastoma and ganglioneuroma in association with neurofibromatosis type I: report of three cases. J Child Neurol 1998 Jul; 13(7):356–8
3. Milovic I, Scekic M, Vujic D, Djurisic S, Djokic D. The characteristics of mediastinal neuroblastoma and perspectives on surgical excision Acta Chir Iugosl 2003; 50(4):103–7
4. Nio M, Nakamura M, Yoshida S, Ishii T, Amae S, Hayashi Y. Thoracoscopic removal of neurogenic mediastinal tumors in children. J Laparoendosc Adv Surg Tech A 2005 Feb; 15(1):80–3
5. Tang KT, Lee HC, Liang DC, Chen SH, Liu HC, Sheu JC. Neural-crest tumor presenting with chronic diarrhea: a report of three cases. J Formos Med Assoc 2002 Dec; 101(12):864–7

Q 40

Giovanni Esposito, Carmelo Romeo, and Ciro Esposito

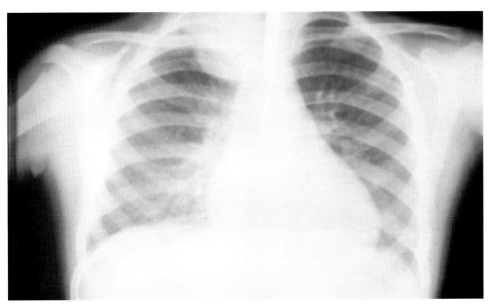

Fig. 1

A 5-year-old girl was admitted to our institution because of a thoracic opacity detected on a chest radiograph which had been acquired to examine a persistent cough after a respiratory infection.

On physical examination, no pathological findings were revealed. Because of the localization of the opacity, other procedures were performed. Subsequently, a surgical intervention was scheduled.

- What does Fig. 1 show?
- Which other procedures were performed and what was their result?
- What was the diagnosis?
- What was the treatment?
- What was the follow-up?

A 40

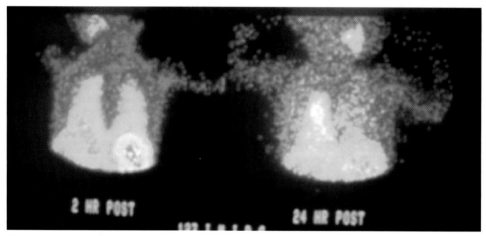

Fig. 2

The thoracic radiograph (Fig. 1) showed an opacity occupying the superior and medial part of the right hemithorax, probably of mediastinal origin.

After a CT scan that confirmed the mediastinal site of the opacity, an MIBG scan was obtained and the vanillylmandelic acid (VMA) and homovanillic acid (HVA) levels were measured.

The MIBG (Fig. 2) test demonstrated an accumulation of the radioisotope in the region of the opacity. The levels of both HVA and of VMA were found to be elevated.

A diagnosis of thoracic neuroblastoma was made.

A posterolateral thoracotomy along the fifth intercostal space was performed, and a paravertebral tumor was excised without many difficulties.

After histologic examination, the diagnosis of neuroblastoma was confirmed.

The postoperative course was uneventful and therefore the child was discharged on the seventh day after the operation. The patient was transferred to a pediatric oncology unit for complementary treatment of the tumor.

At the 2-year follow-up, the girl was doing well without any relapse of the tumor.

Suggested Reading

1. DeCou JM, Schlatter MG, Mitchell DS, Abrams RS. Primary thoracoscopic gross total resection of neuroblastoma. J Laparoendosc Adv Surg Tech A 2005 Oct; 15(5):470–3

2. Diez Jimenez L, Mitjavila Casanovas M. MIBG scintigraphy in neuroblastoma: something more than an image. Rev Esp Med Nucl 2006 Mar–Apr; 25(2):118–43

3. Escobar MA, Grosfeld JL, Powell RL, West KW, Scherer LR 3rd, Fallon RJ, Rescorla FJ. Long-term outcomes in patients with stage IV neuroblastoma. J Pediatr Surg 2006 Feb; 41(2):377–81

4. Kang CH, Kim YT, Jeon SH, Sung SW, Kim JH. Surgical treatment of malignant mediastinal neurogenic tumors in children. Eur J Cardiothorac Surg 2007; 2:321–325

5. Petty JK, Bensard DD, Partrick DA, Hendrickson RJ, Albano EA, Karrer FM. Resection of neurogenic tumors in children: is thoracoscopy superior to thoracotomy? J Am Coll Surg 2006 Nov; 203(5):699–703

Q 41

Giovanni Esposito, Michele Ametrano, and Ciro Esposito

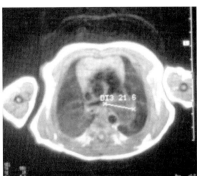 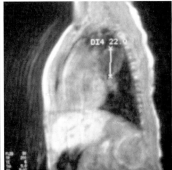

Fig. 1

A 5-year-old boy had a persistent cough that had started a few months earlier. A chest radiograph demonstrated a round opacity in the visceral compartment of the mediastinum. To define the precise nature of the opacity, MR imaging was performed (Fig. 1), which indicated the need for surgical intervention.

- What does the MR image show?
- What is the opacity suggestive of?
- What was found at surgery?
- What was the definitive diagnosis and treatment?
- What was the follow-up?

A 41

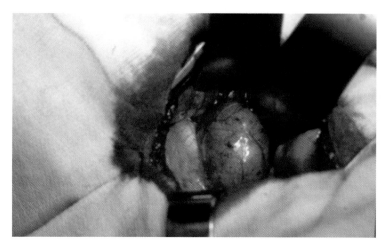

Fig. 2

The MR image (Fig. 1) shows the presence of a cystic area with a high signal on T1- and T2-weighted images that is characteristic of a cyst containing liquid with a high concentration of proteins.

Because of the connection of the cyst with the main left bronchus, the diagnostic suspicion was of a bronchogenic cyst.

At surgery, performed via left posterolateral thoracotomy along the fifth intercostal space, a cyst adherent to the bronchus was found and excised (Fig. 2).

Histological examination confirmed the diagnosis of bronchogenic cyst.

The postoperative course was uneventful and the child was discharged 7 days after surgery. Follow-up consisted in a plain radiograph at 6 and 12 months postoperatively, which was normal.

Suggested Reading

1. Fukasawa C, Ohkusu K, Sanayama Y, Yasufuku K, Ishiwada N, Ezaki T, Kohno Y. A mixed bacterial infection of a bronchogenic lung cyst diagnosed by PCR. J Med Microbiol 2006 Jun; 55(Pt 6):791–4

2. Inzani F, Recusani F, Agozzino M, Cavallero A, De Siena PM, D'Armini A, Vigano M, Arbustini E. Bronchogenic cyst: unexpected finding in a large aneurysm of the pars membranacea septi. J Thorac Cardiovasc Surg 2006 Oct; 132(4):972–4

3. Kunisaki SM, Fauza DO, Barnewolt CE, Estroff JA, Myers LB, Bulich LA, Wong G, Levine D, Wilkins-Haug LE, Benson CB, Jennings RW. Ex utero intrapartum treatment with placement on extracorporeal membrane oxygenation for fetal thoracic masses. J Pediatr Surg 2007 Feb; 42(2):420–5

4. Rubinas TC, Manera R, Newman B, Picken MM. Pneumothorax and pulmonary cyst in a 2-year-old child. Pleuropulmonary blastoma. Arch Pathol Lab Med 2006 Apr; 130(4)

5. Sauvat F, Fusaro F, Jaubert F, Galifer B, Revillon Y. Paraesophageal bronchogenic cyst: first case reports in pediatric. Pediatr Surg Int 2006 Oct; 22(10):849–51

Q 42

Giovanni Esposito and Ciro Esposito

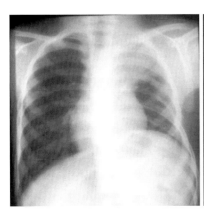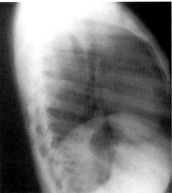

Fig. 1

A 4-year-old boy, without a significant medical history, presented to our department with a respiratory infection accompanied by fever, cough, and light dyspnea that had started 1 week earlier.

The fever disappeared after treatment with antibiotics, whereas the cough and dyspnea continued. After standard radiography of the thorax was carried out (Fig. 1), the child was hospitalized at our institution.

On admission, physical examination of the thorax revealed an anterior hypophonesis in the superior part of the left hemithorax where diffuse humid noises were found.

After other examinations, surgery was scheduled.

- What does the chest radiograph show?
- What other examinations were performed and what were their results?
- What was the diagnostic suspicion?
- What was found at surgery and what was the treatment?
- What was the definitive diagnosis?
- What was the follow-up?

A 42

The chest radiograph of the thorax (Fig. 1) shows an opacity of the superior left hemithorax that resides anteriorly in the lateral position.

MR angiography was performed, which demonstrated that the opacity was located in the anterior mediastinum and presented some cystic areas impregnated with contrast medium.

The diagnosis was of mediastinal lymphangioma.

At surgery, performed via anterolateral thoracotomy at the eighth intercostal space, a lymphangioma was found. The lymphangioma was strongly adherent to the surrounding vascular and nerve structures, and it was isolated after many difficulties. For these reasons, we performed a subtotal excision of the mass. The postoperative course was uneventful and the thoracic drain was removed after 48 h. The child was discharged on postoperative day 8. At the 6-month and 1-year follow-ups, no relapse was observed (Fig. 2).

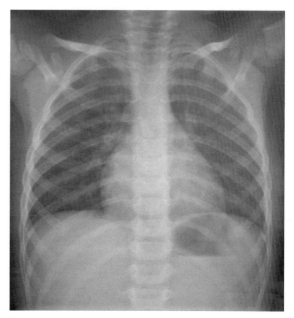

Fig. 2

Suggested Reading

1. Al-Salem AH. Lymphangiomas in infancy and childhood. Saudi Med J 2004 Apr; 25(4):466–9
2. Handa R, Kale R, Upadhyay KK. Isolated mediastinal lymphangioma herniating through the intercostal space. Asian J Surg 2004 Jul; 27(3):241–2
3. Nouri H, Raji A, Rochdi Y, Elhattab Y, M'Barek BA. Cervical cystic lymphangioma in children. Rev Laryngol Otol Rhinol (Bord) 2006; 127(4):263–6
4. Okazaki T, Iwatani S, Yanai T, Kobayashi H, Kato Y, Marusasa T, Lane GJ, Yamataka A. Treatment of lymphangioma in children: our experience of 128 cases. J Pediatr Surg 2007 Feb; 42(2):386–9
5. Tamay Z, Saribeyoglu E, Ones U, Anak S, Guler N, Bilgic B, Yilmazbayhan D, Gun F. Diffuse thoracic lymphangiomatosis with disseminated intravascular coagulation in a child. J Pediatr Hematol Oncol 2005 Dec; 27(12):685–7

Q 43

Giovanni Esposito and Ciro Esposito

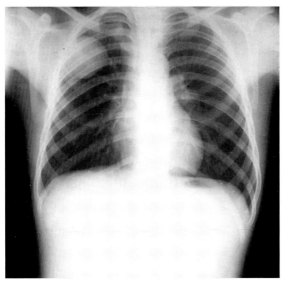

Fig. 1

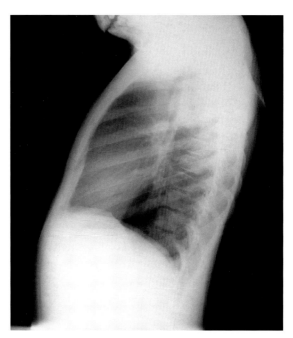

Fig. 2

A 5-year-old child, who was born at term after an uncomplicated delivery, was in good health until 1 month before admission to our hospital when he had a bronchopulmonary infection that was treated with antibiotics. The fever disappeared, but many bouts of nonproductive coughing persisted, and therefore standard radiography of the chest was performed. The radiography findings indicated the need for surgical intervention. On admission, the child, who was in a good general condition, presented many respiratory sounds on auscultation of the left hemithorax. The laboratory test results were normal except for a marked eosinophilia. On the basis of the radiological report, other tests were performed before making the diagnosis and deciding on the type of intervention.

- What do Figs. 1 and 2 show?
- What other examinations were performed and what were their results?
- What was the diagnosis?
- What was the treatment?
- What was the follow-up?

A 43

The radiographs show a single large pulmonary nodule in the superior part of the left hemithorax in the lateral projection.

The other tests performed were: an indirect hemoagglutination assay with the result of 1:152; and an immunoelectrophoresis assay that was positive. Complement fixation test results were both positive. Furthermore, an abdominal ultrasound was performed that was negative for the possible presence of the same lesion.

The diagnosis was of echinococcus cyst of the lung.

Treatment consisted in a posterolateral thoracotomy at the fifth intercostal space and a small pneumotomy of the superior lobe, through which an echinococcus cyst, the size of an orange, was extracted (Fig. 3).

The postoperative course was uneventful and the child was discharged 7 days after the intervention with a prescription of albendazole for 2 weeks.

At the 1-year follow-up, the child was in good condition.

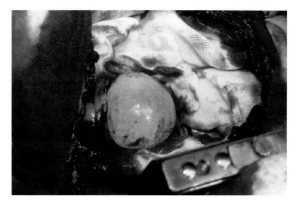

Fig. 3

Suggested Reading

1. Dincer SI, Demir A, Sayar A, Gunluoglu MZ, Kara HV, Gurses A. Surgical treatment of pulmonary hydatid disease: a comparison of children and adults. J Pediatr Surg 2006 Jul; 41(7):1230–6

2. Durakbasa CU, Sander S, Sehiralti V, Tireli GA, Tosyali AN, Mutus M. Pulmonary hydatid disease in children: outcome of surgical treatment combined with perioperative albendazole therapy. Pediatr Surg Int 2006 Feb; 22(2):173–8

3. Erdem CZ, Erdem LO. Radiological characteristics of pulmonary hydatid disease in children: less common radiological appearances. Eur J Radiol 2003 Feb; 45(2):123–8

4. Mallick MS, Al-Qahtani A, Al-Saadi MM, Al-Boukai AA. Thoracoscopic treatment of pulmonary hydatid cyst in a child. J Pediatr Surg 2005 Dec

5. Turkyilmaz Z, Sonmez K, Karabulut R, Demirogullari B, Gol H, Basaklar AC, Kale N. Conservative surgery for treatment of hydatid cysts in children. World J Surg 2004 Jun; 28(6):597–601

Q 44

Giovanni Esposito and Ciro Esposito

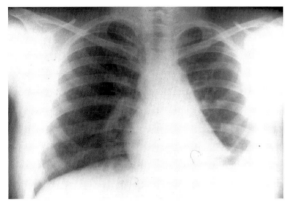

Fig. 1

A 9-year-old boy, born at term after a normal pregnancy and delivery and with no family history of disease, was in good health until the age of 4 years, when he showed dyspnea and cyanosis with some exercise intolerance. Because the symptoms became worse, a radiograph of the chest was acquired after which hospitalization was indicated.

On admission, the physical examination revealed mild cyanosis on the lips and nail beds with marked exercise intolerance.

On auscultation of the left hemithorax, many respiratory murmurs were noted especially inferiorly. Laboratory examination showed an arterial hypoxia with polycythemia.

After other diagnostic procedures, surgery was scheduled.

- What does the radiograph show (Fig. 1)?
- What other procedures were performed and what was their result?
- What was the diagnosis?
- What was the intervention?
- What was the follow-up?

A 44

A standard radiograph of the chest showed a normal cardiac silhouette with a shadow in the inferior part of the left lung that was connected with a spindle-shaped band to the hilum and was interpreted as an enlarged pulmonary artery and vein.

Angioscintigraphy and cardiac catheterization with pulmonary angiography were performed. The angioscintigraphy showed a hypervascularized pulmonary lesion with an arteriovenous shunt, while the cardiac catheterization with pulmonary angiogram showed a large localized arteriovenous fistula of the left lower lobe of the lung (Fig. 2).

The degree of right-to-left shunt was calculated by placing a catheter into the right pulmonary vein (via a retrograde left atrium approach) and measuring the oxygen saturation in the right pulmonary vein, in the left atrium, and in the aorta during basal conditions and after balloon occlusion of the arterial branches of the arteriovenous fistula. The oxygen saturation values were: pulmonary artery 44%, left atrium 58%, right pulmonary vein 86%, aorta 55%, and aorta after occlusion of the fistula 78%.

On the basis of all these procedures the diagnosis was congenital pulmonary arteriovenous fistula.

During surgery, on the surface of the lower lobe many varicose vessels were found. An inferior lobectomy was performed.

The postoperative course showed no complications with prompt relief of symptoms. At 1-year follow-up, the child was in good condition.

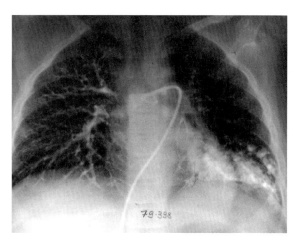

Fig. 2

Suggested Reading

1. Berthezene Y, Howarth NR, Revel D. Pulmonary arteriovenous fistula: detection with magnetic resonance angiography Eur Radiol 1998; 8(8):1403–4
2. Motsch K, Porstmann W. Arteriovenous pulmonary fistula. The differential diagnosis of cyanosis in children. Dtsch Gesundheitsw 1968 Sep 12; 23(37):1750–5
3. Seth RK, Seth S, Kabra SK. Micropulmonary arteriovenous fistula causing cyanosis. Indian J Pediatr 2003 Sep; 70(9):747–9

3

Abdomen

Introduction

Clinical expression of abdominal surgical problems in children comprises a spectrum of symptoms, many of them shared by different diseases. Consequently, a complete and well-oriented medical history and physical examination are the main tools for establishing the diagnosis and the guidelines to request radiological studies.

Sometimes, clinical evaluation is enough to initiate a medical treatment or indicate a surgical therapy, for example, when a patient has vomiting secondary to gastroesophageal reflux or pyloric hypertrophy. In spite of good medical practice, frequently the etiology is not clear and complementary laboratory and/or radiological studies are needed.

There are many studies available to help in the diagnosis of an abdominal problem in childhood. Occasionally, a plain film radiograph alone is sufficient to confirm a diagnosis (appendicolith in acute appendicitis), while in others an expensive and complex examination is needed (MR imaging in cases of tethered cord syndrome). Furthermore, in other cases, radiological studies are not helpful in confirming the diagnosis and an invasive procedure is indicated: pH-metry in a vomiting patient or rectal biopsy in a baby with constipation to rule out a gastroesophageal reflux or Hirschsprung's disease, respectively.

Medical technology has grown quickly in the last few years and pediatricians and pediatric surgeons need to decide on the best option according to the clinical picture and aiming for cost-effective results. Nowadays, for example, examinations that could be used to study a neonate or older child with an upper gastrointestinal problem include, among others, barium esophagogastrogram, ultrasonography, CT scan, MR imaging, PET scan, gammagraphy, endoscopy with or without biopsies, manometry, pH-metry, and electrophysiologic studies.

The approach to an abdominal problem depends on the possible etiology. In this way, for example, "intestinal obstruction syndrome" in neonates and children with no previous laparotomy should be considered a congenital malformation. This syndrome can be approached as "high" or "low" as well as "mechanical" or "functional." The age of presentation is also an important issue when exploring a possible etiology. The radiological study of this syndrome includes in all cases a plain film radiograph; other studies such as a barium enema, barium esophagogram, intestinal transit, ultrasonography, or CT scan depend on the initial clinical and radiological findings.

This section offers over 75 case studies of common congenital or acquired abdominal surgical diseases found in the pediatric population, including abdominal wall, gastrointestinal, hepatic, biliary, pancreatic, and diaphragmatic problems. We hope that these cases will be helpful to the practitioner in the study of their pediatric patients.

Q 45

Salam Yazbeck

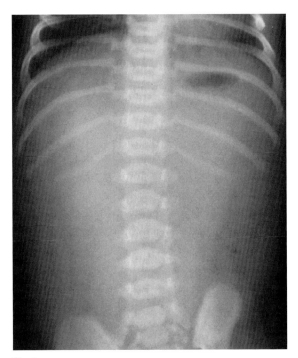

Fig. 1

Fig. 2

A previously healthy 6-month-old boy was brought to the emergency room for bilious vomiting, abdominal distention, and passage of bright red blood per rectum. On physical examination the abdomen was tender and reddish. The abdominal radiograph is shown in Fig. 1.

The emergency room physician asked for an abdominal ultrasound (Fig. 2).

- What are your diagnoses?
- What is your interpretation of the radiograph in Fig. 1?
- Why did the emergency room physician ask for an abdominal ultrasound and what did it show (Fig. 2)?
- What would you do next?

A 45

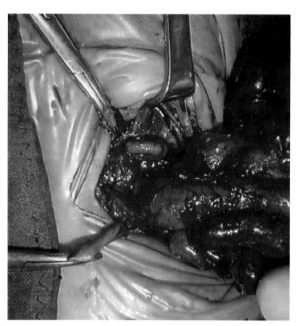

Fig. 3

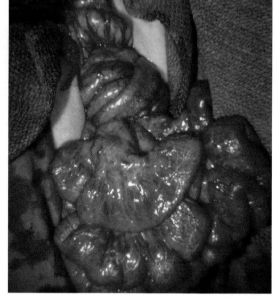

Fig. 4

The diagnosis is any acute bowel obstruction with necrosis.

A gasless abdomen, as that shown in Fig. 1, in a child with bilious vomiting and passage of red blood per rectum should make you suspect a midgut volvulus complicating an intestinal malrotation.

The abdominal ultrasound was requested in order to check the position of the mesenteric vessels. It showed an inversion of these vessels with the mesenteric vein to the left of the superior mesenteric artery, confirming the diagnosis of intestinal malrotation.

An urgent laparotomy is the next step.

In this case, the consultant pediatric surgeon decided to proceed with an immediate laparotomy. There was a midgut volvulus with severe ischemia of the whole bowel that persisted even after reduction of this volvulus and soaking of the bowel loops in warm saline. Only 10–12 cm of the proximal bowel was viable (Fig. 3). It was decided to proceed with the surgical cure of the malrotation (Ladd's procedure) and to close the abdomen and perform a second-look laparotomy the next day. The same findings were noted again and the patient was allowed to die.

Had this patient been brought to our attention earlier, the operative findings could have been like those in Fig. 4, showing a non-ischemic midgut volvulus that could be untwisted in a counter-clockwise direction with the entire bowel intact and ready to undergo the Ladd's procedure.

Q 46

Salam Yazbeck

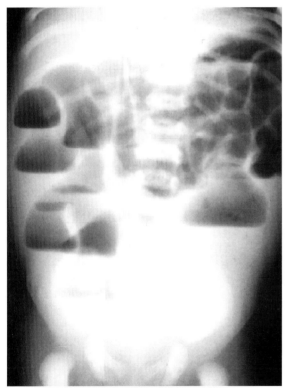

Fig. 1

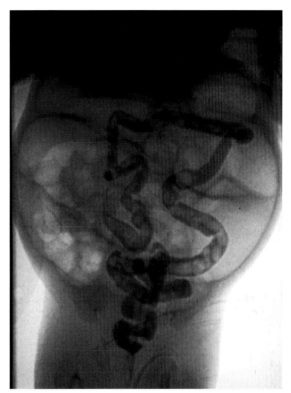

Fig. 2

A 3,000-g male neonate, born in a university hospital, presented with severe abdominal distension, bilious vomiting, and failure to pass meconium in the first 24 h of life. A prenatal ultrasound had shown an important bowel dilatation that lasted for the last trimester.

On physical examination, dilated bowel loops could be recognized. On abdominal inspection the abdomen was tender, and the anus was small but patent.

The abdominal radiograph is shown in Fig. 1.

The consultant pediatric surgeon ordered a barium enema (Fig. 2).

- What is your differential diagnosis?
- What does Fig. 1 show?
- Why did the surgeon order a barium enema?
- How would you manage this patient?
- What is the most likely underlying cause?

A 46

This is a case of bowel obstruction that could be caused by many intrinsic or extrinsic factors (atresias, Hirschsprung's disease, meconium-related diseases, etc.).

Figure 1 is a simple abdominal radiograph showing many dilated bowel loops. It could be associated with any cause of neonatal bowel obstruction.

The contrast enema shows a micro-colon contracted on inspissated meconium pellets. The same aspect could be observed in the terminal ileum.

If there is no perforation, a non-ionic hydrosoluble contrast enema could be therapeutic and relieve the obstruction on the first attempt or after many attempts.

If not, laparotomy is mandatory in order to empty the bowel from its very thick and sticky meconium with or without a temporary ileostomy.

More than 99% of meconium ileus cases are associated with cystic fibrosis of the pancreas. The definitive diagnosis is made with a sweat test that shows a high Cl^- concentration. However, this test may yield normal results in the first month of life, but a genetic mutation of the cystic fibrosis transmembrane regulator protein (CFTR) can be identified on chromosomal studies before birth.

Suggested Reading

1. Del Pin CA, Czyrko C, Ziegler MM, et al. Management and survival of meconium ileus. Ann Surg 1992; 215:179
2. Escobar MA, Grosfeld JL, Burdick JJ, et al. Surgical considerations in cystic fibrosis: a 32-year evaluation of outcomes. Surgery 2005; 138:560–571
3. Noblett HR. Treatment of uncomplicated meconium ileus by gastrograffin enema, a preliminary report. J Pediatr Surg 1969; 4:190–197
4. Rescola F, Grosfeld JL, West KJ, et al. Changing patterns of treatment and survival in neonates with meconium ileus. Arch Surg 1989; 124:837–840

Q 47

Salam Yazbeck

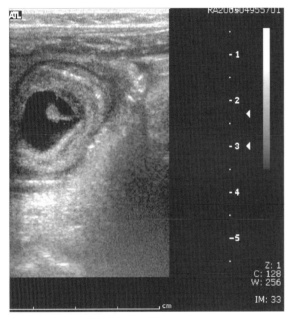

Fig. 1

A 1-month-old boy presented with intermittent vomiting, sometimes of bilious nature. His mother said that he also had 15–30-min episodes of abdominal pain once or twice per day.

Physical examination of the patient was unremarkable.

The treating pediatrician ordered a barium meal that was normal and an abdominal ultrasound (Fig. 1).

- Describe the findings in Fig. 1.
- What is your differential diagnosis?
- Would you order any other test?
- How would you manage this patient?

A 47

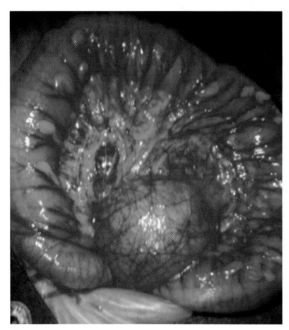

Fig. 2

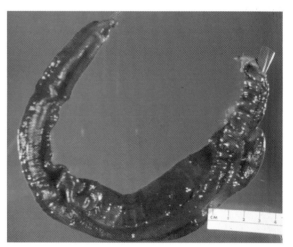

Fig. 3

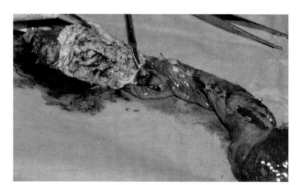

Fig. 4

Figure 1 is an abdominal ultrasound scan that shows a cystic lesion lined by a mucosal inner layer. This is typical of a duplication cyst.

An intra-abdominal cystic lesion could be a mesenteric cyst, a cystic lymphangioma, a Meckel's diverticulum, or a cystic duplication.

A pertechnetate scan could be obtained in order to identify the ectopic gastric mucosa that is frequently present in duplications.

The best treatment is resection of the duplication with its adjacent bowel segment. Figure 2 shows a cystic duplication of the terminal ileum, typically located on the mesenteric side and sharing the same vascular supply with the adjacent bowel.

Gastrointestinal duplications can be found everywhere from the mouth to the anus. Resection of the duplication with the adjacent gastrointestinal segment is not possible if the duplication cyst is located in the duodenal loop or if the duplication is of the tubular type (Fig. 3) and if it extends along a very long segment of the bowel. In these cases marsupialization of the duplication in the adjacent bowel is preferable. If gastric mucosa is present (Fig. 4) within the duplication, it should be resected.

Q 48

Ugo De Luca and Antonino Tramontano

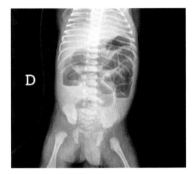

Fig. 1

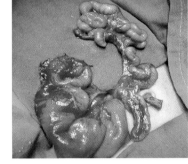

Fig. 2

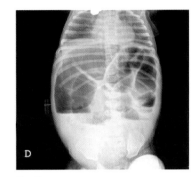

Fig. 3

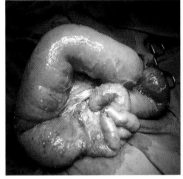

Fig. 4

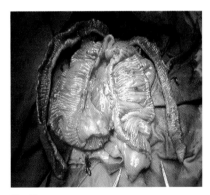

Fig. 5

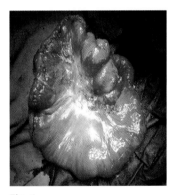

Fig. 6

A 3,050-g (39 weeks) newborn had severe abdominal distension, bile-stained vomiting, and no stool passage at birth.

A plain abdominal radiograph (Fig. 1) was obtained and following this investigation the newborn was operated on.

The surgical specimen is shown in Fig. 2. At surgery, an end-to-end intestinal anastomosis was realized.

The postoperative period was characterized by failure to thrive, abdominal distension, persistent vomiting, and poor stool passage.

Three months postoperatively, the child had another radiograph (Fig. 3) and a second operation was necessary (Figs. 4–6).

- What does Fig. 1 show?
- What is the intraoperative diagnosis?
- What are the surgical options?
- Was postoperative complicated course an expression of which condition?
- What are the surgical options in these reoperations?

A 48

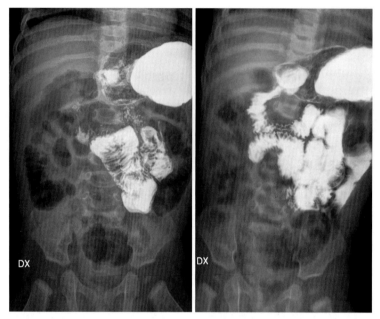

Fig. 7

The radiograph shows neonatal intestinal obstruction. The operative diagnosis is intestinal atresia with a large mesenteric defect (IIIA type). The end-to-end anastomosis without tapering of the large preatresic bowel in the first operation was responsible for the disturbed intestinal transit (DIT) in the postoperative period.

Reoperation, without large intestinal resection in order to avoid small bowel syndrome, was considered with a long antimesenteric tapering of the dilated bowel.

The postoperative course was characterized by good passage of stool, weight gain, and eventually complete recovery. A postoperative barium meal study (Fig. 7) demonstrated a normal appearance of the small intestine and a regular transit time.

Suggested Reading

1. Bianchi A. Longitudinal intestinal lengthening and tailoring: results in 20 children. *J R Soc Med* 1997 Aug; 90(8): 429–432
2. Bueno J., Guiterrez J, Mazariegos GV et al. Analysis of patients with longitudinal intestinal lengthening procedure referred for intestinal transplantation. *J. Ped. Surg* 2001; 36 (1):178–183
3. Miller RC. Complicated Intestinal Atresias. *Ann Surg* 1979 May; 189(5):607–610
4. Thomas CG Jr, Carter JM. Small intestinal atresia: the critical role of a functioning anastomosis. *Ann Surg* 1974 May; 179(5):663–670
5. Thompson JS, Langnas AN, Pinch LW, Kaufman S, Quigley EM, Vanderhoof JA. Surgical approach to short-bowel syndrome. Experience in a population of 160 patients. *Ann Surg* 1995 Oct; 222(4):600–607

Q 49

Ugo De Luca

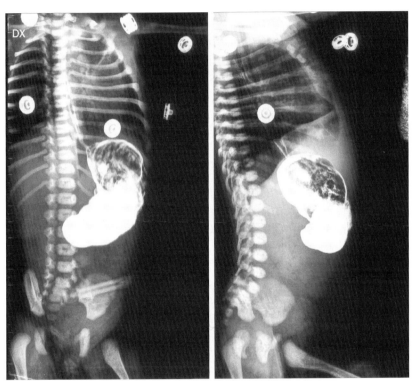

Fig. 1

A 20-day-old preterm female was transferred to our department from another hospital. Initially, the newborn
was on total parenteral nutrition for sepsis. When oral
feeding was started on the 17th day, the baby presented
with vomiting of milk and gastric juice, which was not
bile stained. The vomiting soon became projectile. The
contrast meal study is shown in Fig. 1.

- What is the diagnosis?
- What is the treatment?

A 49

This is a rare case of pyloric atresia with a late presentation of symptoms because of the initial suspension of alimentation.

The treatment is surgical and consists in a Mikulicz pyloroplasty (longitudinal incision and transverse suture; Figs. 2, 3).

The postoperative course was uneventful and alimentation was started on postoperative day 3.

Pyloric atresia is a rare congenital malformation, representing about 1% of all atresias of the gastrointestinal tract. Epidermolysis bullosa is the most common associated abnormality. Familial occurrence of pyloric atresia has been reported. The sex distribution is equal and there is a high proportion of low-birth-weight newborns. Polyhydramnios is encountered in about 50% of all cases of pyloric atresia. The main symptom is vomiting, often projectile and nonbilious. The diagnosis is achieved mainly radiologically by a barium meal study. The particularity of the case presented here is the late diagnosis due to the suspension of alimentation. In other cases the diagnosis may be delayed because the atresia is not complete but represented by a holed web.

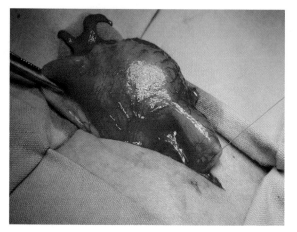

Fig. 2

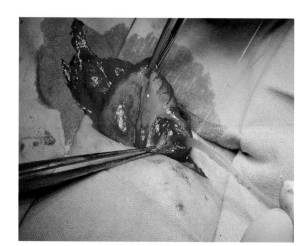

Fig. 3

Suggested Reading

1. Bar-Maor JA, Nissan S, Nevo S Pyloric atresia. J Med Genet 9, 70–72, 1972
2. Ducharme JC, Bensoussan AL Pyloric atresia. J Pediatr Surg 10, 149–150, 1975
3. Grunebaum M, Kornreich L, Ziv N et al. The imaging diagnosis of pyloric atresia. Z Kinderchir 40, 308–311, 1985
4. Muller M, Morger R, Engert J Pyloric atresia. report of four cases and review of the literature. Pediatr Surg Int 5, 276–279, 1990
5. Raffensperger JG, Pyloric and duodenal obstruction. In Swenson's Pediatric Surgery 5th edn, Appleton & Lange, Norwalk, Conn, 509–516, 1990

Q 50

Jürgen Schleef

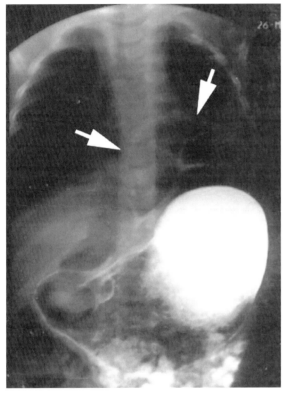

Fig. 1

An 18-month-old boy was brought to our hospital with fever and signs of pulmonary infection.

The mother reported that the boy was growing normally, but had symptoms of vomiting associated with coughing.

The surgeon decided, on the basis of the history reported by the mother, to ask for a barium swallow to rule out gastroesophageal reflux.

- What does Fig. 1 show?
- Why did the surgeon ask for a barium swallow?
- What condition is affecting this child?
- How do you treat this condition?

A 50

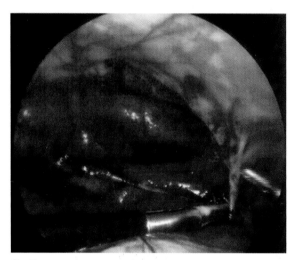

Fig. 2

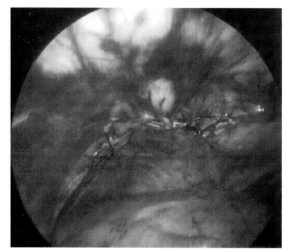

Fig. 3

Figure 1 shows a radiograph of the chest of an 18-month-old boy. The barium swallow showed no evidence of gastroesophageal reflux (the stomach is filled with barium). The small bowel and colon are projected in the thorax, suggestive of a diaphragmatic hernia.

The treatment of this pathological condition is surgical. During laparoscopy, it was noted that the defect in the diaphragm had repositioned the bowel into the abdomen (Fig. 2). The defect was closed at laparoscopy. The final result is shown in Fig. 3: a closed Bochdalek hernia. The child was discharged from hospital 2 days after surgery.

Suggested Reading

1. Eren S, Ciris F. Diaphragmatic hernia: diagnostic approaches with review of the literature. Eur J Radiol 2005; 54(3):448–59
2. Langer JC. Congenital diaphragmatic hernia. Chest Surg Clin N Am 1998; 8(2):295–314
3. Mei-Zahav M, Solomon M, Trachsel D, Langer JC. Bochdalek diaphragmatic hernia: not only a neonatal disease. Arch Dis Child 2003; 88(6):532–5
4. Mullins ME, Saini S. Imaging of incidental Bochdalek hernia. Semin Ultrasound CT MR 2005; 26(1):28–36

Q 51

Nancy Rollins and Korgun Koral

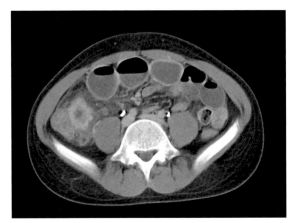

Fig. 1   Fig. 2

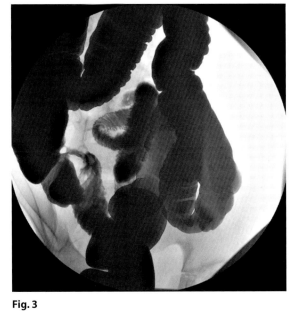

Fig. 3

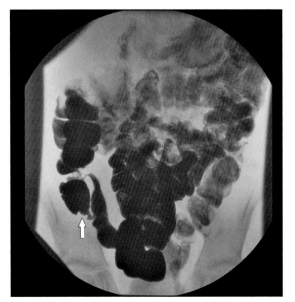

Fig. 4

A 12-year-old boy presented to the emergency room with right upper quadrant pain. A CT scan of the abdomen and pelvis was obtained.
- What are the findings on the CT scan (Figs. 1, 2)?
- What is the differential diagnosis at this point?

After symptoms subsided, a barium enema (Fig. 3) and small-bowel follow-through (Fig. 4) were performed with an interval of 1 week.
- What are the findings?
- What is the differential diagnosis?
- What is the diagnosis?
- What are the complications?

A 51

There is thickening of the walls (*arrow*, Fig. 2) of the cecum and terminal ileum. The terminal ileum is dilated as are the distal small bowel loops. Inflammatory stranding of mesenteric fat is present. No free fluid or abscess is seen.

Wall thickening of the terminal ileum and cecum can be seen in Crohn's disease, ulcerative colitis, infection (Yersinia, tuberculosis), lymphoma, and mesenteric adenitis.

There is luminal narrowing involving the terminal ileum (string sign). The cecum is narrowed with irregular mucosal contours (*arrow*, Fig. 4). The diagnosis is Crohn's disease. Crohn's disease affects the bowel wall in its entirety and results in sinus tracts, fissures, and fistulas; it can present with intra-abdominal abscesses. Skip lesions are characteristic, whereas in ulcerative colitis involvement is continuous. In ulcerative colitis there is only mucosal involvement. In a quarter of patients with ulcerative colitis there is terminal ileum involvement (backwash ileitis).

Suggested Reading

1.   Federle MP. Diagnostic Imaging: Abdomen. Amirsys Ed. 2005

Q 52

Nancy Rollins and Korgun Koral

A 1-month-old boy presented with constipation since birth and failure to thrive.
- What test was performed? How is this test done?
- Which contrast material was used? Why?
- What are the findings?
- How is the definitive diagnosis made?

A 52

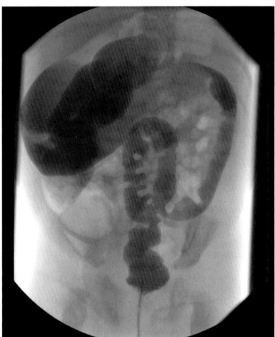

Fig. 1

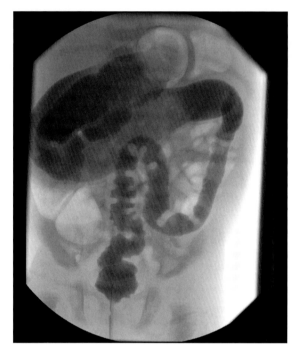

Fig. 2

A contrast enema was performed (Figs. 1, 2). The test was performed without bowel preparation. An enema tip without a balloon was inserted into the distal rectal vault. A balloon may obscure the transition zone.

Water-soluble contrast material was used in this instance to also alleviate constipation. Usually barium provides better anatomical detail.

The transverse colon, hepatic flexure, and ascending colon are markedly dilated. The rectum, sigmoid colon, and descending colon are normal to mildly small in caliber. There is a size discrepancy between the transverse colon and descending colon. The transition zone appears to be in the region of the splenic flexure.

The definitive diagnosis is made with colonic biopsy to assess the presence of ganglion cells in the colonic wall.

Suggested Reading

1. Kuhn JP, Slovis TL, Haller JO. Caffey's Pediatric Diagnostic Imaging. Elsevier Ed. 2004
2. Siegel MJ, Coley BD. Pediatric Imaging. Lippincott Williams & Wilkins Ed. 2006

Q 53

Nancy Rollins and Korgun Koral

A 2-month-old boy presented to the emergency room with bilious vomiting.

- What test should be performed first?
- If a study with contrast medium is performed what should be done? Upper gastrointestinal examination or barium enema?
- What are the findings on the upper gastrointestinal examination?
- Is this condition an emergency?

A 53

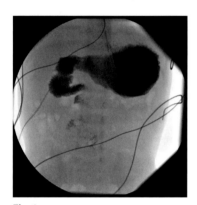

Fig. 1

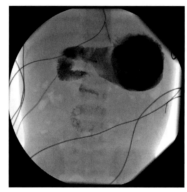

Fig. 2

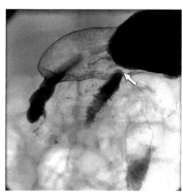

Fig. 3

Plain radiographs of the abdomen should be obtained first to assess for bowel dilatation and presence of free intraperitoneal air.

In a child with bilious vomiting, the test of choice is an upper gastrointestinal (UGI) examination with barium. Bilious vomiting indicates an obstruction distal to the duodenojejunal junction (ligament of Treitz).

A feeding tube is seen in the stomach and proximal duodenum. The ligament of Treitz is to the right of the spine. The proximal jejunum demonstrates the corkscrew appearance (Figs. 1, 2). It is not unusual to place a feeding tube to perform a UGI examination. This provides better control and a shorter procedure time. Every UGI examination should demonstrate the UGI tract, which is normally to the left of the spine at (or about) the level of the duodenal cap (*arrows* in Fig. 3; two different, normal subjects). In this case the duodenojejunal junction and proximal jejunum are to the right of the spine, consistent with a diagnosis of midgut malrotation. This condition constitutes an emergency if the patient is symptomatic.

In malrotation, the attachment of bowel is abnormally short, resulting in an abnormally positioned ligament of Treitz. The peritoneal bands (Ladd bands) cause extrinsic compression and proximal small bowel obstruction. Every effort should be made to obtain a picture of the ligament of Treitz in true frontal projection. If the position of the ligament of Treitz is equivocal, a small bowel follow-through study can be performed; however, demonstrating the normal position of the cecum in the right lower quadrant does not necessarily ensure absence of malrotation.

Suggested Reading

1. Siegel MJ, Coley BD. Pediatric Imaging. Lippincott Williams & Wilkins Ed. 2006
2. Swischuk LE. Imaging of the Newborn, Infant and Young Child. Lippincott Williams & Wilkins Ed. 2004

Q 54

Abdellatif Nouri and Mongi Mekki

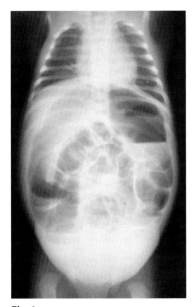

Fig. 1

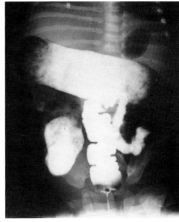

Fig. 2

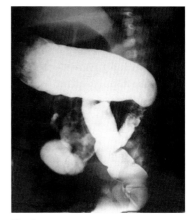

Fig. 3

A 3-day full-term male newborn was hospitalized for abdominal distension, bilious vomiting, and failure to pass meconium.

On examination, he weighed 3800 g, the anus was normal, and withdrawal of the doctor's finger did not produce meconium.

An anteroposterior erect abdominal radiograph was obtained (Fig. 1).

A barium enema was then performed (Figs. 2, 3).

- What does Fig. 1 show?
- What do Figs. 2 and 3 show?
- Which two diagnoses can be suggested on the basis of these figures?

At the end of the enema, the newborn passed meconium and the abdominal distension disappeared. For 6 days, the newborn had normal bowel movements and then presented again with abdominal distension.

- What is the most likely diagnosis and how can you confirm it?
- Which two complications threaten this newborn?
- What treatment do you recommend?

A 54

Figure 1 shows marked dilatation of the large and small bowel loops with air–fluid levels.

The barium enema (Figs. 2, 3) shows significant dilatation of the transverse colon and a small left colon with a transitional zone at the splenic flexure. The rectum does not look narrow.

The first diagnosis is Hirschsprung's disease extended to the splenic flexure. The second diagnosis is small left colon syndrome, which should be suspected when the meconium is not eliminated, the transitional zone is at the splenic flexure, and the rectum is not narrow.

Because of the recurrence of abdominal distension, the most likely diagnosis is Hirschsprung's disease. Anorectal manometry has proved to be a reliable method for diagnosing Hirschsprung's disease in older children by showing the absence of the recto-anal inhibitor reflex, but there is considerable controversy regarding the diagnostic accuracy of manometry in neonates. The diagnosis of Hirschsprung's disease is based on the histological examination of rectal wall biopsy specimens.

The two serious complications that threaten this newborn are enterocolitis, which remains the most common cause of death in Hirschsprung's disease patients, and spontaneous perforation of the intestinal tract that occurs particularly with long-segment aganglionosis.

After rectal irrigations for 5 days (Nursing), the abdominal distension disappeared completely and the newborn was operated on at the age of 14 days. The procedure was a one-stage primary transanal Soave carried out under laparoscopic assistance. Laparoscopy is necessary to adequately mobilize the descending colon, the splenic flexure and the transverse colon, to perform safe ligations of the vessels, and to ensure that there is no intra-abdominal twisting of the pull-through bowel. Figure 4 is the operative view of the transanal Soave. Biopsy of the frozen sections confirmed the presence of ganglionic cells at the pull-through bowel. Figure 5 shows the surgical specimen, which was 31 cm long and showed a long narrow colon, the transitional zone, and the dilated colon.

The child had an increased frequency of defecation (eight times daily) with peri-anal irritation during the first four postoperative months. After a 2-year follow-up, the child has two bowel movements daily and he is free of symptoms.

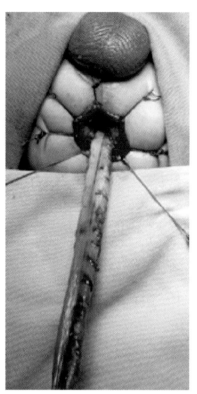

Fig. 4

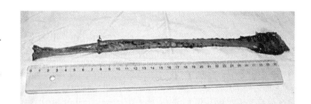

Fig. 5

Suggested Reading

1. Lister J, Tam PKH (1990) Hirschsprung's disease. In: neonatal surgery (eds J Lister and IM Irving). Butterworths, London, 523–546
2. Nunez R, Cabrera R, Moreno C, Agulla E, Vargas I, Blesa E. Usefulness of anorectal manometry in the neonatal diagnosis of Hirschsprung disease. Cir Pediatr 2000; 13:16–9
3. Puri P (1996) Hirschsprung's disease. In: newborn surgery (edited by P. Puri). Butterworths-Heinemann, Oxford, 363–378

Q 55

Abdellatif Nouri and Mongi Mekki

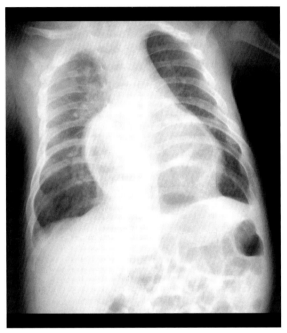

Fig. 1

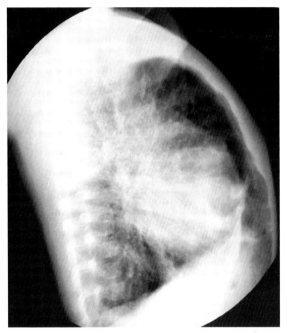

Fig. 2

A 4-month-old boy had a history of alimentary vomiting and recurrent bronchopneumopathy since birth.

The mother reported that a medical treatment for supposed gastroesophageal reflux had been prescribed to her infant without any improvement in his symptoms.

The physical examination revealed Down syndrome with a cutis excavatum and inspiratory crackles on pulmonary auscultation.

The pediatrician obtained a postero-anterior recumbent chest radiograph (Fig. 1) and completed the investigation with a lateral recumbent chest radiograph (Fig. 2).

- What does Fig. 1 show?
- Why did the pediatrician ask for the second chest radiograph?
- What does Fig. 2 show?
- What diagnosis is suspected?
- Which investigation can confirm the diagnosis?
- How do you explain the alimentary vomiting?
- Which other malformations can be associated with this pathological condition?
- How do you manage this condition?

A 55

Figure 1 shows a gas-filled mediastinum which is continuous with abdominal gas.

The pediatrician obtained a lateral recumbent chest radiograph (Fig. 2) to determine whether the air-filled appearance is posterior, suggesting a hiatal hernia, anterior suggesting a retrosternal hernia, or anterior and posterior, generally suggesting a large posterolateral hernia.

Figure 2 shows that the abdominal gut loops are in continuity, just behind the xiphoid process and the sternum, with the anterior air-filled mediastinum.

A retrosternal hernia is suspected.

This diagnosis can be confirmed by rectocolic opacification, because a hernia usually contains the transverse colon. This is shown in Fig. 3. If the colon is not involved with the hernia, the best radiological exploration is three-dimensional CT.

Other malformations that can be associated with retrosternal hernia are pericardium defect, cardiac malformations, sternum malformations, epigastric diastases or omphalocele (Cantrell's pentalogy), and trisomy 21.

The alimentary vomiting was explored by a barium meal. It showed no gastroesophageal reflux, no intestinal malrotation, and no supravaterian duodenal stenosis. Vomiting may be explained by the compression of the herniated intestine.

Surgical repair is indicated because of the risk of incarceration. Operative repair is easily performed through an upper abdominal incision or by laparoscopy.

Figure 4 is a laparoscopic view of the retrosternal hernia. It shows the diaphragmatic defect after reduction of the transverse colon.

The herniated viscera are easily reduced, the sac should be resected, and the defect closed.

After the 3-year follow-up, the child was well and free of symptoms.

Suggested Reading

1. Ipek T, Altinli E, Yuceyar S. Laparoscopic repair of Morgani Larrey hernia: report of three cases. Surgery Today 2002; 32:902–5

2. Sahnoun L, Ksia A, Jouini R, Maazoun K, Mekki M, Krichene I, Belghith M, Nouri A. Pediatric retro sternal hernia. Arch Pediatr 2006; 13:1316–9

3. Yamashita K, Tsunoda T. Three dimensional computer images of Morgani hernia. Am J Surg 2004; 187:109–110

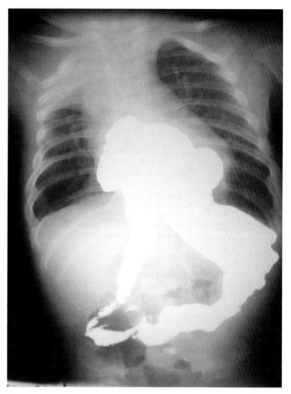

Fig. 3

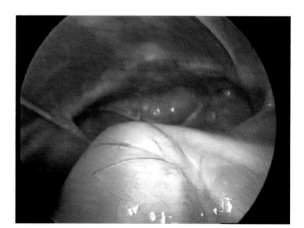

Fig. 4

Q 56

Abdellatif Nouri and Mongi Mekki

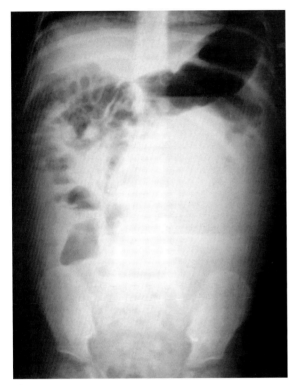

Fig. 1

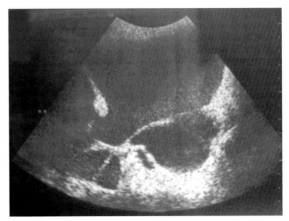

Fig. 2

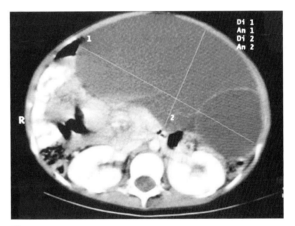

Fig. 3

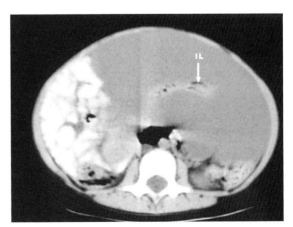

Fig. 4

A 4-year-old girl presented with a 1-month history of umbilical pain and abdominal distension without vomiting.

The physical examination revealed a protuberant nontender abdominal mass that was dull to percussion and mobile at palpation.

The surgeon performed the examinations shown in Figs. 1–4.

- What does the recumbent abdominal radiograph (Fig. 1) show?
- What does the abdominal ultrasound (Fig. 2) show?
- What does the abdominal CT scan (Figs. 3, 4) show?
- Which diagnosis can be suggested?
- How do you manage this pathological condition?

A 56

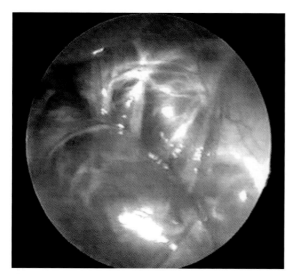

Fig. 5

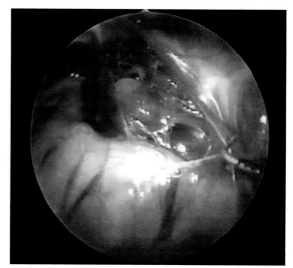

Fig. 6

Figure 1 shows an abnormal bulbing and opaque abdomen with an intestinal gas pattern pushed to the right.

The abdominal ultrasound (Fig. 2) shows a multilocular pelvi-abdominal intraperitoneal cyst with multiple hypoechoic zones separated by echogenic septa.

The abdominal CT scan (Fig. 3) confirms the presence of a multilocular intraperitoneal cyst which contains vascularized septa and pushes the intestine backward and to the right. This cyst contains an intestinal structure (Fig. 4).

An intraperitoneal multicystic lymphangioma is suspected, especially because the cyst contains an intestinal structure and its septa are vascularized. The mobilization of the cyst by palpation and the vascularization of the septa refute the diagnosis of compartmentalized ascites. If the ultrasound and/or CT scan show(s) two normal ovaries, the diagnosis of ovarian cyst can be ruled out. The aspect of a thin wall delimiting the cyst refutes the diagnosis of intestinal duplication.

Ultrasound and CT are highly sensitive in the diagnosis and preoperative evaluation of an abdominal multilocular cyst. For an abdominal localization in children, MRI is indicated only in the case of hemorrhagic complications of the cyst.

The most serious acute complication of this cyst is intestinal volvulus.

Laparoscopy confirmed the diagnosis of mesenteric multicystic lymphangioma (Fig. 5) holding an ileal loop

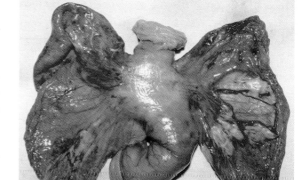

Fig. 7

(Fig. 6). Aspiration of the cyst permitted exteriorization of the lymphangioma and the ileal loop via an umbilical opening and complete removal of the lymphangioma and the ileal loop with intestinal anastomosis.

The surgical specimen (Fig. 7) shows a "butterfly aspect." The pathology report confirmed the diagnosis of cystic lymphangioma.

After a 2-year follow-up, the child is well and free of symptoms.

Q 57

Abdellatif Nouri and Mongi Mekki

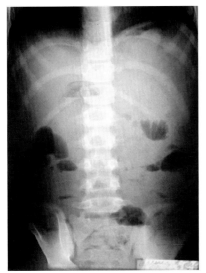

Fig. 1

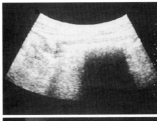
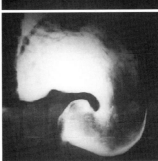

Fig. 2, 3

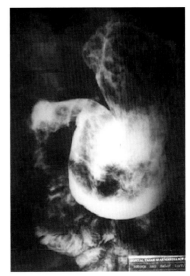

Fig. 4

An 11-year-old girl presented with a 6-month history of alimentary vomiting, abdominal pain, anorexia, and weight loss.

The mother has noticed epigastric distension, which had gradually increased in size. Four days before consultation, the patient experienced intolerance to food with bilious vomiting and abdominal pain.

The physical examination revealed a nervous and pale patient with a large, firm, relatively mobile and tender mass located in the left upper quadrant of the abdomen.

Laboratory test results showed iron-deficiency anemia (hemoglobin, 6 g/dl) and hyperleukocytosis (WBC, 15.6 10^3/mm^3).

The surgeon performed the examinations shown in Figs. 1–4.

- What do Figs. 1 and 2 show?
- What do Figs. 3 and 4 show?
- What are the three important clinical signs that should be sought systematically for the diagnosis?
- Is there any other investigation that will help confirm the diagnosis?
- How can you explain the iron-deficiency anemia?
- Are there any differential diagnoses?
- How is this condition best managed?

A 57

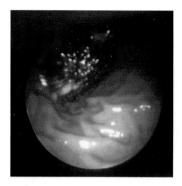

Fig. 5

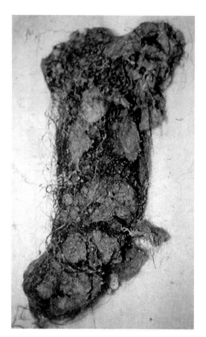

Fig. 6

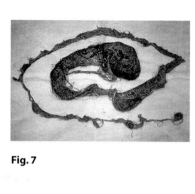

Fig. 7

This girl is affected by trichobezoar, which is a conglomerate of swallowed hair because of a mental disturbance.

The abdominal plain radiograph (Fig. 1) shows the absence of gastric bubble and the presence of air–fluid intestinal levels. In association with bilious vomiting, these levels confirm the intestinal occlusion. The abdominal ultrasonography (Fig. 2) shows an echogenic, dense, solid mass in the stomach with posterior clean sonic shadowing.

Figures 3 and 4 show a large bezoar outlined by barium, occupying the stomach and extending to the pylorus and the duodenum.

The three important clinical signs which should be sought systematically are a history of active trichophagia, a patchy baldness from hair pulling, and an emotional disturbance.

When trichophagia is denied by the patient, gastroscopy can show the trichobezoar and confirm the diagnosis (Fig. 5).

The iron-deficiency anemia can be explained by malnutrition and chronic blood loss from erosions and ulcerations of the gastric mucosa.

The differential diagnosis includes gastric duplication, gastric tumor, and pancreatic pseudocyst. All these diagnoses are easily ruled out by ultrasound and barium meal study.

After correction of the hydro-electrolytic disorders and transfusion, laparotomy revealed a huge dilation of the stomach containing a bezoar. The intestinal occlusion was due to a prolongation of the bezoar to the duodenum and the proximal jejunum, which was dilated and necrotic because of a large hair ball (10 cm in diameter). A longitudinal gastrotomy allowed removal of the bezoar (Fig. 6). Resection of the necrotic proximal jejunum allowed removal of the hair ball with a 60-cm tail (Fig. 7). After jejunal anastomosis and closure of the gastrotomy, the evolution was uneventful.

No attempt should be made to disrupt a large bezoar endoscopically because of the risk of detaching fragments and forming satellite intestinal lesions. For the same reasons, the prescription of pancreatic enzymes to dissolve a bezoar is not recommended. Psychiatric care is often indicated for the long term in the case of psychological problems so as to avoid recurrence.

At the 8-year follow-up, the patient was well and free of symptoms; her psychiatrist still recommended psychotherapeutic measures.

Q 58

Luciano Mastroianni and Alba Cruccetti

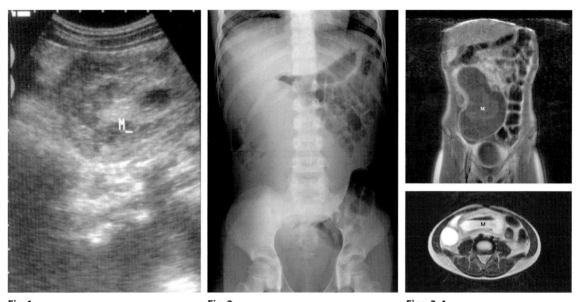

Fig. 1   Fig. 2   Figs. 3, 4

An 8-year-old boy was brought to the emergency department complaining of abdominal pain and high temperature which had started a few hours earlier.

On examination, the abdomen was not distended, a palpable mass was present and it was movable and tender. Rectal examination was normal.

The first radiological investigations performed are shown in Figs. 1 and 2.

- What do Figs. 1 and 2 show?

The patient was transferred to the department of surgery where he had loose stools and melena.

- What would you do next?
- What do Figs. 3 and 4 show?
- What pathological condition is affecting this child?
- What is the best way to manage this condition?

A 58

This child had an ileal intestinal duplication. Figure 1 is an abdominal ultrasound scan revealing a large mass with an inhomogeneous structure measuring 18×10×7 cm and was located in the abdomen.

Figure 2 shows an abdominal radiograph with dislocation of the bowel because of the presence of an abdominal mass without calcification.

The MR imaging scan showed a large mass located in the pelvis and in the central abdomen (Fig. 3) with an inhomogeneous signal, a mixed mass with predominantly liquid structure, and the presence in the lesion of an air–fluid level (Fig. 4).

The child underwent laparotomy. An ileal duplication (Fig. 5) was found. Subsequently, resection of the duplication and the adjacent bowel with end-to-end anastomosis of the remaining bowel was performed.

The postoperative period was uneventful and 9 months after surgery the child was doing well.

Intestinal duplication is a rare congenital anomaly that may arise anywhere along the gastrointestinal tract. Most duplications cause symptoms in infancy or early childhood, but some present as an incidental finding. The symptoms and signs of presentation depend on the type and location of the duplications, which include obstruction, hemorrhage, infection, perforation, and an asymptomatic mass. It is important to include intestinal duplications in the differential diagnosis of gastrointestinal bleeding, especially in children and when associated with an abdominal mass.

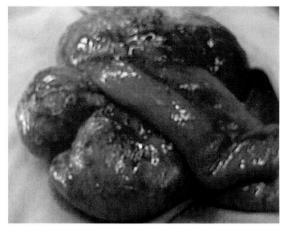

Fig. 5

Suggested Reading

1. Brown RL, Azizkhan RG. Gastrointestinal bleeding in infants and children: Meckel's diverticulum and intestinal duplication. Semin Pediatr Surg 1999; 8:202–209
2. Iyer CP, Mahour GH. Duplications of the alimentary tract in infants and children. J Pediatr Surg 1995; 30:1267–70
3. Long L, Zhang JZ and Wang YX. Vascular classification for small intestinal duplications: Experience with 80 cases. J Pediatr Surg 1998; 33:1243–1245
4. Pinter AB, Schubert W, Szemledy F, Gobel P, Schafer J, Kustos G. Alimentary tract duplications in infants and children. Eur J Pediatr Surg 1992; 2:8–12
5. Wardell S, Vidican DE. Ileal duplication cyst causing massive bleeding in a child. J Clin Gastroenterol 1990; 12:681–4

Q 59

Luciano Mastroianni and Alba Cruccetti

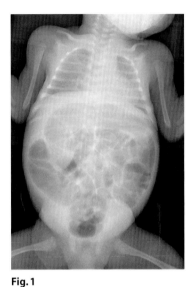

Fig. 1

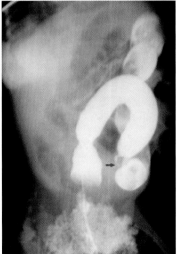

Fig. 2

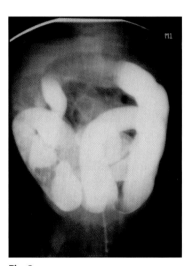

Fig. 3

A 49-day-old boy without a significant medical history developed abdominal distension and vomiting. He was a preterm infant of 30 weeks' gestational age and a birth weight of 1,700 g.

On examination, distended loops of gut were visible and palpable, bowel sounds were present, and the abdomen was slightly tender.

The first radiological investigation performed is shown in Fig. 1.

- What does Fig. 1 show?

Eight hours after abdominal decompression with a nasogastric tube and a rectal probe, the patient showed no improvement in symptoms.

- What would you do next?
- Why did the surgeon perform the second examination?
- What do Figs. 2 and 3 show?
- What pathological condition is affecting this child?
- What is the best way to manage this condition?

A 59

This infant is affected by intestinal obstruction. In particular, he is affected by a distal intestinal obstruction; the lower the obstruction, the greater the distended loops of bowel observed.

Figure 1 is an abdominal radiograph showing with several markedly distended loops of bowel and few air–fluid levels.

Figures 2 and 3 show the second investigation performed to distinguish between the different causes of low intestinal obstruction: a contrast enema with Gastrografin, demonstrating a narrowing between the sigmoid colon and the descending colon with distended bowel proximal to the narrowed bowel, reflux of contrast through the ileocecal valve and into the terminal ileum, filling several dilated loops.

The infant underwent laparotomy. A Meckel's diverticulum attached to the abdominal wall through a cord-like fibrous remnant was found obstructing the sigmoid colon where a stenosis was present (Figs. 4, 5). Diverticulectomy and intestinal resection with anastomosis of the stenotic bowel segment were performed.

The postoperative period was uneventful and 1 year after surgery the child was well.

Meckel's diverticulum should be considered in the differential diagnosis of any previously healthy infant without a history of surgery who develops a bowel obstruction.

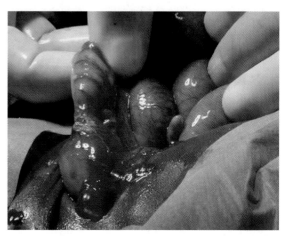

Fig. 4

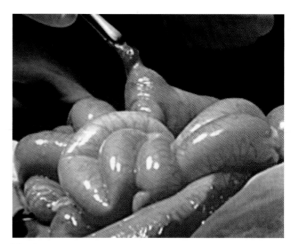

Fig. 5

Suggested Reading

1. Al-Zahem A, Arbuckle S, Cohen R. Combined ileal heterotopic pancreatic and gastric tissues causing ileocolic intussusception in an infant. Pediatr Surg Int 2006; 22:297–9
2. Ameh EA, Mshelbwala PM, Dauda MM, Sabiu L, Nmadu PT. Symptomatic vitelline duct anomalies in children. S Afr J Surg 2005; 43:84–5
3. Martinez Biarge M, Garcia-Alix A, Luisa del Hoyo M, Alarcon A, Saenz de Pipaon M, Hernandez F, Perez J, Quero J. Intussusception in a preterm neonate; a very rare, major intestinal problem—systematic review of cases. J Perinat Med 2004; 32:190–4
4. Moore TC. Omphalomesenteric duct malformations. Semin Pediatr Surg 1996; 5:116–23
5. Sy ED, Shan YS, Tsai HM, Lin CH. Meckel's diverticulum associated with ileal volvulus in a neonate. Pediatr Surg Int 2002; 18:529–31

Q 60

François Luks

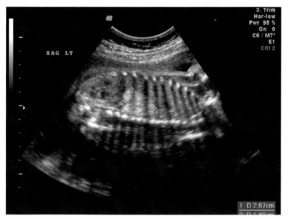

Fig. 1

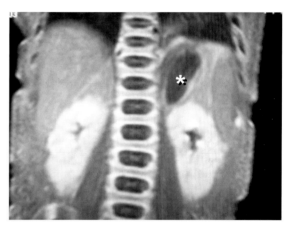

Fig. 2

A left adrenal mass was found on routine ultrasound in a 24-week-old fetus. The remainder of the examination was unremarkable (Fig. 1).

A fetal MR imaging study was performed, which confirmed the presence of a left adrenal lesion of uncertain origin and of heterogeneous consistency (cystic elements in a largely solid mass).

- What is the differential diagnosis?
- What further diagnostic and therapeutic measures, if any, would be indicated?

The mass remains unchanged on three further ultrasound examinations, each 4 weeks apart.

The infant is delivered at term in a tertiary center. Ultrasound on day 1 of life confirms the presence of the lesion, which is unchanged from the prenatal images. MR imaging at 2 weeks of life confirms the persistence of a lesion above the left kidney, possibly separate from the adrenal gland (Fig. 2).

- What are the other diagnostic and therapeutic options after birth?
- If surgical intervention is indicated, what are the different approaches?
- Is there a place for nonoperative management of this lesion?

A 60

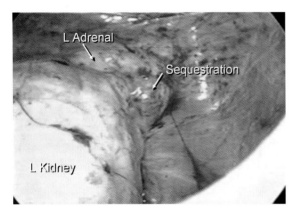

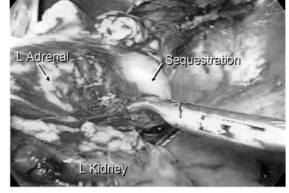

Fig. 3   **Fig. 4**

The differential diagnosis of a fetal adrenal mass is relatively narrow. The most common lesion of the fetal adrenal gland is a neuroblastoma. Adrenal hemorrhage can resemble a lesion, and a cause for the hemorrhage is often not found. However, the appearance of an adrenal hemorrhage tends to change over time as the hematoma is reabsorbed, showing more cystic features as it decreases in size. The third and possibly most common lesion in that region is an intra-abdominal pulmonary sequestration. This is a variant of an extralobar sequestration, typically found in the basal region of the thoracic cavity. As the diaphragm closes, a sequestration may become encased in the posterior mediastinum or even become separated from the thoracic cavity altogether.

If there are no other fetal anomalies, further testing is not strictly speaking necessary. However, close follow-up may be indicated: as mentioned, an adrenal hemorrhage will tend to decrease in size through the remainder of the pregnancy. Fetal neuroblastomas almost always behave in a nonaggressive fashion (similar to neuroblastomas in infants), but rapid growth and fetal or placental metastases have been described.

A fetal MR imaging study may help further define the lesion, although cystic elements can be seen in all three conditions (including cystic neuroblastoma). Finding a normal adrenal gland adjacent to the lesion essentially rules out adrenal hemorrhage of neuroblastoma, but an MR image is usually not very sensitive for small lesions or glands.

With a working diagnosis of neuroblastoma, two therapeutic approaches are possible. Adrenalectomy in the newborn period is feasible and can be performed through a retroperitoneal approach (open or laparoscopy). However, the "benign" course of most infant neuroblastomas has paved the way for a nonoperative approach to congenital neuroblastoma, on the assumption that these lesions will spontaneously regress.

If a conservative approach is used, it is important to follow up the infant closely (ultrasound every 3–4 weeks and at least two MR imaging studies) and to measure urinary catecholamines (VMA and HVA).

Intra-abdominal pulmonary sequestrations are obviously benign lesions. However, up to 50% of sequestrations contain elements of cystic adenomatoid malformation (CCAM), which may have a potential for malignant degeneration. The exact incidence of malignancies developing into a CCAM is unknown and is likely very small, but real. Therefore, several authors advocate elective resection if the lesion does not spontaneously regress.

This child was followed up for 6 months, at which time an ultrasound showed persistence of the lesion. He underwent a retroperitoneal laparoscopic resection of the mass at 9 months of age (Figs. 3, 4). In Fig. 3, the relationship between the left kidney, the adrenal gland, and the sequestration can be seen. The lesion was dissected off the left adrenal gland, as shown in Fig. 4.

On pathological examination, a diagnosis of pulmonary sequestration with CCAM elements (hybrid lesion) was confirmed.

Q 61

François Luks

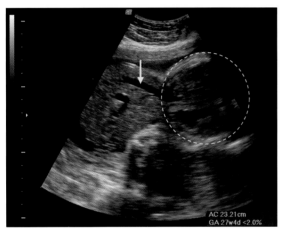

Fig. 1

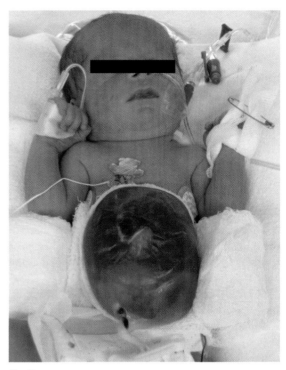

Fig. 2

On a routine second-trimester ultrasound (Fig. 1), an abdominal wall defect was noted.

- How can the main types of abdominal wall defects be differentiated by prenatal examination?
- What additional testing would you recommend if the lesion appears to be gastroschisis? And if the lesion is an omphalocele?
- How would you counsel the future parents if the lesion is an omphalocele?
- What would you estimate the mortality rate to be, and what degree of morbidity would you predict?

On subsequent ultrasound examination, the lesion is confirmed to be a giant omphalocele, and approximately 85% of the liver mass is seen outside the abdominal cavity.

- How does this information affect your counseling, and what precautions would you recommend at the time of delivery?

The infant is born at 36 weeks (Fig. 2).

- What immediate and medium-term therapeutic measures would you recommend?

A 61

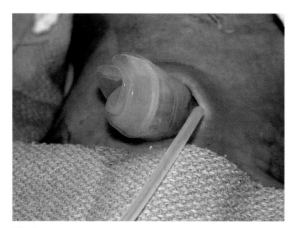

Fig. 3

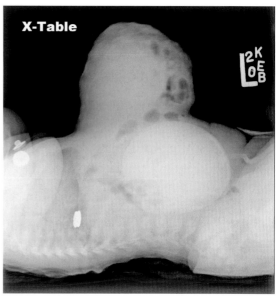

Fig. 4

With current ultrasound technology, it is possible to determine whether the umbilical cord insertion is lateral to the abdominal wall defect (in which case the diagnosis is gastroschisis) or whether the cord is inserted at the apex of the defect itself (omphalocele).

Typically, gastroschisis is an isolated lesion, and no further work-up is required, except for a complete ultrasound assessment of the fetus. Omphalocele, however, is associated with other anomalies in about 70% of cases. These anomalies can be chromosomal (trisomy 18 is the most common) or part of a complex syndrome (Pentalogy of Cantrell, from a fusion defect in the upper, or epigastric, abdominal fold; cloacal exstrophy, a lower abdominal folding defect). In more than a third of omphaloceles, there is an associated cardiac malformation. The prognosis of infants born with an omphalocele depends for the most part on the associated anomalies.

If a large portion of the liver is exteriorized, these lesions are called "giant" omphaloceles. They are not associated with a higher mortality, but difficulties in reducing the viscera may lead to significant morbidity in the first 6–18 months of life. Although a cesarean section is no longer mandatory for abdominal wall defects, the presence of a large portion of the liver in the defect could increase the risk of rupture and hemorrhage with vaginal delivery. Most centers will therefore recommend C-section.

Management of a giant omphalocele can be challenging, and immediate reduction of the liver may lead to acute kinking of the hepatic veins and the vena cava. A more gradual approach is therefore necessary.

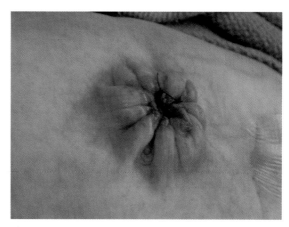

Fig. 5

In the present case, the intact membrane offered a natural barrier. Wrapping of the abdomen with an elastic bandage offered graded pressure on the defect, to start reduction of the viscera.

At 2 weeks of life, a tissue expander was inserted in the pelvis through a small Pfannenstiel incision (Fig. 3). The expander was enlarged by 10 ml each day through an external reservoir (Fig. 4). At 4 weeks of life, surgical reduction of the defect was achieved and the abdominal wall fascia could be closed (Fig. 5).

Q 62

Mario Lima and Giovanni Ruggeri

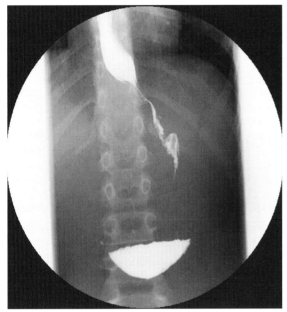

Fig. 1

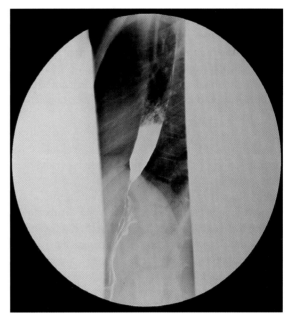

Fig. 2

An 8-year-old girl had a 6-month history of progressive dysphagia, at first for liquids and then for solid, associated with frequent regurgitations, substernal pain, and weight loss. She did not have any respiratory symptoms. At another hospital medical, therapy was initiated to relieve the dysphagia, but without any improvement.

The girl came to our attention because her symptoms worsened.

A barium swallow was performed (Figs. 1, 2).
- What do Figs. 1 and 2 show?
- Which other examinations were performed to reach a diagnosis?
- What do these examinations show?
- What is the differential diagnosis of this disease?
- What kind of therapy would be possible for this disease?
- How did we treat this girl?

A 62

This girl is affected by esophageal achalasia.

Achalasia consists in a failure of relaxation in the distal esophagus and esophagogastric junction. The cause is unknown, but most studies point to a primary neurogenic abnormality with lack of inhibitory innervation and progressive degeneration or loss of ganglion cells in the myenteric plexus.

The barium swallow (Figs. 1, 2) shows a markedly dilated esophagus with a tapering at the lower end, which has the appearance of a "rat tail." There is no evidence of gastroesophageal reflux.

Esophagoscopy was performed (see Fig. 3), which showed lots of retained undigested food; in the lower part of the esophagus a stenosis was seen, but the instrument could easily pass through. A congenital stenosis could be excluded.

Esophageal manometry is the diagnostic examination of choice for this disease: it shows hypertension of the lower esophageal sphincter (LES) and incomplete or absent relaxation of the LES together with disordered, weak, or absent peristaltic contractions in the body of the esophagus after swallowing.

The differential diagnosis of achalasia includes Chagas' disease, a South American parasitic infection caused by *Trypanosoma cruzi.*.

Pharmacologic management (nifedipine) of achalasia is almost always unsuccessful. Pneumatic dilation under endoscopic guidance is an alternative to surgical treatment; it is seldom successful and the risk of major complications (esophageal perforation, mediastinitis) is high.

We performed laparoscopic Heller myotomy (Fig. 4) associated with a Dor anterior hemifundoplication. We added pharmacological antireflux therapy (ranitidine) in the immediate postoperative period.

After 1 year, we performed endoscopy, which showed a patent esophagus, no supracardial dilation, and no difficulty in instrument insertion. At the time of writing, the girl was feeding regularly, without any problems, had a good weight gain, and was well and free of symptoms.

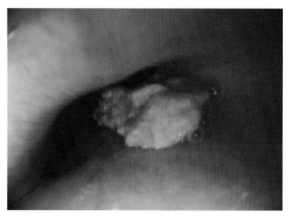

Fig. 3

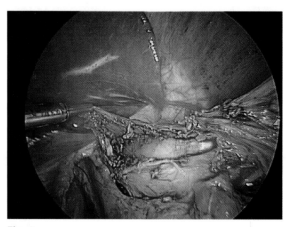

Fig. 4

Suggested Reading

1. Boeckxstaens GE et al. Achalasia: from new insights in pathophysiology to treatment. J Pediatr gastroenterol Nutr 2005; 41:S36–7

2. Mattioli G et al. Results of the laparoscopic Heller-Dor procedure for pediatric esophageal achalasia. Surg Endosc 2003; 17:1650–52

3. Smith CD et al. Endoscopic therapy for achalasia before Heller myotomy results in worse outcomes than Heller myotomy alone.Ann Surg 2006; 243:579–84

Q 63

Mario Lima and Giovanni Ruggeri

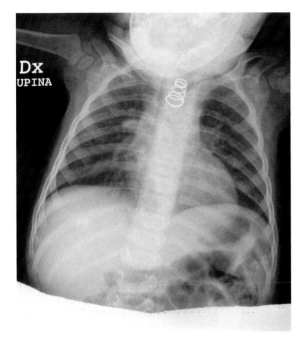

Fig. 1

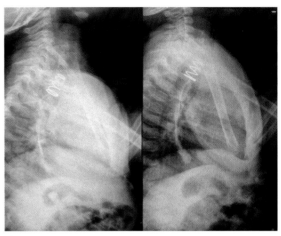

Fig. 2

A 1-year-old child suffered from dyspnea, cough, mucous secretions, and regurgitations for 2 weeks.

The pediatrician, suspecting a pulmonary infection, administered antibiotic therapy. Because the symptoms persisted, the child was taken to the emergency department where a chest radiograph was obtained (Fig. 1).

- What does Fig. 1 show?
- What other diagnostic examinations could be useful?
- What examinations are to be avoided and why?
- What did the surgeon do?
- What are the risks of this procedure?
- What are the possible surgical alternatives?
- How can possible complications be managed?

A 63

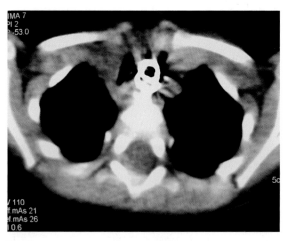

Fig. 3

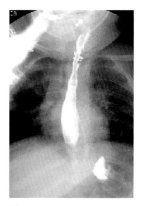

Fig. 4

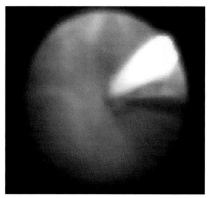

Fig. 5

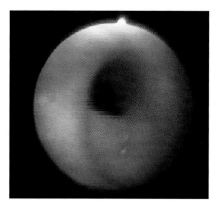

Fig. 6

The girl had ingested a spring. Her parents had not realized that their daughter had ingested a part of a small toy she was playing with; in fact, this toy was later found to be broken and some parts were missing.

The radiograph (Fig. 1) clearly shows the spiral shape of a radiopaque, ingested foreign body (a spring); especially in lateral view (Fig. 2), it is clear that the foreign body is in the proximal part of the esophagus.

Before attempting removal, it is important to study the relationships between the foreign body and the other structures of the mediastinum, in particular the aortic arch. For this reason, a CT scan (see Fig. 3) was performed. It shows the radiopaque body in the proximal part of the esophagus; it seems to lean on the aortic arch but there is an intact esophageal wall. Obviously, MR imaging, although less detrimental to health, could not be performed because the radiopaque body was metallic, and this is an absolute contraindication to MR imaging.

The surgeon removed the foreign body endoscopically with a rigid endoscope. The procedure was not without difficulties, because the spring was strongly embedded in the esophageal mucosa and part of the inflamed mucosa stuck out through the loops of the spiral.

The removal procedure is not free of possible complications; the risk of causing an esophageal laceration is high, as well as of creating a fistula between the esophagus and the aorta.

If removal had not been possible, or in the case of a major complication, the surgeon would have been ready to perform a thoracotomy to open the esophagus, reach and remove the foreign body, and/or to repair any complication. Luckily, this was not our case.

In the postoperative period, the child developed an esophageal stricture, which was documented by a barium swallow (see Fig. 4). This stricture was managed with periodical dilations with Savary's bougies (Fig. 5) and corticosteroid therapy. The dilations were successful (Fig. 6), and at the time of writing the child was feeding without any problems.

Q 64

Vincenzo Jasonni, Girolamo Mattioli, and Alessio Pini Prato

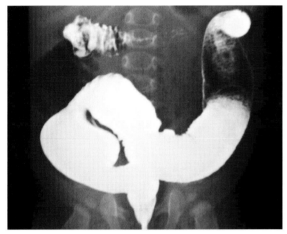

Fig. 1

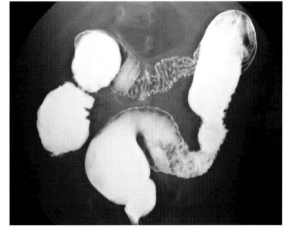

Fig. 2

A 3-month-old girl had a history of chronic constipation dating back to birth and delayed meconium passage.

She was in a good general condition with a slightly distended belly. Up to the time of referral, she was managed with daily enemas for regular bowel emptying. Her family history was unremarkable.

Figures 1 and 2 show an investigation performed on this infant.

- What investigation was performed? What do Figs. 1 and 2 show?
- What should the first diagnostic step be in a case like this one?
- What are the second-line investigations?
- What are possible explanations of severe chronic constipation? What is the disease?
- What other diagnostic investigations can be performed in the work-up of such a patient?
- What is the suggested treatment and are there different therapeutic options?
- What are the long-term implications of the disease?

A 64

This patient is affected by Hirschsprung's disease (HSCR). In particular, the infant is affected by a classic form of HSCR extending up to the sigmoid colon, as confirmed by the intraoperative histochemical study of seromuscular biopsy specimens taken during surgery. HSCR disease occurs in up to 1:5,000 live births and is due to an abnormal development of the enteric nervous system (absence of migration of ganglion cells in the Auerbach and Meissner plexuses—aganglionosis). It can present early after birth or later in childhood.

This infant underwent a barium enema study that showed an unclear picture: slightly dilated sigmoid colon and absence of stenosis or atresia. There are no clear transition zones to allow a diagnosis of intestinal dysganglionosis (Hirschsprung's disease) to be made.

The first diagnostic step should have been a rectal suction biopsy that permits a reliable diagnosis to be made or exclusion of intestinal dysganglionosis (Hirschsprung's disease and intestinal neuronal dysplasia). Figure 3 is a typical histogram of HSCR, where the rectal suction biopsy specimen is stained in acetylcholinesterase (AChE; histochemical stains for parasympathetic fibers and ganglion cells). A dramatic increase of AChE activity in the lamina propria and in the submucosa along with the absence of ganglion cells permits one to diagnose HSCR.

A barium enema should follow the rectal suction biopsy for any possible bowel involvement of aganglionosis to be identified.

Severe chronic constipation in patients younger than 6 months of age can occur also in cases of cystic fibrosis, hypothyroidism, electrolyte disturbance, anorectal malformations (rectoperineal fistula), and infant dischezia (functional disorder).

In this case, there is no need for further investigations as the diagnosis is complete. However, searching

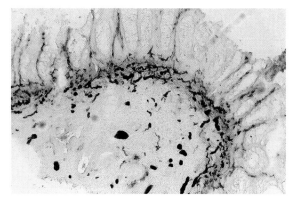

Fig. 3

for Ret mutations allows one to discriminate between sporadic HSCR and inherited HSCR. This can be helpful in the counseling of parents who fear recurrence of the disease. Cardiac anomalies can be associated with HSCR in up to 10% of patients and these anomalies should be ruled out. HSCR will not resolve on its own. Therefore, surgery is the only treatment. There are many available pull-through procedures to resect the affected bowel and to re-establish bowel continuity. Laparoscopic, laparotomic, and transanorectal approaches are safe and effective in experienced hands.

Although HSCR has an excellent prognosis, parents should be aware of the possible occurrence of long-term complications such as constipation, enterocolitis, and soiling. These complications (mainly soiling) usually improve with time. Overall quality of life is very good in these patients.

Suggested Reading

1. Martucciello G, Pini Prato A, Puri P, Holschneider AM, Meier-Ruge W, Jasonni V, Tovar JA, Grosfeld JA. Controversies concerning diagnostic guidelines for anomalies of the enteric nervous system: a report from the fourth International Symposium on Hirschsprung's disease and related neurocristopathies. J Ped Surg 2005; 40(10):1527–1531

2. Martucciello G, Ceccherini I, Lerone M, Jasonni V. Pathogenesis of Hirschsprung's disease. J Ped Surg 2000; 35(7): 1017–1025

Q 65

Vincenzo Jasonni, Girolamo Mattioli, and Alessio Pini Prato

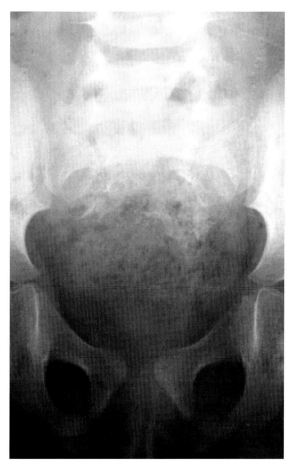

Fig. 1

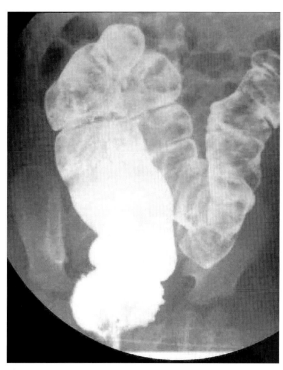

Fig. 2

A 2-year-old girl had a history of chronic constipation dating back to birth. She was sent to a specialist pediatric surgeon at the age of 2.5 years for a suspected anorectal malformation with rectoperineal fistula.

Her mother had an anterior meningocele that had been treated conservatively (observation and cesarean section). A cousin (mother's side) had undergone surgery for a mild form of anorectal malformation. Nothing else was described in her family history.

- What was the first investigation performed by the pediatric surgeon?
- What does Fig. 1 show?
- Why did the surgeon perform the second investigation?
- What does Fig. 2 show?
- What other diagnostic examinations should be performed in this specific case?
- What is the right timing for the treatment of this disease?
- What is the long-term outcome of these patients?

A 65

This girl is affected by Currarino syndrome (CS). CS is a congenital disease, frequently inherited, due to a mutation on the long arm of chromosome 7 (gene *HLXB9*). It is a peculiar form of caudal regression syndrome that involves the last lumbar vertebral bodies and the sacrum/coccyx. It is characterized by the association of hemisacrum, anorectal malformation, and presacral mass (anterior meningocele or teratoma). Patients with this disease often present with isolated severe chronic constipation dating back to birth. Frequently, there is a family history of spinal dysraphism or anorectal malformations. The disease is extremely rare.

On the grounds of the suggestive family history and clinical examination, the pediatric surgeon acquired a sacral radiograph (two projections).

Figure 1 shows the hypoplastic hemisacrum (complete absence of right portion of sacral bone). The lateral projection is used to quantify the degree of sacral hypoplasia in symmetric forms of caudal regression syndrome. This investigation alone is sufficient for the diagnosis of CS, since this feature is pathognomonic.

CS can be associated (more than 50% of patients) with Hirschsprung's disease. Furthermore, the presence of an associated anorectal malformation (rectoperineal fistula in this patient) makes the development of severe rectosigmoid dilatation possible, which sometimes needs enterostomy. Barium enema is mainly required to exclude rectosigmoid dilatation and to assess colonic shape.

Figure 2 shows mild rectosigmoid dilatation and no sign of Hirschsprung's disease.

Rectal suction biopsy (exclusion of Hirschsprung's disease), *spinal MR imaging* (to look for anterior meningocele), *pelvic CT* (presacral teratoma), *neurophysiological tests, cardiac US, thoracic radiography, and abdominal US* (to exclude associated anomalies) should be performed to complete the diagnostic work-up.

In cases of associated anterior meningocele, neurosurgical treatment should be performed first, with or without protective colostomy. This patient had anterior meningocele, spinal tethering lipoma, and presacral teratoma. She did not undergo colostomy, but underwent closure of the meningocele and untethering first. Afterward, she underwent teratoma resection and posterior sagittal anorectoplasty.

The long-term outcome of these patients is excellent, provided the teratoma is completely removed and no malignancy is detected. Strict neurological follow-up is required, at least in the early postoperative period, for early detection of neurological deterioration. In cases of associated anorectal malformations, constipation is very common but it can be dealt with effectively.

Suggested Reading

1. Martucciello G, Torre M, Belloni E, Lerone M, Pini Prato A, Cama A, Jasonni V. Currarino syndrome: proposal of a diagnostic and therapeutic protocol. J Pediatr Surg 2004; 39(9):1305–11

2. Merello E, De Marco P, Mascelli S, et al. HLXB9 homeobox gene and caudal regression syndrome. Birth Defects Res A Clin Mol Teratol 2006; 76(3):205–9

Q 66

Vincenzo Jasonni, Girolamo Mattioli, and Alessio Pini Prato

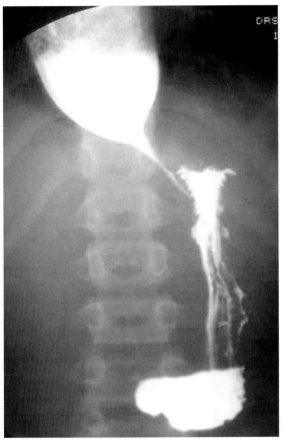

Fig. 1

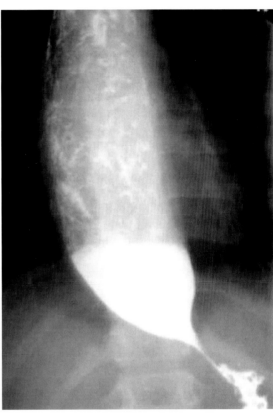

Fig. 2

An 8-year-old boy had a long-standing history of vomiting, regurgitation, recurrent respiratory infections, and failure to thrive. The onset of his symptoms dated back to the age of 5 years.

The patient's mother told the doctors that her child underwent repeated cycles of antireflux medical therapy (PPI and prokinetics) with partial and transient benefit.

He was brought to the emergency department after an episode of acute respiratory distress. The pediatrician obtained a chest radiograph that showed a right lobar pneumonia. The patient was treated accordingly and afterwards he was referred to a pulmonologist for his recurrent symptoms.

The pulmonologist performed the examination shown in Figs. 1 and 2.

- What do Figs. 1 and 2 show?
- The patient was subsequently referred to a surgeon. What is the second examination performed?
- What should be included in the diagnostic work-up of this condition?
- What are the main etiological considerations of this condition?
- How should this condition be managed?
- Are there any therapeutic options?

A 66

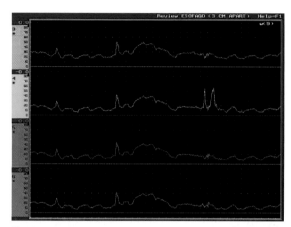

Fig. 3

The patient is affected by esophageal achalasia (EA). This disease is characterized by abnormal synchronous motor activity of the esophageal body, associated with an absence of postdeglutive relaxation of the lower esophageal sphincter (LES). The achalasia of the LES determines the progressive dilatation of the esophageal body and deterioration of the esophageal clearing capacity.

This boy is affected by a severe form of AE, as the symptoms date back to early childhood. The previous episodes of respiratory symptoms are suggestive of the severity of the disease. Gastroesophageal reflux (GER) is not the cause of this condition. Therefore, EA does not respond to antireflux therapy.

EA can present with dysphagia. Alternatively, respiratory symptoms can occur. Aspiration pneumonia usually involves the right lung due to the predisposing anatomy.

In the case of suspected GER, the barium meal is one of the main examinations to be performed in order to detect GER and to study the GE junction and any possible anatomical abnormalities.

Figures 1 and 2 show the barium meal test. The esophagus is extremely dilated, with the typical mouse-tail sign (narrowing of the distal esophagus at the esophagogastric junction). Moreover, the esophagus is clearly depicted, as demonstrated by the contrast level in the lumen.

When EA is suspected, one should immediately perform esophageal manometry in order to assess esophageal motility. Figure 3 shows the typical manometric findings in patients with EA: low-amplitude synchronous esophageal contractions and absence of postdeglutive LES relaxations.

To rule out GER, 24-h pH monitoring should be performed. Moreover, these patients should always undergo esophago-gastroduodenoscopy to rule out the presence of stenosis or strictures and to confirm the diagnosis. Endoscopic assessment is typically unremarkable and the tube easily passes from the esophagus to the stomach. This is pathognomonic, as the cause of EA is functional and not anatomic.

EA is a rare condition in childhood. Only 5% of the patients suffering from this disease are younger than 15 years of age. Although EA is usually considered an acquired esophageal motility disorder, several studies suggested that genetic background may play a role, at least in children. The etiology and pathogenesis remain controversial; however, the abnormal esophageal motility in EA seems to result from defects or an imbalance between the excitatory and inhibitory neuromuscular transmitters.

Different treatments have been proposed for EA: pharmacological treatments, pneumatic dilatations, removable self-expanding metal stents, and injection of Botulinum toxin. The results are transitory and repeated treatments are frequently required. The only way to definitively relieve symptoms is surgery. Anterior extramucosal myectomy according to Heller, in association with a partial anterior fundoplication according to Dor, is the most effective option. At present the laparoscopically modified Heller–Dor procedure is the treatment of choice for EA.

Suggested Reading

1. Mattioli G, Esposito C, Pini Prato A, Doldo P, Castagnetti M, Barabino A,Gandullia P, Staiano AM, Settimi A, Cucchiara S, Montobbio G, Jasonni V. Results of the laparoscopic Heller-Dor procedure for pediatric esophageal achalasia. Surg Endosc 2003; 17(10):1650–2

2. Mattioli G, Cagnazzo A, Barabino A, Caffarena PE, Ivani G, Jasonni V. The surgical approach to esophageal achalasia. Eur J Pediatr Surg 1997; 7:323–7

Q 67

Vincenzo Jasonni, Girolamo Mattioli, and Alessio Pini Prato

An 18-year-old girl had been operated on at the age of 10 years for total colonic Hirschsprung's disease. She had an uneventful course and grew properly up to the time of presentation. Five moths before referral, she experienced an episode of bowel obstruction related to intestinal adhesions. She underwent laparotomy but did not recover completely.

She presented to the emergency department with bilious vomiting, soft and nondistended abdomen, and absence of bowel movement that had started 5 days earlier.

The pediatric surgeon at the emergency department acquired an abdominal radiograph.

- What does Fig. 1 show?
- What was the next investigation?
- What are the possible diagnoses?
- What is a possible treatment?
- What was the course of this girl?

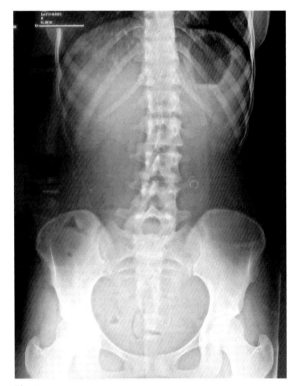

Fig. 1

A 67

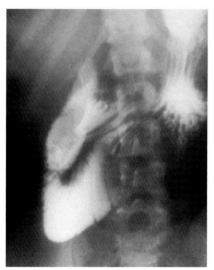 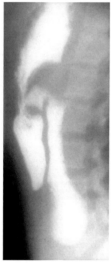 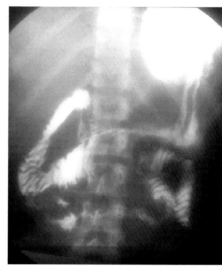

Fig. 2   **Fig. 3**   **Fig. 4**

Figure 1 shows the patient, who had undergone a colectomy and ileal pull-through carrying an ileal loop stretched down to the lower rectum. During growth the stretched loop and its vessels can press and fall onto the duodenum, thus producing a clinical picture that resembles that of aortomesenteric compression.

This girl is affected by an upper gastrointestinal (GI) obstruction. Bilious vomiting without abdominal distension supports this suspicion. The previous laparotomies could also suggest the possibility of a proximal adhesion.

An abdominal radiograph with the patient standing is the most useful investigation to be performed in cases of intestinal obstruction as it gives information regarding the level and degree of obstruction.

Figure 1 does not show any air-filled levels and looks almost normal. The only abnormality is the presence of poor air content. The rectum is empty and the stomach contains a normal amount of air.

An upper GI barium meal was performed in order to better understand the level of the obstruction. Figures 2 and 3 show an enormous dilated duodenum with no passage of contrast medium distally to the Treitz ligament. Figure 2 is an anterior–posterior projection and Fig. 3 is a latero-lateral view of the same situation.

There are different possibilities to explain this situation: proximal adhesions, previously asymptomatic web, aortomesenteric compression, expanding lesion, and neurogenic abnormalities (the patient was previously operated on for Hirschsprung's disease).

The child kept on vomiting and became dehydrated. The surgeon therefore decided to perform a laparotomy, which confirmed the suspicion of aortomesenteric compression (normal progression of a tube through the duodenum—the obstruction was functional more that extrinsic or anatomic). A duodenojejunal anastomosis was effectively performed on the extremely dilated duodenum. Alternatively, a gastrojejunal anastomosis could have been performed.

The girl recovered very slowly. Figure 4 shows the passage of contrast medium down in the small bowel, distal to the anastomosis, and the significant improvement of the duodenal dilatation.

Q 68

Vincenzo Jasonni, Girolamo Mattioli, and Alessio Pini Prato

An 8-year-old boy had a recent onset of recurrent abdominal pain. In the past, he had experienced some episodes of vomiting and regurgitation, but everything else
was normal. Growth was within the normal range. His
family and personal history was unremarkable.

He was brought to the pediatrician because of recurrent abdominal pain and constipation. The doctor asked
for an abdominal US.

- What do Figs. 1 and 2 show?
- What was done next?
- What does Fig. 3 show?
- What should be done next?
- What condition is affecting this child?
- What are the risks and implications of the disease?

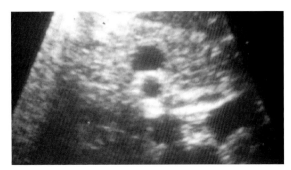

Fig. 1

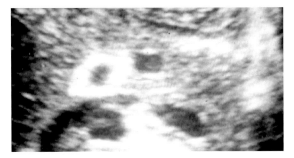

Fig. 2

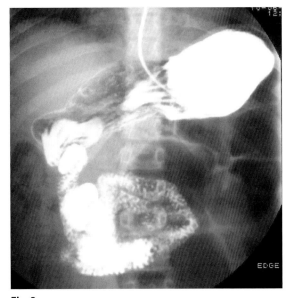

Fig. 3

A 68

This child is affected by intestinal malrotation. Intestinal malrotation is the result of a failure of the 270-degree anticlockwise rotation the usually occurs prenatally. If this rotation does not occur, different forms of malrotation can develop (non-rotation, partial malrotation, etc.). Malrotation can represent a dramatic acute problem in the newborn period but also afterwards if midgut volvulus occurs. Its occurrence is facilitated by the predisposing anatomy of the gut in this subset of patients. Moreover, malrotation is associated with the persistence of the Ladd's band that can cause duodenal obstructive symptoms and secondary GER. Therefore, malrotation can produce chronic GER-like symptoms, recurrent abdominal pain, or represent a dramatic emergency.

It is well known that asymptomatic intestinal abnormalities occur in up to 10% of healthy subjects and that they are frequently incidental findings. This is one of the possible ways to diagnose malrotation.

The most frequent incidental diagnosis of malrotation is made during a routine abdominal US (performed for abdominal pain, trauma, or urinary infections). Abdominal US and color-Doppler demonstrate the abnormal orientation of the mesenteric vein and artery, which is pathognomonic for the disease.

Figures 1 and 2 show the abnormal US findings in this patient with malrotation.

A barium meal is the next diagnostic step to verify the degree of malrotation.

In the case, the barium meal was performed after US in order to assess the degree of malrotation and to exclude torsion of the mesenteric vessels. Figure 3 shows the typical radiological picture of a patient with malrotation. The duodenum is malpositioned and fails to bend on the left hand side. This situation can be associated to different anomalies of cecal fixation.

Once the diagnosis is reached, surgery should be performed (also in asymptomatic patients) in order to avoid and prevent the possible occurrence of midgut volvulus, a potentially fatal complication (if not promptly recognized and treated). The surgical treatment of malrotation involves division of Ladd's band, appendectomy, widening of the mesentery, and positioning of the colon on the left hand side and ileum on the right hand side.

Midgut volvulus is rare but represents one of the most serious and severe emergencies in abdominal surgery. When misdiagnosed, it can be fatal or it results in short bowel syndrome. Although a percentage of patients with unknown malrotation will not experience such a complication, it is wise and safe to prevent it with proper surgical treatment.

Suggested Reading

1.   Applegate KE, Anderson JM, Klatte EC. Intestinal malrotation in children: a problem-solving approach to the upper gastrointestinal series. Radiographics 2006; 26(5):1485–500

2.   Palmas G, Maxia L, Fanos V. Volvulus and intestinal malrotation in the newborn. Pediatr Med Chir 2005; 27(1-2):62–6

Q 69

Frédéric Gauthier, Sophie Branchereau, and Chiara Grimaldi

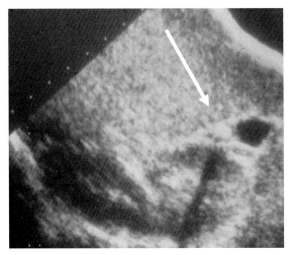

Fig. 1

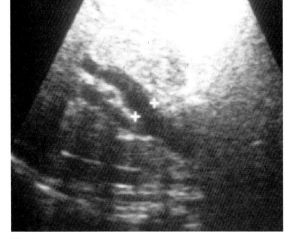

Fig. 2

A 5-month-old infant with no significant medical history presented to the pediatric emergency department with abdominal pain, fever, jaundice, dark urine, and white stools. Blood tests showed an aspartate aminotransferase level of 203 U/l, an alanine aminotransferase level of 142 U/l, a gamma-glutamyl transferase level of 608, and increased levels of bilirubin.

- What do Figs. 1 and 2 show?
- The jaundice and AP did not resolve in the following days. What is the next step?
- What procedure would you perform?
- Is there a surgical indication, and which procedure should be carried out?

A 69

This boy has cholestasis with increased conjugated bilirubin.

Abdominal US shows intra- and extrahepatic biliary dilatation, with one stone in the gallbladder and one in the main biliary duct.

The patient underwent cutaneous cholangiography, which shows the persistence of lithiasis in the main biliary duct (Fig. 3).

Biliary lavage was carried out and the choledocal lithiasis was eliminated. The stone in the gallbladder was still present at the end of the lavage.

There was a risk of a second episode of stone migration, and therefore this child was scheduled to undergo cholecystectomy.

Suggested Reading

1. Debray D, Pariente D, Gauthier F, Myara A, Bernard O. Cholelithiasis in infancy: a study of 40 cases. J Pediatr 1993; 122(3):385–91

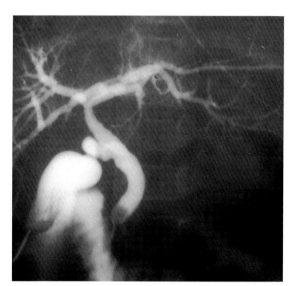

Fig. 3

Q 70

Frédéric Gauthier, Sophie Branchereau, and Chiara Grimaldi

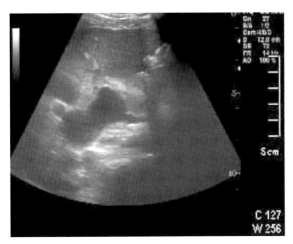

Fig. 1

A 2-year-old girl with a history of recurrent abdominal pain presented to the pediatric emergency department with acute abdominal pain with vomiting. There was no jaundice and her hepatic enzyme levels were normal: amylase was 264 (2.5 N) and lipase 1,533 (25 N).

- What examination did the surgeon perform?
- What do you see on the US scan (Fig. 1)?
- What is your diagnosis and how can you confirm it?
- What is the surgical management?

A 70

The diagnosis is acute pancreatitis. The US examination performed in the ER is shown in Fig. 1.

The US image shows a cystic dilatation of the biliary ducts with intrahepatic duct dilatation.

The US findings are suggestive of a congenital dilatation of the main biliary duct. This diagnosis is confirmed by cholangiography (Fig. 2) or MR cholangiography, which shows a common biliopancreatic duct, and a high level of amylase and lipase in the gallbladder bile sample.

The surgical management consists of resection of the gallbladder and of the cystic main bile duct.

In this case, a biliodigestive anastomosis with a Roux-en-Y loop was performed.

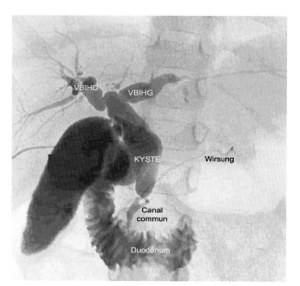

Fig. 2

Suggested Reading

1. Branchereau S, Valayer J: Malformations kystiques de la voie biliaire chez l'enfant: dilatation congenitale de la voie biliaire principale. Traitement chirurgical; En Encyclopedie Medico-Chirurgicale, Editions Scientifique et Medicales Elsevier SAS, 2002

2. O'Neill J. Choledochal Cyst; In O'Neill J, Grosfeld J, Fonkalsrud E, Coran A, Caldamone A. Principles of Pediatric Surgery, Second Edition, Mosby 2003

Q 71

Frédéric Gauthier, Sophie Branchereau, and Chiara Grimaldi

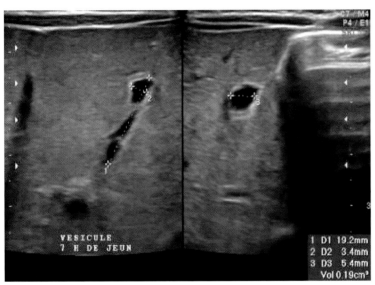

Fig. 1

A 19-day-old infant presented with a history of jaundice, white stools, dark urine, and hepatomegaly. The results of a series of blood tests showed an aspartate amino-transferase level of 237 U/l, an alanine aminotransferase level of 171 U/l, and a gamma-glutamyl transferase level of 1,004 U/L. There were no signs of infection.

- What is the differential diagnosis?
- Which examinations would you perform?
- The US study is shown in Fig. 1. What is your diagnosis?
- What should be done to confirm the diagnosis?
- Which procedure would you perform?

A 71

In neonatal cholestasis, you must rule out maternofetal infection, metabolic disease, hemolytic disease, toxicity, certain genetic syndromes, Alagille's syndrome, and biliary atresia.

The following examinations should be performed: hepatobiliary US, A1AT measurements, viral serology for hepatitis, liver enzyme test, bilirubin test, sweat test, and protein electrophoresis.

The US shows a small and irregular gallbladder (volume of 0.19 cc after 7 h of strict nil by mouth) and a small cyst at the hepatic hilum. These findings are in favor of a diagnosis of biliary atresia.

The examination that confirms this diagnosis is an explorative laparotomy. The ponction of the gallbladder shows limpid bile. An operative cholangiography via a gallbladder catheter shows nonopacification of the intrahepatic biliary ducts. In this case, cholangiography shows a patent gallbladder, the duodenum is opacified via the common bile duct, and the hepatic ducts and intrahepatic biliary ducts are not opacified (Fig. 2).

Since the gallbladder and the common hepatic ducts are patent, a cholecystoportoenterostomy is done.

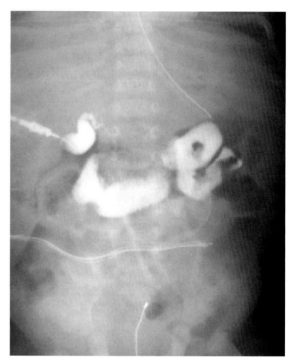

Fig. 2

Suggested Reading

1. Alagille D. Extrahepatic biliary atresia. Hepatology, Vol. 4, 1984
2. Kasai M, Kimura S, Asakura Y, Suzuki Y, Taira Y . Surgical treatment of biliary atresia. J Pediatr Surg 1968; 3:665–675
3. Lykavieris P, Chardot C, Sokhn M, Gauthier F, Valayer J, Bernard O. Outcome in Adulthood of Biliary Atresia: a Study of 63 patients Who Survived for Over 20 Years With Their Native Liver. Hepatology, Vol. 41, No. 2, 2005

Q 72

Donald Frush

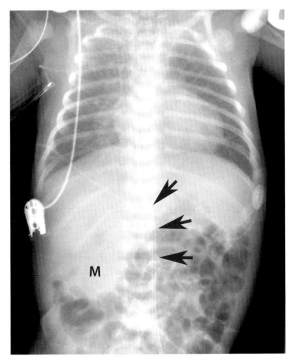

Fig. 1

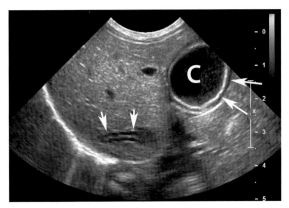

Fig. 2

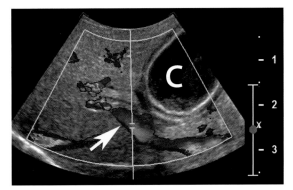

Fig. 3

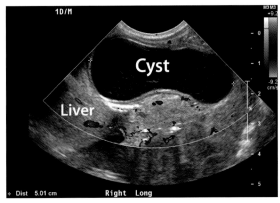

Fig. 4

A 1-day-old male infant had an abdominal mass that was identified on a prenatal sonogram. At the time of imaging, the neonate was asymptomatic.

Initially, an abdominal radiograph was obtained followed by an abdominal sonogram.

- What does the radiograph (Fig. 1) show?
- What do Figs. 2–4 show?
- What is the differential diagnosis?
- What other imaging, if any, should be performed?
- What is the management in this case?

A 72

This neonate has a gastrointestinal duplication cyst, which was suspected on prenatal sonography and confirmed by a sonographic evaluation in the immediate postnatal period.

The anteroposterior chest and abdomen radiograph ("babygram"; Fig. 1) obtained to assess umbilical catheter positions shows the region of the mass (*M*) in the right upper quadrant displacing the hepatic flexure and proximal transverse colon inferiorly and possibly displacing the umbilical venous catheter slightly to the left (*arrows*). No bowel obstruction is evident.

The sonographic evaluations are shown in Figs. 2–4. Figure 2 is a transverse epigastric view showing the duplication cyst (*C*) adjacent to the liver, and containing dependent intraluminal debris. Note the normal neonatal prominent limb of the adrenal gland (*arrows*). The bowel signature sign is evident consisting of echogenic mucosal lining and subjacent hypoechoic muscularis (*long arrows*). Together these layers are virtually only seen with hollow viscus and, when seen with a cystic mass, are usually diagnostic of gastrointestinal duplica-

tion. In Fig. 3, the cyst (*C*) is displayed relative to the portal vein (*arrow*). Figure 4 is a longitudinal sonographic view showing the 5-cm extent of this cyst, beginning in the sub-hepatic region (*Liver*).

In addition to gastrointestinal duplication, differential considerations include a choledochal abnormality (including choledochal cyst and choledochocele), and omental cyst or mesenteric cyst (i.e., lymphatic malformation), loculated fluid such as ascitis or abscess, and meconium pseudocyst; other less likely considerations would include abnormalities of regional organs such as a mesenchymal hamartoma of the liver, duplication or other cystic abnormality of the kidney, or ectopic gallbladder.

With these sonographic findings, a duplication cyst is strongly suspected. Other cross-sectional imaging such as MR and CT could be performed as part of the preoperative evaluation but are not necessary.

The surgical procedure is generally to remove these lesions since there is a high frequency of symptoms caused by pain (due to secretion of enzymes into the cyst), bleeding, or mass effect.

Suggested Reading

1. Carachi R, Azmy A. Foregut duplications. Pediatr Surg Int 2002; 18:371–374
2. Macpherson RI. Gastrointestinal tract duplications: clinical, pathologic, etiologic, and radiologic considerations. RadioGraphics 1993; 13:1063–1080
3. Puligandla PS, Nguyen LT, St-Vil D, Flageole H, Bensoussan AL, Nguyen VH, Laberge JM. Gastrointestinal duplications 2003; 38(5):740–744
4. Tong SC, Pitman M, Anupindi SA. Ileocecal enteric duplication cyst: radiologic-pathologic correlation. RadioGraphics 2002; 22:1217–1222

Q 73

Donald Frush

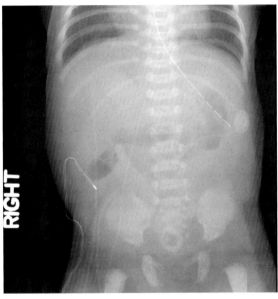

Fig. 1

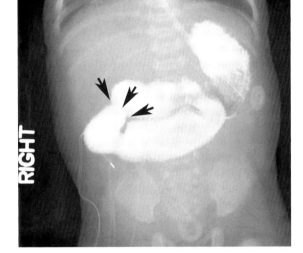

Fig. 2

A 2-week-old neonate presented with bilious vomiting. The neonate was brought to the radiology department to rule out malrotation with midgut volvulus.

An abdominal radiographic series (Fig. 1) was obtained and an upper gastrointestinal (GI) series was performed (Fig. 2).

- What are the findings in Fig. 1?
- What are the findings in Fig. 2?

Subsequently, an enema (Fig. 3) was performed to assess for possible additional anomalies of the colon.

- What is demonstrated in Fig. 3?
- What are the diagnostic considerations?
- What study, if any, should be performed next?

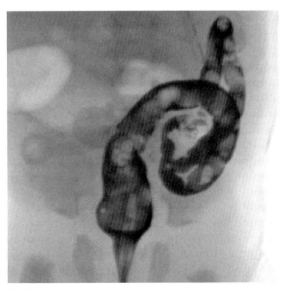

Fig. 3

A 73

This neonate has a proximal bowel obstruction. The obstruction is in the proximal jejunum and its appearance is not the classic double bubble, but given the gas pattern with gas seen in the proximal bowel on the radiograph, this does represent a proximal obstruction.

The upper GI series demonstrated a normal duodenal jejunal junction but there was a complete obstruction of the proximal jejunum (*arrows*) with dilation of the proximal bowel.

Figure 3 obtained early in the enema examination does not show a microcolon, which would be present with distal small bowel or colonic abnormalities. The remainder of the enema was likewise normal.

Given the clinical history of bilious vomiting, and the findings of proximal obstruction, operative intervention is indicated. Further imaging would not be of additional use.

At operation, several segments of proximal jejunal atresia were encountered.

For proximal obstructions, such as those causing a double bubble (Fig. 4; including midgut volvulus, duodenal atresia, duodenal web, duodenal stenosis, duodenal diaphragm, annular pancreas, pre-duodenal portal vein, extrinsic mass causing proximal duodenal obstruction), if the radiographic examination demonstrates typical features of dilated duodenum with no bilious vomiting then a gastrointestinal series is not necessary; the child undergoes surgical exploration, but not emergent as with suspected volvulus.

For distal obstruction, with gas filling the small bowel, initially, a limited upper GI series is performed to rule out malrotation (since this can mimic a distal obstruction) with a subsequent contrast enema (usually water-soluble contrast material) performed to assess for the etiologies. The major etiologies consist of Hirschsprung's disease, immature colon syndrome (small left colon)—which may be associated with meconium plug or meconium plug may be an independent process—meconium ileus, or ilea atresia.

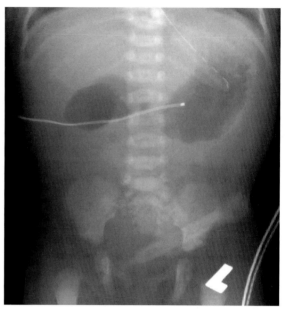

Fig. 4

Suggested Reading

1. Berrocal T, Lamas M, Gutierrez J, Torres I, Prieto C, del Hoyo ML. Congenital anomalies of the small intestine, colon, and rectum. RadioGraphics 1999; 19:1219–1236
2. Dalla Vecchia LK et al. Intestinal atresia and stenosis: a 25-year experience with 277 cases. Arch Surg 1998; 133:490–6
3. Hajivassiliou C. Intestinal obstruction in neonatal/pediatric surgery. Semin Pediatr Surg 2003; 12:241–53

Q 74

Donald Frush

A 5-week-old male infant presented with nonbilious, projectile vomiting.

The neonate was seen in the emergency department. His past medical history was unremarkable.

- What does the abdominal radiograph in Fig. 1 demonstrate?
- What do the sonographic images in Figs. 2 and 3 demonstrate?
- What other imaging, if any, is indicated in this situation?

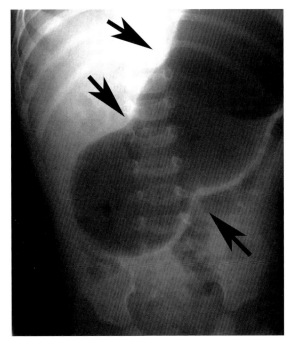

Fig. 1

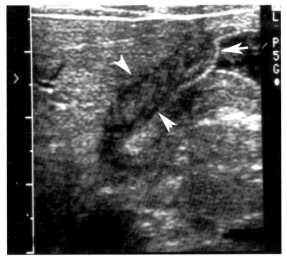

Fig. 2

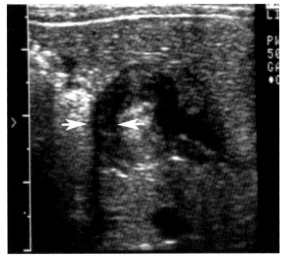

Fig. 3

A 74

The diagnosis is hypertrophic pyloric stenosis.

The abdominal radiograph (Fig. 1) shows a markedly gas-distended stomach with areas of slight constriction due to active peristaltic contractions (*arrows*).

Longitudinal (Fig. 2) and transverse (Fig. 3) views in the epigastric region show an elongated pylorus with a thickened muscularis measuring over 3 mm on the transverse (*arrows*) and longitudinal (*arrowheads*) views. Note that this hypertrophied muscularis causes a "shoulder" effect, projecting into the gastric antrum (*arrow* in Fig. 2).

On an upper gastrointestinal series performed in another infant with hypertrophic pyloric stenosis (Fig. 4), the pyloric channel is narrowed (*arrows*). A contrast upper gastrointestinal series for pyloric stenosis is no longer the primary imaging modality given the sensitivity and specificity of sonography.

Pyloric stenosis is an entity of uncertain etiology. Differential considerations include pyloric stenosis due to other conditions (for example, pylorospasm, infiltrative disorder such as eosinophilic gastritis, and use of prostaglandins), as well as extrinsic processes which may compress the pylorus and inflammatory changes such as in severe gastritis.

While this is a self-limited disease, nonsurgical management is complicated. Pyloromyotomy is in general recommended.

While palpation of an "olive" has traditionally been the method of diagnosis on a physical examination, the ability of sonography to accurately assess for the presence of hypertrophic pyloric stenosis has placed much less emphasis on both physical findings and other imaging evaluation (i.e., gastrointestinal series) in the appropriate clinical situation.

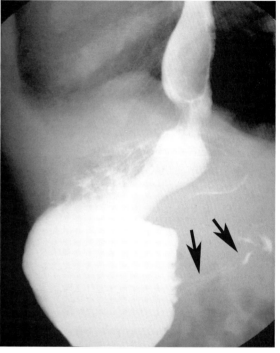

Fig. 4

Suggested Reading

1. Hernanz-Schulman M. Infantile hypertrophic pyloric stenosis. Radiology 2003; 227:319–331
2. Hernanz-Schulman M et al. Hypertrophic pyloric stenosis in infants: US evaluation of vascularity of the pyloric canal. Radiology 2003; 229:389–93
3. Hernanz-Schulman et al. In vivo visualization of pyloric mucosal hypertrophy in infants with hypertrophic pyloric stenosis: is there an etiologic role? AJR Am J Roentgenol 2001; 177:843–8
4. Ito BS, Tamura K, Nagae I, Yagyu M, Tanabe Y, Aoki T, Koyanagi Y. Ultrasonographic diagnosis criteria using scoring for hypertrophic pyloric stenosis. J Pediatr Radiol 2000; 35(12):1714–1718

Q 75

Donald Frush

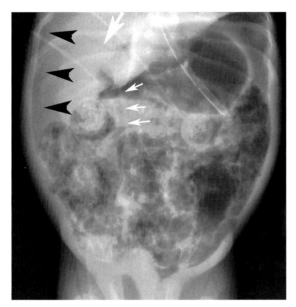

Fig. 1

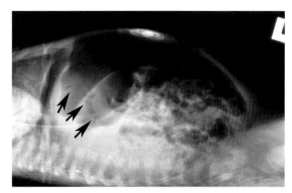

Fig. 2

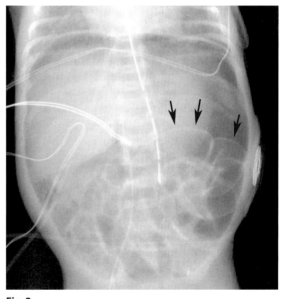

Fig. 3

A 3-week-old infant presented with heme-positive stools and abdomen distention. The infant was 31 weeks at gestation age.

- What are the findings on the frontal abdominal radiograph?
- What are the findings on the lateral abdominal radiograph?
- What is the most likely diagnosis in this case?
- What are the differential considerations?
- What other imaging, if any, should be performed?

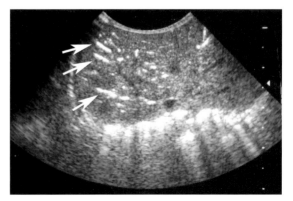

Fig. 4

A 75

The diagnosis is necrotizing enterocolitis.

The frontal abdominal radiograph (Fig. 1) demonstrates multiple cystic lucencies representing pneumatosis intestinalis as well as portal venous gas (*white arrows*). Note the abnormal lucency in the right upper quadrant due to pneumoperitoneum adjacent to the abdominal wall (*arrowheads*). In Fig. 2, portal venous gas (*arrows*) is also seen. The pneumoperitoneum is more obvious on the lateral examination.

The differential considerations in this case are limited given the pneumatosis intestinalis and portal venous gas, which are hallmarks of necrotizing enterocolitis. Without the portal venous gas, there are situations in which benign pneumatosis can be present, but virtually all cases seen in the intensive care nursery in preterm infants are not this benign variety. Mottled lucency from stool or meconium can sometimes mimic pneumatosis intestinalis; pneumatosis, however, is seen as cystic or linear lucencies in the bowel wall.

When there is a clinical suspicion of necrotizing enterocolitis (for example, gastric residuals, heme-positive stools, abdominal distention), radiographic evaluation is obtained. If a certain feature is present such as fixed, featureless segments of bowel, or wall thickening, further radiographic evaluation is generally warranted, but the interval should be based on clinical concern. When pneumatosis intestinalis is present, images are usually obtained in 6–12-hour intervals in order to assess for perforation. Portal venous gas is a more ominous sign. When perforation with pneumoperitoneum is present, the cross-table lateral view is more sensitive than the anteroposterior view. Small amounts of air may be evident as triangular lucencies between bowel segments on the lateral view. When pneumoperitoneum is large, this will be evident as a central lucency in the mid-abdomen, may outline both sides of the bowel wall (Rigler's sign; *arrows* in Fig. 4) and, when very large, pneumoperitoneum may constitute the "football" sign where gas fills the entire abdominal pelvic cavity (Fig. 3) also outlining the falciform ligament.

In the setting of necrotizing enterocolitis, radiographic surveillance is all that is warranted. Given the disruption of mucosal integrity, contrast examinations are not indicated. Sonography is more sensitive at detecting both portal venous gas (*arrows* in Fig. 4) and pneumatosis intestinalis.

In the setting of perforation, and in a relatively stable infant, a laparotomy is generally warranted. In extremely sick preterm infants, catheter drainage can be performed as an intermediate step.

Suggested Reading

1. Butter BY, Flageole H, Laberge JM. The changing face of surgical indications for necrotizing enterocolitis. J Pediatr Surg 2002; 37(3):496–499
2. Kim WY, Kim WS, Kim IO, Kwon TH, Chang W, Lee EK. Sonographic evaluation of neonates with early-stage necrotizing enterocolitis. Pediatr Radiol 2005; 35:1056–1061
3. Pierro A. The surgical management of necrotizing enterocolitis. Early Human Development 2005; 81:79–85

Q 76

Donald Frush

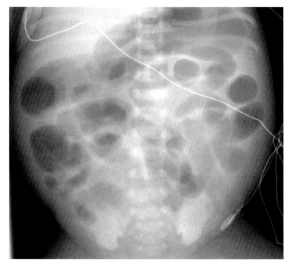

Fig. 1

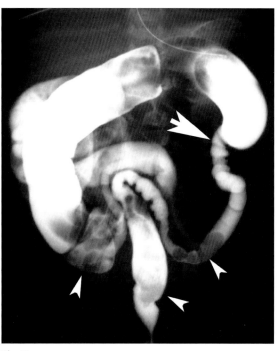

Fig. 2

A newborn female patient had abdominal distention and there was failure to pass meconium.

- What does the anteroposterior abdominal radiograph in Fig. 1 show?
- What are the possible causes of the appearance of the abdominal radiograph in Fig. 1?

- What is the principal finding in Fig. 2?
- What are the two major possible etiologies for this finding?

A 76

The diagnosis is distal bowel obstruction due to immature colon syndrome (small left colon syndrome).

The anteroposterior radiograph shows multiple distended to mildly dilated segments of bowel which, given the number of segments that are affected, indicate a distal obstruction.

When a distal obstruction is suspected, a contrast enema is indicated. One should consider doing a limited upper gastrointestinal series just to make sure that there is no malrotation since this may present, rarely, as a distal bowel obstruction.

The contrast enema demonstrates a caliber change between the descending colon (*arrows*) compared with the more proximal colon at the splenic flexure (Fig. 2). Note the gas-filled distended bowel proximal to this and multiple filling defects indicating meconium in scattered segments of the distal colon (*arrowheads*).

No further imaging evaluation is necessary when these findings are encountered.

A distal obstruction could be due to a number of etiologies including imperforate anus/anorectal malformations (these could be diagnosed clinically), immature colon syndrome (small left colon syndrome), Hirschsprung's disease, meconium ileus, or ileal atresia. Given the change in caliber, the two major considerations are long-segment Hirschsprung's disease (Fig. 3, different neonate) and small left colon syndrome. A suction biopsy is the appropriate next step to assess Hirschsprung's disease.

Immature colon syndrome (small left colon) is associated with maternal diabetes. The etiology is unclear. Hirschsprung's disease must be ruled out. Immature colon syndrome is self-limited and no further imaging evaluation is generally indicated.

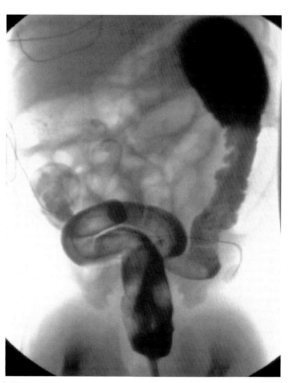

Fig. 3

Suggested Reading

1. Burge D, Drewett M. Meconium plug obstruction. Pediatr Surg Int 2004; 20:108–110
2. Dalla Vecchia LK et al. Intestinal atresia and stenosis: a 25-year experience with 277 cases. Arch Surg 1998; 133:490–6
3. Hajivassiliou C. Intestinal obstruction in neonatal/pediatric surgery. Semin Pediatr Surg 2003; 12:241–53

Q 77

Ciro Esposito, Carla Settimi, and Michele Ametrano

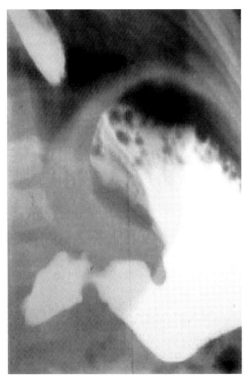
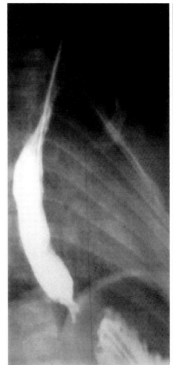
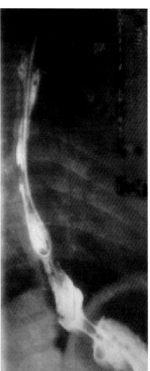

Fig. 1   **Fig. 2**

A 5-year-old boy had a history of vomiting, recurrent respiratory infections from the age of 18 months, asthma, and cough, especially during the night.

The mother told the doctor that her child had undergone several types of medical therapy without any improvement in his symptoms. The boy came to our attention after a significant episode of apnea.

The surgeon in the emergency department performed the examinations shown in Figs. 1, 2.

- What do Figs. 1 and 2 show?
- Why did the surgeon perform the second examination?
- What other diagnostic examinations are necessary in this case?
- What condition is affecting this child?
- How should this condition be managed?

A 77

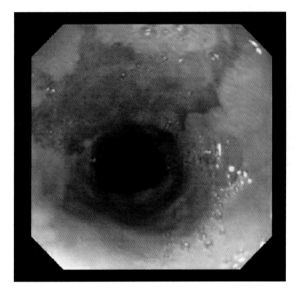

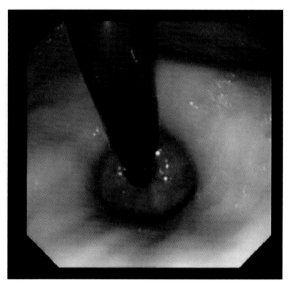

Fig. 3

Fig. 4

This child is affected by a gastroesophageal reflux (GER).

In particular, this child is affected by a gastroesophageal reflux disease (GERD), considering that he is resistant to medical therapy, as reported by the mother.

Figures 1 and 2 show a barium esophagogram (BE) that is considered, by pediatric surgeons, one of the main examinations for the detection of GER and for studying the GE junction.

After the introduction of an adequate amount of barium (equal to a normal meal; Fig. 1), the BE demonstrates GER and a sliding hernia with the esophago-gastric junction above the diaphragm (Fig. 2). Considering that many patients with GERD have delayed gastric emptying, the surgeon in the emergency department asked for ultrasonography to be performed to check the gastric emptying.

To complete the work-up of this patient, it is necessary to perform two more examinations: a 24-h pH-metry and an esophago-gastroscopy (Figs. 3, 4).

The pH tracing (Fig. 5) shows a 24-h recording period. Clusters of numerous episodes of GER are evident in the post-prandial period (*black vertical lines* indicate feeding time). A long-lasting episode of GER is also recorded during the nocturnal period (recording between 1:00 and 5:00), which accounts for the child's symptoms and the episode of apnea, due to aspiration of gastric content.

Figures 3 and 4 show the results of the endoscopy. In Fig. 3 the presence of extensive esophagitis is remarkably clear in the lower part of the esophagus.

Figure 4 shows a hiatal hernia after the U-turn of the endoscope, already clear on the barium swallow study in Fig. 2. In view of the child's symptoms, as well as the fact that he was refractory to the medical therapy with proton pump inhibitors, he was referred to a surgeon for an antireflux procedure. One month later, he underwent a 360-degree laparoscopic fundoplication according to Nissen.

After 3 years of follow-up, the child was well and free of symptoms.

Suggested Reading

1. Esposito C, Montupet Ph, Rothenberg S. Gastroesophageal Reflux in Infants and Children. Springer Ed. 2004
2. Esposito C, Montupet P, Reinberg O. Laparoscopic surgery for gastroesophageal reflux disease during the first year of life. J Pediatr Surg 2001; 36:715–717
3. Esposito C, Langer J, Schaarschmidt K, Mattioli G, Centonze A, Cigliano B, Settimi A, Jasonni V. Efficacy of laparoscopic antireflux procedures in the management of gastroesophageal reflux following esophageal atresia repair J Ped Gastroenterol Nutr 2005; 40:349–351

Q 78

Ciro Esposito and Alaa El-Ghoneimi

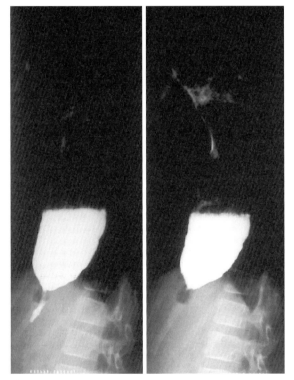

Fig. 1

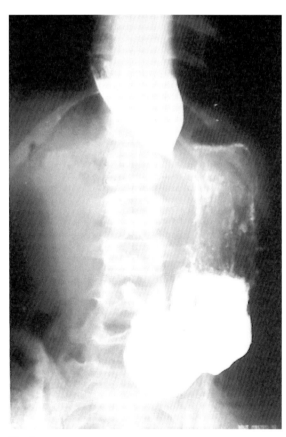

Fig. 2

A 9-year-old child without any previous illness came to our attention because of feeding-related vomiting that had started when he was 7 years old.

In the last 3 months the vomiting had become more frequent with regurgitation and the child had lost weight. The child was hospitalized and a radiological examination was performed (Figs. 1, 2).

At physical examination, the child had signs of mild malnutrition.

- What kind of examination was performed?
- What does this examination show?
- What was the suspected diagnosis?
- What is the diagnostic work-up in this pathological condition?
- What is the management of this condition and what other possible therapies are there?
- What is the follow-up?

A 78

This child is affected by esophageal achalasia. The barium radiograph shows (Figs. 1, 2) a dilated large proximal esophagus without proper peristalsis and without complete relaxation of the distal part of the esophagus, and therefore the contrast material stagnates in its distal part. In Figs. 1 and 2 it is possible to see a small amount of contrast material passing in the stomach. This is a typical radiological image of the so-called rat-tail sign in esophageal achalasia.

To complete the diagnostic work-up for this pathology, endoscopy could be performed to find any anatomic anomalies and manometry (Fig. 3), which will show disordered and weak peristaltic waves at the level of the esophageal body with high pressure at the level of the lower esophageal sphincter (LES) and no relaxation of the latter.

Esophageal achalasia is a functional disorder characterized by impaired motility of the distal esophagus and failure of the lower sphincter to relax in response to swallowing. The incidence of this pathological condition is about five cases per million people per year and only 5% of these patients are children. In clinical terms, the patient complains of rumination, substernal pain, burning, and dysphagia. Pharmacological management of achalasia in children is almost always unsuccessful, pneumatic dilatation is rarely carried out in the pediatric age, and treatment usually consists of surgery. The surgical approach seems to be the treatment of choice and most pediatric surgeons prefer to perform an esophagomyotomy according to Heller's procedure.

In this case, we performed a laparoscopic esophagomyotomy according to Heller (Fig. 4). To reduce the risk of postoperative GER, we performed an antireflux procedure according to Dor after the myotomy.

Long-term follow-up in these patients is essential, and it includes manometric and barium upper GI studies.

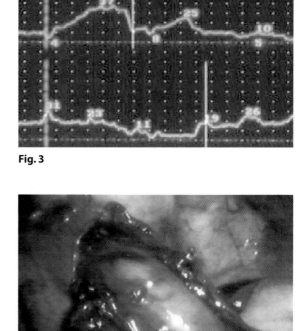

Fig. 3

Fig. 4

Suggested Reading

1. Esposito C, Cucchiara S, Borrelli O, Roblot-Maigret B, Desruelle P, Montupet P. Laparoscopic esophagomyotomy for the treatment of achalasia in children: a preliminary report of eight cases. Surg Endosc 2000; 14(2):110–3

2. Esposito C, Mendoza-Sagaon M, Roblot-Maigret B, Amici G, Desruelle P, Montupet P. Complications of laparoscopic treatment of esophageal achalasia in children. J Pediatr Surg 2000; 35(5):680–3

3. Tovar JA, Prieto G, Molina M, Arana J. Esophageal function in achalasia: preoperative and postoperative manometric studies. J Pediatr Surg 1998; 33:834–838

Q 79

Ciro Esposito, Antonella Centonze, and Carolina De Fazio

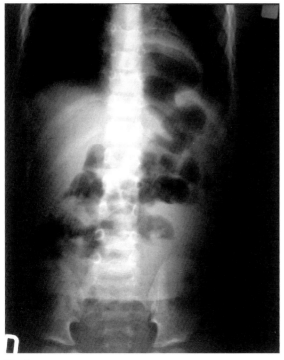

Fig. 1

A 9-year-old boy had undergone surgery 1 year previously at a different institution for GER with an open fundoplication.

He came to our attention after a car accident because he experienced vomiting, retrosternal pain, and difficulties in swallowing. The surgeon at the emergency department performed the examination shown Fig. 1.

- What is the suspected pathological condition affecting this child?
- What does Fig. 1 show?
- Which other diagnostic examinations are necessary in this case?
- What is the best way to manage this condition?

A 79

This child has a migration of the fundoplication into the thorax. Figure 1, a plain film radiograph, shows clearly that part of the stomach is dislocated above the diaphragm. To confirm this diagnosis, you can give the patient a small contrast meal (Fig. 2).

In the case of GER recurrence after surgery, symptoms are typical: substernal pain, vomiting, difficulty to swallow; however, sometimes the presentation may be variable according to the age of the patient and to other factors such as the anatomic condition.

In this case no other diagnostic examinations are necessary and the only therapeutic option is a redo surgery that can be performed laparoscopically.

The first step of the laparoscopy consists in lysis of the adhesions, which are particularly strong after an open procedure, in particular between the epiploon and the abdominal wall (Fig. 3) and between the liver and the stomach. Thereafter, the old antireflux mechanism is dismounted, the anatomic structures identified, and a new fundoplication performed. In our case we performed a new Nissen procedure after reducing the stomach into the abdomen and after having performed a hiatoplasty with two figure of "8" stitches of nonresorbable material.

The differential diagnosis in this case should include failure of an antireflux procedure with recurrence of symptoms but without migration of the valve. Recurrence of GER after surgery can affect about 3%–7% of patients.

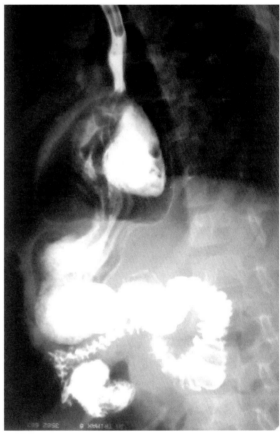

Fig. 2

Suggested Reading

1. O'Reilly MJ, Mullins S, Reddick EJ. Laparoscopic management of failed antireflux surgery. Surg Laparosc Endosc Apr 1997; 7(2):90–93
2. Pointner R, Bammer T, Then P, Kamolz T. Laparoscopic refundoplications after failed antireflux surgery. Am J Surg Dec 1999; 178(6):541–544
3. Simpson B, Ricketts RR, Parker PM. Prosthetic patch stabilization of crural repair in antireflux surgery in children. Am Surg Jan 1998; 64(1):67–9; discussion 69–70

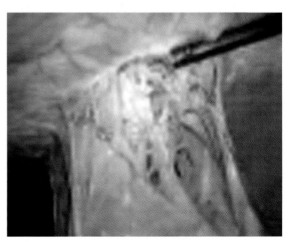

Fig. 3

Q 80

Ciro Esposito, Antonella Centonze, and Aurelie Chiappinelli

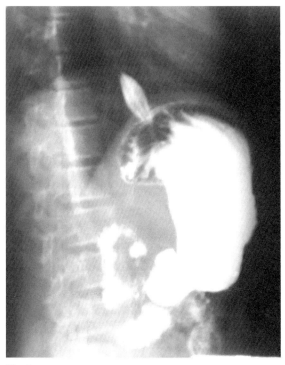

Fig. 1

A 6-year-old boy was operated on by our team 19 months previously for GERD with a laparoscopic Nissen fundoplication.

He presented with vomiting and retrosternal pain that had started 1 week earlier. We performed the examination shown in Fig. 1.

- What is the suspected diagnosis?
- What does Fig. 1 show?
- Which other diagnostic examinations are necessary in this case?
- Which other examinations must be performed on a child who has undergone laparoscopic fundoplication?

A 80

Figure 1 shows a radiographic barium swallow study, which is absolutely normal. The radiograph clearly shows the fundoplication profile under the diaphragm, without signs of GER. To confirm that this child does not have GER you can perform GI endoscopy (Fig. 2). This examination can show in retroversion the aspect of the cardia (perfectly closed, as Fig. 2 shows). Additionally, you can assess the situation of the gastric mucosa and perform gastric biopsy to search for *Helicobacter pylori* (HP). In fact, this child had gastritis caused by HP. He was referred to our pediatric gastroenterologist, who treated him with proton pump inhibitors and antibiotics. At the 1-year follow-up, the boy was free of symptoms.

The differential diagnosis in this case should include failure of an antireflux procedure or migration of the valve into the thorax. These events are reported in about 3%–7% of operated patients and can be due to recurrence of GERD or to migration of the valve to the thorax.

Postoperative follow-up for a child who has undergone laparoscopic fundoplication comprises clinical check-ups 7 days, 1, 3, and 6 months after surgery, and then annual check-ups for the first 5 years. We also perform a barium swallow 1, 2, and 5 years postoperatively. If there are more symptoms, other examinations can be scheduled.

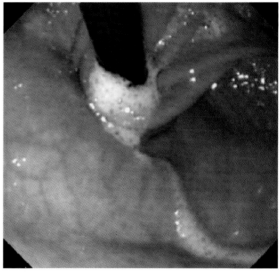

Fig. 2

Suggested Reading

1. Esposito C, Montupet P, Amici G, Desruelle P. Complications of laparoscopic antireflux surgery in childhood. Surg Endosc 2000; 622–624
2. Steyaert H, Al Mohaidly M, Lembo MA, Carfagna L, Tursini S, Valla JS. Long-term outcome of laparoscopic Nissen and Toupet fundoplication in normal and neurologically impaired children. Surg Endosc 2003; 543–546
3. Sydorak RM, Albanese CT. Laparoscopic antireflux procedures in children: evaluating the evidence. Semin Laparosc Surg 2002; 9:133–138
4. van der Zee DC, Arends NJT, Bax NMA. The value of 24-h Ph study in evaluating the results of laparoscopic antireflux surgery in children. Surg Endosc 1999; 13:918–21

Q 81

Deepika Nehra, Samuel Rice-Townsend, and Sanjeev Dutta

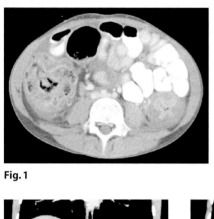

Fig. 1

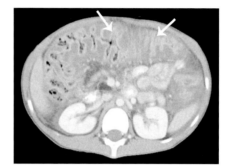

Fig. 2

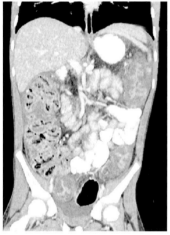

Fig. 3

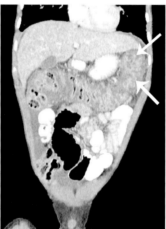

Fig. 4

A 10-year-old boy with cystic fibrosis (CF) complicated by severe obstructive lung disease, pancreatic insufficiency, and sinusitis presented with a 2-day history of increasing abdominal pain localizing to the lower abdomen associated with nausea, reduced oral intake, and loose stools. He was on trimethoprim-sulfamethoxazole (TMP-SMX) for *Pneumocystis carinii* pneumonia (PCP) prophylaxis.

He was tachycardic and appeared acutely ill with generalized abdominal tenderness and peritoneal signs.

His white blood cell count was 39.4×10³ cells/μl with >20% bands; the amylase level was 33 U/l and lipase 11 U/l.

CT was performed (Figs. 1–4).

- What are the salient findings of the CT scan?

- What possible etiologies could account for these findings?
- What laboratory study would confirm the most likely diagnosis in this particular case?
- What radiographic findings are typical of this condition? What unique sign do the *arrows* indicate?

After 6 days of intravenous ciprofloxacin, metronidazole, TMP-SMX, and oral vancomycin, the patient's pain and abdominal girth continued to worsen.

- What are the indications for surgery in this condition?
- Why is this a surgical emergency?
- What is the surgical procedure of choice?
- How might this condition present differently in a CF patient?

A 81

The CT scan shows a grossly dilated colon with bowel wall thickening. The submucosal edema and enhancement are consistent with colitis.

Potential etiologies include infectious causes (pseudomembranous colitis with *Clostridium difficile* overgrowth, *Salmonella*, *Shigella*, certain viruses, etc.) and inflammatory causes (ulcerative colitis, Crohn's disease). Ischemic colitis, uncommonly seen in children, is a result of vasculopathy and usually displays segmental involvement.

Based on the history of CF with long-term antibiotic use, the most likely etiology in this case is pseudomembranous colitis. The diagnosis can be confirmed with a stool test for the *C. difficile* toxin B. A positive stool test is confirmatory for *C. difficile* colitis, but a negative result does not rule it out. Even in cases of fulminant colitis, the stool toxin test has a false-negative rate of 12.5%.

The boy had a positive stool test, confirming the suspected diagnosis.

In a case of pseudomembranous colitis, a dilated colon with haustral thickening and a "thumbprinting" pattern may be seen on plain radiographs. On a CT scan, colonic wall thickening and a "target sign" may be seen. The "target sign" is a nonspecific finding that can be seen on a contrast-enhanced CT scan, when a hyperemic mucosa is surrounded by a relatively hypodense submucosa resulting in a bull's eye or target appearance. In more advanced cases, trapping of oral contrast material between edematous folds or the "gas accordion sign" may be seen (*arrows*). This sign is highly suggestive of pseudomembranous colitis.

Surgery is indicated for lack of response to maximal medical therapy and in cases of life-threatening complications (peritonitis, progressing toxic megacolon, uncontrolled bleeding, and colonic perforation). Generally, 1% of all patients with *C. difficile* colitis require a colectomy.

The boy's condition was refractory to medical management and his preexisting CF significantly increased his mortality risk from this condition, therefore emergent operation was performed

The preferred surgical procedure for fulminant *C. difficile* colitis is a subtotal colectomy with an ileostomy. The colon may appear deceptively normal at surgery, tempting the surgeon to perform less than the required subtotal colectomy. Patients with a segmental colectomy have higher mortality and later often require subtotal colectomy.

Patients with CF are more likely to be colonized by *C. difficile* from repeated hospitalizations and frequent antibiotic use. Diagnosis may be delayed as they may have constipation instead of the characteristic diarrhea. The surgeon must have a low threshold for ordering imaging studies in a CF patient with abdominal complaints.

The patient had a quick and uneventful postoperative recovery.

Suggested Reading

1. Binkovitz LA, Allen E, Bloom D, Long F, Hammond S, Buonomo C, Donnelly LF. Atypical presentation of Clostridium difficile colitis in patients with cystic fibrosis. AJR 1999; 172(2):517–521
2. Bradbury AW, Barrett S. Surgical aspects of Clostridium difficile colitis. Br J Surg 1997; 84:150–159
3. Brook I. Pseudomembranous colitis in children. Journal of Gastroenterology and Hepatology 2005; 20(2):182–186
4. Dallal RM, Harbrecht BG, Boujoukas AJ, Sirio CA, Farkas L, Lee KK, Simmons RL. Fulminant Clostridium difficile: an underappreciated and increasing cause of death and complications. Ann Surg 2002; 235:363–372
5. Klingler PJ, Metzger PP, Seelig MH, Pettit PD, Knudesen JM, Alvarez SA. Clostridium difficile infection: risk factors, medical and surgical management. Dig Dis 2000; 18: 147–160

Q 82

Luis de la Torre

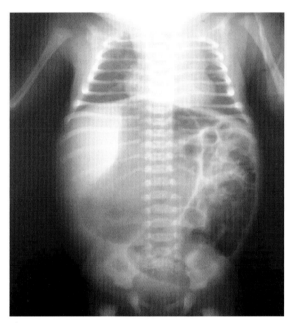

Fig. 1

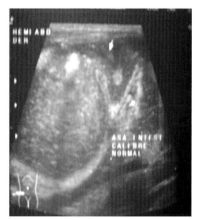

Fig. 2

A 36-h-old term newborn delivered by cesarean section and weighing 2.7 kg had abdominal distension, biliary vomiting, and no stools. Radiographic and ultrasound examinations were performed.

An intestinal duplication was suspected and a pediatric surgeon was called to evaluate the patient.

- What do Figs. 1 and 2 show?
- What is the diagnosis?
- What other diagnostic examination do you recommend to establish a diagnosis?
- What is the most appropriate surgical management in this case?
- What pathological condition should be investigated in this case?

A 82

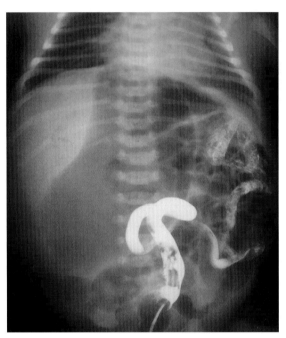

Fig. 3

Fig. 4

This boy has a "congenital low intestinal obstruction syndrome."

The most common surgical causes are intestinal atresia, anorectal malformation and Hirschsprung's disease.

Figure 1 shows big dilated loops without air at the rectum.

The sonogram in Fig. 2 shows dilated intestinal loops filled with hyperechogenic material. To compare, you can see a normal loop (*arrow*). An intestinal duplication was suspected because this image looks like a cyst.

The colon enema is a very effective study in patients with congenital low intestinal obstruction syndrome for differentiating functional vs. mechanical obstruction.

Figure 3 shows a defunctionalized distal colon until the splenic flexure where the contrast stops and the big dilated loop is not filled.

Colonic atresia was suspected and laparotomy was performed confirming this condition (Fig. 4).

Figure 4 shows the dilated proximal colon and the distal hypoplastic segment (in Babcock forceps). A 10:1 disproportion was found and a colostomy was performed. A rectal biopsy was performed and Hirschsprung's disease was confirmed in this patient.

After 3 years, an ileal pull-through was performed. Because of the severe hypoplastic distal colon, a posterior sagittal approach was used during the pull-through.

A colon enema in patients with low intestinal obstruction syndrome and rectal biopsy in patients with colonic atresia are mandatory.

Q 83

Luis de la Torre

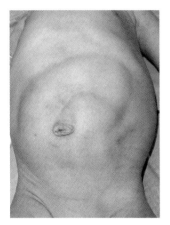

Fig. 1

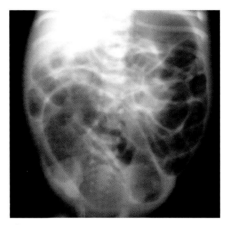

Fig. 2

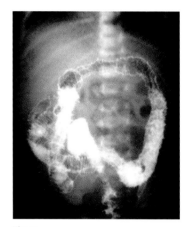

Fig. 3

A 43-day-old boy was admitted to hospital with acute abdominal distension and gastric vomiting.

The mother told the doctor she had been using a glycerin suppository daily to facilitate her baby's bowel movements since his birth.

Physical examination showed a normal anus. The abdomen is shown in Fig. 1.

In the ER an abdominal radiograph was obtained (Fig. 2).

A rectal tube was inserted, resulting in an explosive evacuation with abundant gas; the baby improved noticeably within hours.

A pediatric surgical evaluation was considered and a colon enema was indicated (Figs. 3, 4).

- What does Fig. 1 show?
- What does Fig. 2 show?
- What do Figs. 3 and 4 show?
- What is the diagnosis?
- What is the initial management in this case?
- What pathological condition should be investigated in this case?
- How do you confirm the diagnosis?
- Which medical or surgical option is better to resolve this problem?

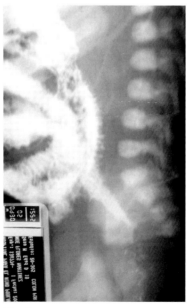

Fig. 4

A 83

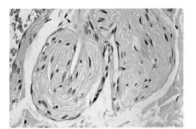

Fig. 5

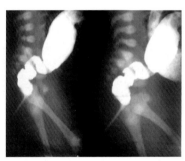

Fig. 6

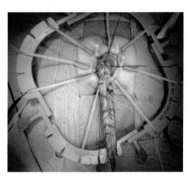

Fig. 7

This boy had "constipation syndrome" since birth and Hirschsprung's disease should be suspected.

He was well with suppositories for 43 days, but suddenly developed acute intestinal obstruction with visible dilated loops (Fig. 1).

Figure 2 shows greatly dilated loops in the lower abdomen correlating with low intestinal obstruction.

Figures 3 and 4 show a whole spastic colon with an inflamed spike-like mucosa indicating Hirschsprung's colitis. In this condition, the transitional zone cannot be demonstrated.

Colon enema is suggested as the first study for Hirschsprung's disease; however, we recommend performing it after histopathological confirmation.

Forty-eight hours after admission, the baby was much better, with rectal irrigations through the rectal tube and IV antibiotics allowing oral feeding.

All Hirschsprung's disease patients have rectal aganglionosis, *regardless of the length of the aganglionic segment*, therefore the disease must be sought in the rectum. A definitive diagnosis of Hirschsprung's disease can be made by demonstrating the absence of ganglion cells and nerve hypertrophy on histopathological examination of the rectal biopsy specimen.

A rectal suction biopsy was performed 1 week after admission and the histopathological hallmarks of Hirschsprung's disease were confirmed (Fig. 5).

Once the inflammatory process was resolved, a new colon enema was performed easily demonstrating the transitional zone (Fig. 6).

One-stage transanal colectomy with endorectal pullthrough resolved this length of aganglionosis, avoiding a colostomy. The baby underwent this procedure 9 days after admission and 28 cm of colon was resected (Fig. 7). The baby was discharged 3 days after surgery.

Suggested Reading

1. Dasgupta R, Langer JC. Transanal pullthrough for Hirschsprung disease. Sem Pediatr Sur 2005; 14:64–71
2. De la Torre ML, Ortega SJ. Transanal endorectal pullthrough for Hirschsprung's disease. J Pediatr Surg 1998; 33:1283–1286
3. IPEG Guidelines for surgical treatment of Hirschsprung's disease. J Laparoendosc Adv Surg Tech 2005; 15:89–91
4. Marty TL et al. Rectal irrigations for the prevention of postoperative enterocolitis in Hirschsprung's disease. J Pediatr Surg 1995; 30:652–654

Q 84

Luis de la Torre

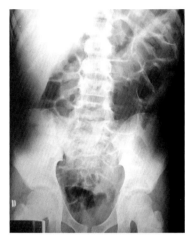 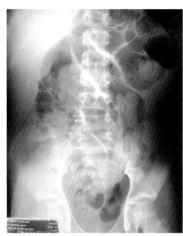 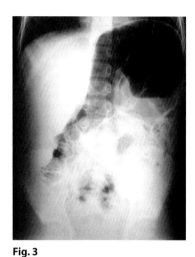

Fig. 1 **Fig. 2** **Fig. 3**

A 9-year-old boy, weighing 25 kg, was admitted to the emergency department because of acute abdominal pain, nausea, abdominal distension, and visible intestinal loops. These symptoms had been recurrent for 8 years with asymptomatic periods, but they had been more frequent during the last 2 years after the ingestion of laxatives. A plain film radiograph was obtained (Fig. 1).

The patient had an 8-year history of mild constipation and multiple visits to several pediatricians, gastroenterologists, and pediatric surgeons. The mother recalled using suppositories occasionally when he was a baby, and since then she had given him different diets, analgesics, laxatives, and enemas.

A rectoscopy showed lymphoid follicular hyperplasia and the results of a rectal biopsy revealed nonspecific colitis with follicular hyperplasia; no abscess and no submucosa were observed. Tegaserod was administered orally, but no clinical response was observed.

Two weeks after rectoscopy, he presented with nausea and a new episode of abdominal pain with 5 days of no bowel movements. The plain film radiograph is shown in Fig. 2.

The patient was admitted to our department and another rectal biopsy was performed. There were no ulcers, no abscess, and normal ganglion cells in the submucosa. A new radiograph was obtained, shown in Fig. 3.

- What do Figs. 1–3 show?
- What is the diagnosis?
- Do you continue with the laxatives?
- Which studies would you perform in this case?
- What medical or surgical option is better to resolve this problem?
- Does this patient have constipation or chronic low intestinal obstruction?
- Does this boy have constipation or inflammatory bowel disease?

A 84

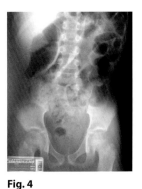

Fig. 4

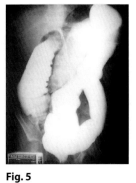

Fig. 5

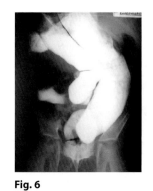

Fig. 6

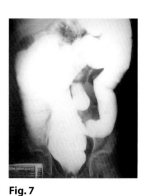

Fig. 7

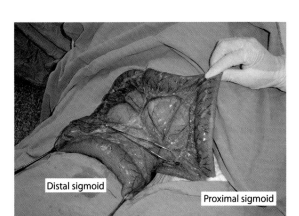

Distal sigmoid

Proximal sigmoid

Fig. 8

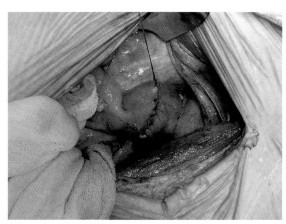

Fig. 9

Figures 1 and 2 show distended loops of small intestine, due to low "chronic" intestinal obstruction rather than constipation.

Hirschsprung's disease and inflammatory bowel disease should be considered.

A history of constipation and the left colon dilatation with an air-fluid level in the splenic flexure (Fig. 3) ruled out aganglionosis of the rectum.

A colon enema was redone.

The initial radiograph (Fig. 4) shows similar findings to those in Figs. 1 and 2. Figures 5 and 6 show a very large and tortuous sigmoid. Figure 7 shows a transverse and right dilated colon. These finding are characteristics of dolichocolon.

A colonoscopy showed follicular hyperplasia and an extraordinary large sigmoid. The whole colonoscope reached the splenic flexure.

During laparotomy 110 cm of sigmoid (Fig. 8) came out through the incision. A sigmoidectomy and primary colorectal anastomosis were made (Fig. 9). After surgery the patient was well and asymptomatic.

Dolichocolon is a rare disorder in the pediatric population characterized by elongation of the colon, especially the sigmoid. It can cause constipation and recurrent chronic volvulus expressed as abdominal pain and distension, as in this case.

Dolichocolon (long colon) should be distinguished from megarectosigmoid (a wide colon and sigmoid) that is far more common.

Q 85

Luis de la Torre

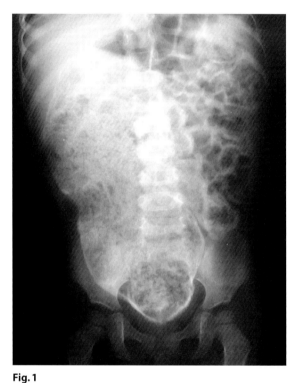

Fig. 1

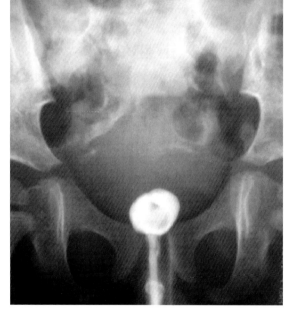

Fig. 2

A 20-month-old boy presented to the emergency department because of severe abdominal distension, gastric vomiting, and dehydration. The initial radiograph is shown in Fig. 1.

On physical examination, a large abdominal mass was palpated and a well-positioned surgical anus was observed.

The boy had undergone anorectoplasty because of a rectoperineal fistula.

The mother reported that the boy had not had bowel movements for the last 17 months, but his diapers always had fecal soiling. A physician had prescribed loperamide, but the mother discontinued this medication. For the last 10 months, she had used laxatives and enemas without any improvement.

A colon enema with hydrosoluble contrast medium was performed, shown in Figs. 2, 3.

- What is the diagnosis?
- What do Figs. 1–3 show?
- Would you request other studies?
- What treatment would you propose?

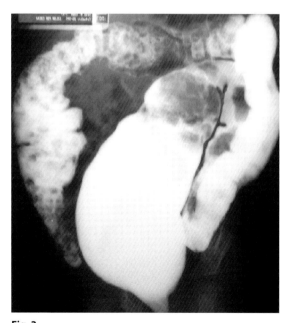

Fig. 3

A 85

This patient was born with one of the most common anorectal malformations (ARMs), a rectoperineal fistula, treated surgically with anorectoplasty in the newborn period. A common outcome in this type of ARM is constipation, which should be treated from birth to avoid complications.

The patient has chronic constipation, fecal soiling, and an abdominal mass. This triad should be suggestive of a megarectosigmoid.

Figure 1 shows a megafecaloma. Figure 2 demonstrates a hemivertebra. Figure 3 shows a huge megarectosigmoid with a proximal normal descending colon.

Fecal soiling and megarectosigmoid (fecal pseudoincontinence) can be managed medically; however, some cases will need a sigmoidectomy to resolve the problem.

Moreover, in this patient with ARM and hemivertebra, it is necessary to rule out a presacral mass. These three defects are called Currarino triad.

MR imaging was performed and an anterior meningocele was found (Fig. 4). The patient underwent colostomy followed by a plasty of the meningocele via a posterior sagittal approach and 2 months later sigmoidectomy was performed. Figure 5 shows the resected megasigmoid; note the normal caliber of the descending proximal colon.

At the time of writing, the patient was fecally continent and clean using 10 ml of lactulose per day.

This case illustrates two entities that should be borne in mind when treating patients with ARM: (1) a megarectosigmoid as a source of fecal pseudoincontinence and (2) Currarino's triad, whose frequency is underestimated.

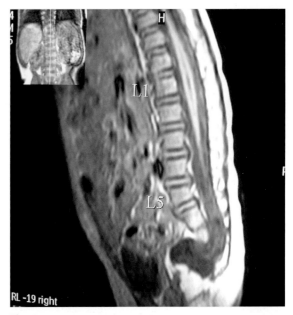

Fig. 4

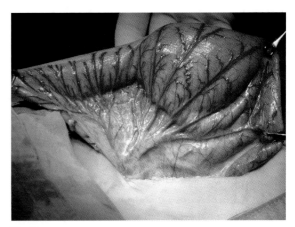

Fig. 5

Suggested Reading

1. Currarino G, Coln D, Votteler TP. Triad of anorectal, sacral and presacral anomalies. Am J Roentg 1981; 137:395–398
2. Peña A, el Behery M. Megasigmoid: a source of pseudoincontinence in children with repaired anorectal malformations. J Pediatr Surg 1993; 28:199–203
3. Swamy S, et al. Anterior sacral meningocele as part of the Currarino triad. Ind J Radiol Imag 2003; 13:207–208

Q 86

Luis de la Torre

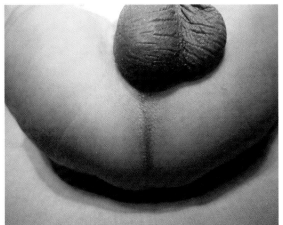

Fig. 1

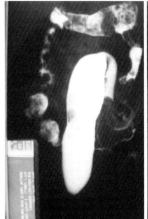
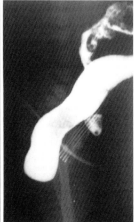

Fig. 2

A 3-month-old boy with imperforate anus was admitted to hospital because of a 2-day history of fever, lethargy, intolerance to oral intake, and three episodes of gastric vomiting.

On admission, his temperature was 38.7°C. Down syndrome was eliminated, and an intestinal stoma on the right side of the abdomen was observed. The perineum is shown in Fig. 1.

An initial laboratory evaluation showed 12.4 g/dl of hemoglobin, 15,300 white blood cells, 79% neutrophils, and 2% bands. A urine examination showed abundant bacteria, uncountable leukocytes, and positive nitrites.

The mother showed us a contrast radiological study performed for the nonfunctional stoma, which demonstrated an anorectal malformation without fistula (Fig. 2).

- What does Fig. 1 show?
- What does Fig. 2 show?
- What is the diagnosis?
- What surgical procedure is indicated in this case?
- What radiological studies would you order for this patient?

A 86

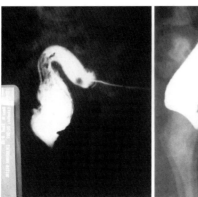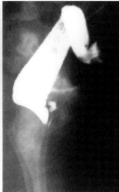

Fig. 3

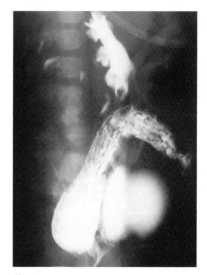

Fig. 4

The patient has an anorectal malformation (ARM) with urinary tract infection; consequently, a urinary fistula or urinary malformation should be ruled out.

Figure 1 shows a flat perineum. This is characteristic of a perineum in a child without Down syndrome and suggests clinically an ARM with a urinary fistula.

To demonstrate the anatomy of an ARM a *high-pressure distal colostogram with hydrosoluble contrast* is mandatory. This study allows one to define: (a) the length of the distal (defunctionalized) segment, (b) the distance between the distal pouch and the perineum, and (c) whether or not there is an associated fistula.

Figure 2 shows the distal cologram of this patient. We can observe a right colostomy that defunctionalized most of the colon, therefore the boy has a distal colon that is too long; the distal pouch seems to be far from the perineum and without an associated fistula. However, because it is almost impossible to generate high pressure during the cologram in a right colostomy—which would allow opening of the elevator muscle and consequently demonstrating a recto-urinary fistula and the rectal pouch—we must not assume that this patient does not have a fistula.

After treating the urinary tract infection, closure of the right colostomy and a new (left) descendent colostomy were performed. Subsequently, renal ultrasonography was performed, which was normal.

A new high-pressure distal colostogram with hydrosoluble contrast medium was obtained 1 month after the second operation. Figure 3 is an anteroposterior view demonstrating the distal segment with an adequate length for the pull-through; in the lateral view a recto-urethral bulbar fistula is identified.

When performing colostography, it is not rare for the contrast medium to pass from the urethra to the bladder. This situation should be kept in mind, because if barium is used for the colostogram, it can be introduced into the urinary tract with grave consequences.

In this patient, during the colostography the contrast medium passed to the bladder and refluxed to the ureter. Figure 4 illustrates the vesicoureteral reflux in this case.

The patient underwent anorectoplasty and closure of the urethral fistula by a posterior sagittal approach, anal dilatations, closure of the colostomy, and ureter reimplantation.

Q 87

Bruno Cigliano

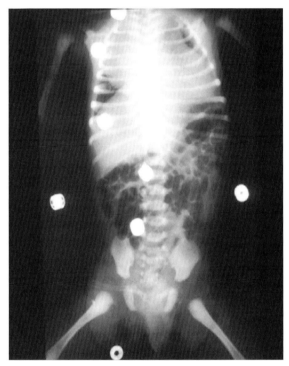

Fig. 1

A full-term neonate with prenatal diagnosis of dextro-cardia was admitted to hospital on the first day of life. The general condition of the infant was good and only a mild polypnea was present. An ECG was performed and a radiograph (Fig. 1) was obtained. The ECG was compatible with the prenatal diagnosis of dextrocardia.

- What does Fig. 1 show?
- Which is the possible diagnosis?
- Which other diagnostic procedures are needed to confirm the diagnosis?
- What is the treatment?

A 87

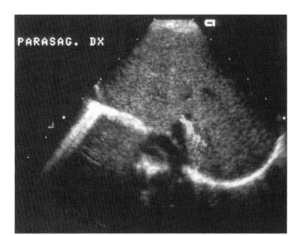

Fig. 2

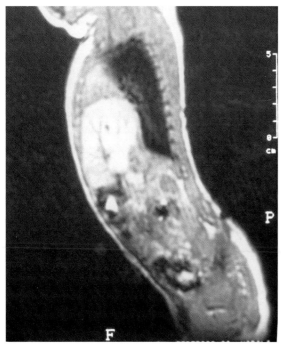

Fig. 3

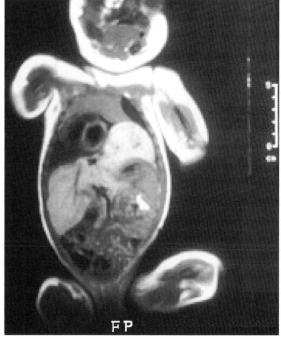

Fig. 4

Figure 1 shows a mass in the right hemithorax that moves down and left to the heart or a right displacement of the heart caused by a solid mass in the left lung.

A cardiologic consultation and an echocardiography are mandatory.

The cardiologic consultation and ultrasonography showed a normal heart but positioned to the right with a normal atrioventricular ratio. The examinations also revealed a structure in the middle left pulmonary field with a parenchymal aspect caused by anomalous liver development, probably due to a left eventration of the diaphragm (Fig. 2).

MR imaging (Figs. 3, 4) confirmed the diagnosis, showing anomalous development of the left liver lobe caused by a congenital elevated left hemidiaphragm.

The treatment of diaphragmatic eventration can be conservative or surgical. The choice is based on clinical and radiological assessment.

Q 88

Bruno Cigliano

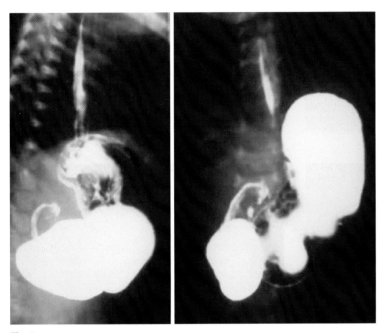

Fig. 1

A 26-day-old newborn, who had been breastfed, presented with vomiting that had started since the tenth day of life and had progressively worsened. The vomit was never bile-stained, but sometimes contained fresh blood. Constipation was also present. Abdominal examination revealed an abdominal fullness in the epigastric region. Laboratory studies showed some degree of hypochloremic alkalosis.

A barium meal (Fig. 1) was performed, and the baby was referred to our unit.

- Do you believe that the diagnostic study was correct?
- What is the most appropriate management in this case?
- What is the differential diagnosis?
- What are the complications of the surgical treatment?

A 88

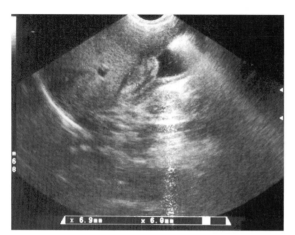

Fig. 2

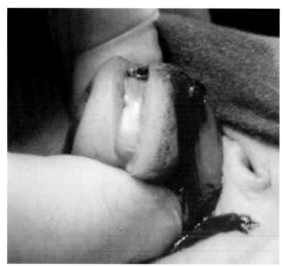

Fig. 3

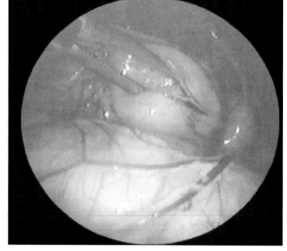

Fig. 4

Infantile hypertrophic pyloric stenosis (IHPS) has interested investigators for several decades; the cause is now thought to be a mechanism other than a developmental defect, but no definitive cause has been found. There is evidence of a genetic predisposition. The pylorus appears enlarged, measuring 2–2.5 cm in length and 1–1.5 cm in diameter. The mucosa is normal, while marked muscle hypertrophy primarily involving the circular layer produces partial or complete luminal occlusion.

The diagnosis is based on careful physical examination, laboratory examinations, and ultrasonography (Fig. 2). Rarely is a barium upper GI examination or endoscopy necessary.

The differential diagnosis includes milk intolerance, gastroesophageal reflux, pyloric atresia, duodenal stenosis, infections, and neurological diseases.

The therapy of IHPS is surgical correction. It is important to prepare the infant appropriately for anesthesia and operation.

The operative procedure is extramucosal pyloromyotomy that can be performed either during laparotomy (Fig. 3) or laparoscopy (Fig. 4).

The complications are minimal if the procedure is performed by an experienced surgeon but include: persistent vomiting (incomplete myotomy), wound infection, laparocele, and damage of the duodenal mucosa.

Q 89

Bruno Cigliano

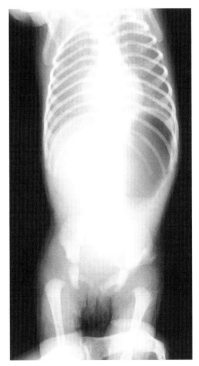

Fig. 1

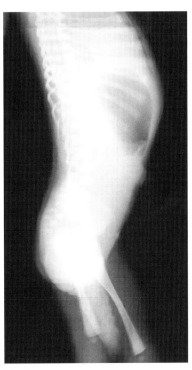

Fig. 2

A neonate with vomiting of gastric content without bile was hospitalized on his second day of life.

An upper abdominal distension with visible peristalsis was found.

A plain thoracoabdominal radiograph was obtained with the patient in the clinostatic position (Figs. 1, 2).

- Which anomalies can be observed on these radiographs?
- What is the possible diagnosis?
- Which other diagnostic procedures can be useful for the diagnosis?
- What should be done in this case?

A 89

The anteroposterior radiograph (Fig. 1) shows an enlarged stomach distended by swallowed air with absence of gas beyond the stomach.

This radiological findings are confirmed by the radiograph obtained in the latero-lateral position (Fig. 2), which shows a stomach distended by gas that does not pass into the duodenum.

In this case, the possible diagnosis can be a high-degree gastric outlet obstruction due to either pyloric aplasia or atresia or even caused by the presence of a complete antral or pyloric diaphragm.

To differentiate these forms, gastroscopy can be very useful, whereas barium swallow can be contraindicated because of possible vomiting and consequent inhalation of contrast material.

In this case, the gastroscopy showed the presence of congenital pyloric atresia (CPA). Laparotomy confirmed this diagnosis.

CPA is a very rare malformation occurring in 1 of 100,000 live births. It can occur as an isolated lesion or in association with other genetically determined conditions such as epidermolysis bullosa or congenital aplasia cutis, or form part of the hereditary multiple intestinal atresias syndrome.

Excision or incision of the diaphragm with pyloroplasty and gastroduodenostomy are the procedures of choice. Gastrojejunostomy should be avoided because of its high mortality rate. In our case the surgical procedure consisted in excising the atresic pylorus and in performing an end-to-end gastroduodenostomy.

Suggested Reading

1. Dessanti A, Di Benedetto V, Iannuccelli M, Balata A, Cossu Rocca P, Di Benedetto A. Pyloric atresia: a new operation to reconstruct the pyloric sphincter. J Pediatr Surg 2004 Mar; 39(3):297–301
2. Nawaz A, Matta H, Jacobsz A, Al-Salem A. Congenital pyloric atresia and junctional epidermolysis bullosa: a report of two cases. Pediatr Surg Int 2000; 16(3):206–8
3. Okoye BO, Parikh DH, Buick RG, Lander AD. Pyloric atresia: five new cases, a new association, and a review of the literature with guidelines. J Pediatr Surg 2000 Aug; 35(8):1242–5
4. Toma P, Mengozzi E, Dell'Acqua A, Mattioli G, Pieroni G, Fabrizzi G. Pyloric atresia: report of two cases (one associated with epidermolysis bullosa and one associated with multiple intestinal atresias). Pediatr Radiol 2002 Aug; 32(8): 552–5

Q 90

Giovanni Esposito and Ciro Esposito

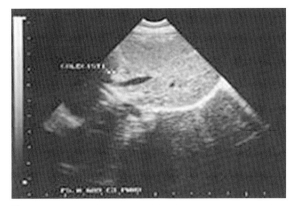

Fig. 1

The patient was a 6-week-old infant, born at full term after a spontaneous delivery and normal pregnancy. He was breastfed and his initial development was normal. When he was 35 days old, his mother noticed darkening of the urine and lightened feces color, which became completely acholic after a few days. At the same time the baby began showing signs of jaundice, initially limited to the sclera and afterward to the entire body.

On hospitalization the jaundiced baby was in good condition. On palpation of the abdomen the liver, moderately enlarged, had a firm consistency. There was no splenomegaly.

Laboratory test results were normal except for the total bilirubin level that was over 9 mg/dl with a direct fraction of 6.8 and an indirect one of 2.2; the serum alkaline phosphatase levels were also elevated.

An abdominal US was performed (Fig. 1). On the basis of the US data, other examinations were performed, and subsequently a surgical intervention was scheduled.

- What does the US show?
- What was the diagnostic suspicion?
- Which other examinations were performed to define the diagnosis and what were their results?
- On the basis of illness evaluation, laboratory tests, and all other examinations, what was the diagnosis?
- What is the treatment for this disease?
- What was the follow-up?
- What is the prognosis?

A 90

The abdominal US shows an enlarged liver with a moderate increase in its echogenicity and the absence of any visible biliary structures.

On the basis of the clinical features and laboratory data, biliary atresia was suspected.

To confirm this diagnosis and to exclude other jaundice conditions, especially neonatal hepatitis, 99mTc-dimethyl-iminodiacetic acid scintigraphy (HIDA), hepatic biopsy, and laparoscopy were performed. The HIDA (Figs. 2, 3) showed lack of excretion of the contrast material thought the biliary tree. The hepatic biopsy highlighted the characteristics of biliary atresia, with proliferating bile ducts and without giant cells and focal areas of necrosis which, on the contrary, are characteristic of neonatal hepatitis. Lastly, the laparoscopy confirmed the diagnosis of biliary atresia, with the characteristic aspect of biliary cirrhosis and absence of the gallbladder that was replaced by fibrous cords.

The treatment consists in an anastomosis between the porta hepatis, conveniently prepared to expose the intrahepatic biliary ductules, and a segment of intestinal tract. In this case a portohepatic appendicoduodenostomy was performed (Fig. 4).

The follow-up was normal and the infant was discharged 15 days after surgery when the jaundice regressed. At 1 year the jaundice disappeared and the total bilirubin level was 1.6.

The prognosis of biliary atresia depends on the successful outcome of the operation which, when performed before the age of 2 months, achieves good results only in about 30% of cases. In the rest of the cases, liver transplantation is necessary.

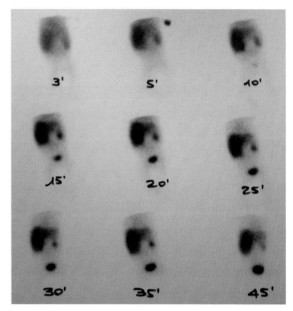

Fig. 2

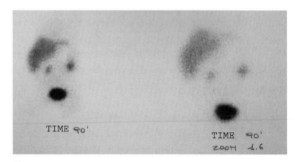

Fig. 3

Suggested Reading

1. Casaccia G, Catalano OA, Marcellini M, Bagolan P. Biliary atresia associated with multiple unrelated anomalies: what about it? Pediatr Surg Int 2006; 20:345–348
2. Dehghani SM, Haghighat M, Imanieh MH, Geramizadeh B. Comparison of different diagnostic methods in infants with Cholestasis. World J Gastroenterol 2006 Sep 28; 12(36):5893–6

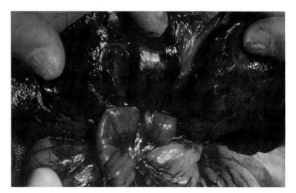

Fig. 4

Q 91

Giovanni Esposito and Ciro Esposito

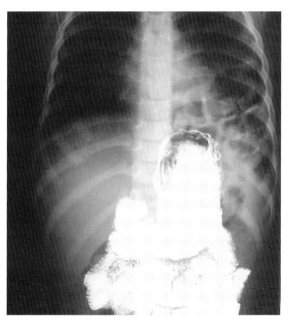

Fig. 1

A 3-year-old boy, in good general condition, presented with sudden abdominal pain localized in the epigastric and left upper regions, which appeared a few hours after a meal. Sometimes, the child had stipsis. At the same time, the patient presented respiratory symptoms such as a cough.

A gastric disease was suspected, and therefore a simple chest radiograph series and a barium meal were performed. On physical examination the abdomen was normal, while auscultation of the left hemithorax revealed humid rales.

- What do the thoracic radiograph and barium meal (Fig. 1) show?
- Which other examinations were performed to define the diagnosis and what were their results?
- What was the diagnosis?
- What was the surgical treatment?
- What was the follow-up?

A 91

The barium meal showed a normal stomach, duodenum, and first jejunal segment, while in the inferior left hemithorax there were some gaseous irregular images. This finding was confirmed by the chest radiograph.

Based on the clinical and radiological features, a gastrografin enema was performed, which revealed the presence of the colon in the left hemithorax (Fig. 2). The diagnosis was Bochdalek diaphragmatic hernia. This is a congenital malformation due to an agenesis of the diaphragm's dorsal part; through this hole, one or more abdominal organs may move into the thorax. This hernia is more frequent on the left site, and it may have a real hernial sac. Because of the presence of abdominal viscera in the thorax, the lung becomes more or less hypoplastic. Clinically, congenital diaphragmatic hernia (CDH) may occur, outside the more frequent neonatal period, in the first years of life. Because of the different clinicoradiological features of these conditions from the classic findings of congenital hernia (tachypnea, cyanosis, respiratory failure, and presence of the polycyclic hyperlucent endothoracic blebs with a shift of the mediastinum on the right seen on chest radiographs), the diagnosis is often missed and it may be discovered incidentally on chest radiographs.

At surgery, a large defect of the left posterior diaphragm was found. The herniated colon was replaced in the abdomen and the diaphragm defect was closed. Today it is possible to perform this operation with laparoscopy, and if there is a prenatal diagnosis of a very large defect, fetal surgery may be considered.

The postoperative course was uneventful with good lung expansion. The child was discharged 7 days after surgery and at follow-up was growing well.

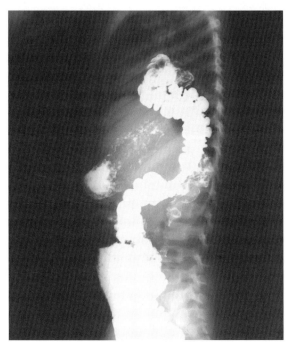

Fig. 2

Suggested Reading

1. Baeza-Herrera C, Velasco-Soria L, Garcia-Cabello LM, Osorio-Aguero CD. Bochdalek hernia with late manifestation. Relevant clinico-surgical features Gac Med Mex 2000 Jul–Aug; 136(4):311

2. Elhalaby EA, Abo Sikena. Delayed presentation of congenital diaphragmatic hernia. Pediatr Surg Int 2002 Sep; 18(5–6):480–5

3. Mei-Zahav M, Solomon M, Trachsel D, Langer JC. Bochdalek diaphragmatic hernia: not only a neonatal disease. Arch Dis Child 2003 Jun; 88(6):532–5

4. Newman BM, Afshani E, Karp MP, Jewett TC Jr, Cooney DR. Presentation of congenital diaphragmatic hernia past the neonatal period. Arch Surg 1986 Jul; 121(7):813–6

5. Ozturk H, Karnak I, Sakarya MT, Cetinkursun S. Late presentation of Bochdalek hernia: clinical and radiological aspects. Pediatr Pulmonol 2001 Apr; 31(4):306–10

Q 92

Giovanni Esposito and Ciro Esposito

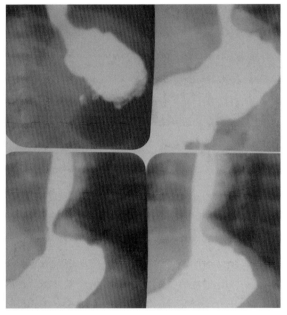

Fig. 1

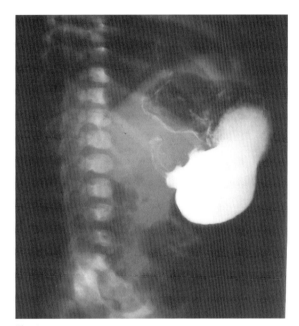

Fig. 2

A full-term newborn, with normal breast-feeding since the third week of life, suddenly presented with post-feeding vomiting. The vomiting became more frequent and severe. On physical examination, the child had severe signs of dehydration without any abdominal problems. A radiological examination, shown in Figs. 1 and 2, was carried out. After more examinations the infant was operated on.

- What do the radiographs show (Figs. 1, 2)?
- Which other examinations were performed?
- What was the diagnosis?
- What was the treatment?
- What was the follow-up?

A 92

The barium swallow reveals some episodes of gastro-esophageal reflux (GER) and significant gastric dilatation and a large air–fluid level. There is a hypertrophic stenosis of the pylorus, with the typical sign of a double railroad.

Laboratory tests showed a hydroelectrolitic imbalance with hypocloremia, hyperpotassemia, and metabolic alkalosis.

The diagnosis was hypertrophic stenosis of the pylorus associated with GER. This disease is known as phreno-pyloric syndrome or Roviralta's syndrome. Roviralta's syndrome is rare, affecting 3% of pyloric stenosis cases.

The treatment consists in correcting the dehydration and then surgery in order to perform a Fredet–Ramstedt-type pyloromyotomy. In our case the operation was open, but today some surgeons prefer to do it laparoscopically. There was no indication for reflux correction because the GER was due to hyperpressure inside the stomach.

The follow-up was normal and the patient's prognosis good.

Suggested Reading

1. Rode H, Cywes S, Davies MR. The phreno-pyloric syndrome in symptomatic gastroesophageal reflux. J Pediatr Surg 1982 Apr; 17(2):152–7

Q 93

Alessandro Settimi and Ciro Esposito

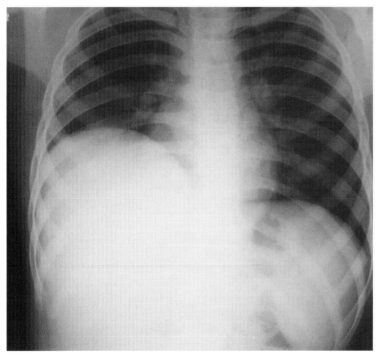

Fig. 1

A 4-year-old boy, without any respiratory problems, underwent chest radiography (Fig. 1) before an operation for hypospadias. Physical examination was normal, except for the finding of an elevation of hepatic dullness found on percussion of the right hemithorax.

- What does the radiograph show?
- What was the suspected diagnosis and what should it be differentiated from?
- Which examinations are necessary to confirm the diagnosis?
- What is this pathological condition and what is the treatment?
- What did the surgeon perform in this case?
- What is the prognosis?

A 93

The chest radiograph shows a remarkable elevation of the right diaphragm with one reduced respiratory area.

The suspected diagnosis was diaphragmatic eventration, which must be differentiated from other thoracic disease (collapse of inferior pulmonary lobe or pulmonary hypoplasia) or abdominal hepatic pathologies (inflammatory, cancer, Echinococcus cyst) and extrahepatic pathologies (subphrenic abscess, retroperitoneal tumors).

In the past, to confirm the diagnosis, pneumoperitoneum was created and peritoneography was performed. Today it is useful to perform ultrasound and fluoroscopy; for left eventration, a barium swallow with upper gastrointestinal series followed by pulmonary scanning are recommended. In this case, fluoroscopy revealed a paradoxical motion of the right diaphragm during respiration that confirmed the diagnosis of diaphragmatic eventration.

Diaphragmatic eventration consists in diaphragm elevation of different degrees, and is congenital or acquired. The congenital form is characterized by hypoplasia or atrophy of the diaphragmatic muscle, formed only by pleural and peritoneal layers (Fig. 2). The acquired type is a result of phrenic nerve paralysis due to different etiologies (traumatic, surgery, extrinsic compression). Clinically, the patients may present with respiratory problems of varied degree in connection with

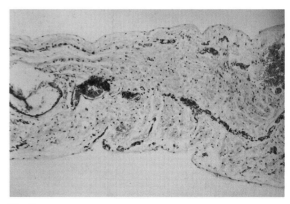

Fig. 2

compression of the lung caused by displacement of the diaphragm. The treatment in symptomatic patients is surgery, and it can be performed via open surgery (laparotomy or thoracotomy) or videosurgery (laparoscopy or thoracoscopy). The operation consists in reducing the diaphragm with partial resection or plication.

Conservative treatment is indicated in asymptomatic patients, as in our case, and periodical follow-ups are necessary. The prognosis is generally very good in both cases.

Suggested Reading

1. Becmeur F, Talon I, Schaarschmidt K, Philippe P, Moog R, Kauffmann I, Schultz A, Grandadam S, Toledano D. Thoracoscopic diaphragmatic eventration repair in children: about 10 cases. J Pediatr Surg 2005 Nov; 40(11):1712–5
2. Gierada DS, Slone RM, Fleishman MJ. Imaging evaluation of the diaphragm. Chest Surg Clin N Am 1998 May; 8(2):237–80
3. Tiryaki T, Livanelioglu Z, Atayurt H. Eventration of the diaphragm. Asian J Surg 2006 Jan; 29(1):8–10
4. Tsugawa C, Kimura K, Nishijima E, Muraji T, Yamaguchi M. Diaphragmatic eventration in infants and children: is conservative treatment justified? J Pediatr Surg 1997 Nov; 32(11):1643–4
5. Yazici M, Karaca I, Arikan A, Erikci V, Etensel B, Temir G, Sencan A, Ural Z, Mutaf O. Congenital eventration of the diaphragm in children: 25 years' experience in three pediatric surgery centers. Eur J Pediatr Surg 2003 Oct; 13(5):298–301

Q 94

Giovanni Esposito, Alessandro Settimi, and Ciro Esposito

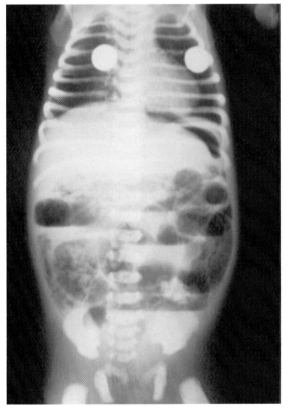

Fig. 1

A 2-year-old boy had undergone pyeloplasty for ureteropelvic junction obstruction via a retroperitoneal approach. The initial postoperative course was uneventful with removal of the drainage device on postoperative day 2.

Six days after surgery the patient began vomiting. Feeding was stopped and a nasogastric tube was inserted in the stomach from which a large quantity of bile-stained liquid came out. Based on the findings of an abdominal radiograph, explorative laparotomy was performed (Fig. 1).

- What does the abdominal radiograph show?
- What was found at surgery?
- What type of surgery was undertaken?
- What was the follow-up?

A 94

This boy had jejunojejunal intussusception. The abdominal radiograph shows some air–fluid levels, indicative of an intestinal occlusion.

Ultrasonography was performed (Fig. 2), confirming the diagnosis.

We performed a laparotomy and at operation a small amount of peritoneal liquid was found with a significant degree of high intestinal occlusion caused by a jejunojejunal intussusception.

Because of the good appearance of the intestinal loops involved, the surgery consisted in an easy reduction of the intussusception. Palpation of the invaginated loops did not reveal any anomaly causing the intussusception.

The postoperative course was uneventful with rapid normalization of the intestinal canalization. The boy was discharged 14 days after the pyeloplasty. Six months later the boy's growth was normal.

In general, intussusceptions are located at the ileocecal segment and their treatment consists in a barium or air enema, which is able to solve the problem in more than 75% of cases. When the intussusception involves the upper intestinal loops, as in our case, surgery is the best option.

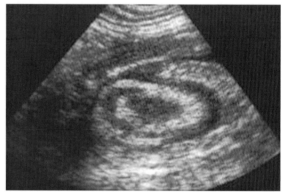

Fig. 2

Suggested Reading

1.   Erichsen D, Sellstrom H, Andersson H. Small bowel intussusception after blunt abdominal trauma in a 6-year-old boy: case report and review of 6 cases reported in the literature. J Pediatr Surg 2006; 11:1930–1932

2.   Grimprel E, de La Rocque F, Romain O, Minodier P, Dommergues MA, Laporte-Turpin E, Lorrot M, Parez N, Caulin E, Robert M, Lehors H, Cheron G, Levy C, Haas H. Management of intussusception in France in 2004: investigation of the Paediatric Infectious Diseases Group, the French Group of Paediatric Emergency and Reanimation, and the French Society of Paediatric Surgery Arch Pediatr 2006; 12:1581–1588

3.   Munden MM, Bruzzi JF, Coley BD, Munden RF. Sonography of pediatric small-bowel intussusception: differentiating surgical from nonsurgical cases. AJR Am J Roentgenol 2007; 1:275–279

4.   Simanovsky N, Hiller N, Koplewitz BZ, Eliahou R, Udassin R. Is non-operative intussusception reduction effective in older children? Ten-year experience in a university affiliated medical center. Pediatr Surg Int 2006; 19:345–347

5.   Wiersma F, Allema JH, Holscher HC Ileoileal intussusception in children: ultrasonographic differentiation from ileocolic intussusception. Pediatr Radiol 2006; 11:1177–1181

Q 95

Giovanni Esposito and Ciro Esposito

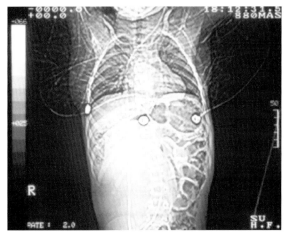

Fig. 1

The patient was a 7-year-old child, born at term after an uncomplicated pregnancy. At 3 months of age he was affected by meningitis, due to *Escherichia coli* and *Pseudomonas*, and complicated by hydrocephalus that was treated with a ventriculoperitoneal shunt (VPS). After 1 year, a simple revision of the shunt was carried out because of malfunctioning, and 6 years later, because of skin ulceration along its pressure points, the shunt was replaced in the abdomen. Three days before admission to our hospital, the child had an abdominal colic episode complicated by convulsions. On admission, the child complained of abdominal pain. His abdomen was enlarged and at percussion a dull sound was revealed on the right site of the abdomen. Abdominal CT was performed (Figs. 1, 2), followed by other procedures before planning the treatment.

- What does the CT scan show?
- Which other procedures were performed?
- What was the diagnosis?
- What was the treatment?
- What was the follow-up?

A 95

The CT shows a large intra-abdominal cyst with a diameter of 10.7×9.7 that displaces the intestinal loops connecting the right kidney.

Laparoscopy was performed and a large pseudocyst was found where the catheter shunt entered.

Laparoscopy treatment was decided consisting in opening the pseudocyst, voiding its content, pulling the catheter out, and replacing it in the abdomen (Fig. 3).

The follow-up was uncomplicated and a CT scan showed the disappearance of the cyst.

At 2 years the child was doing well.

VPSs are frequently used to treat hydrocephalic children. The frequency of complications in children with VPS varies from 5% to 47%, and in the majority of the cases involves the abdominal part of the catheter. Any obstruction of the ventriculoperitoneal derivation system will lead to endocranial hypertension; this should be considered an emergency requiring immediate surgery. Recently, laparoscopy using three ports has been reported for the treatment of VPS complications.

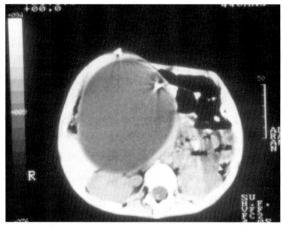

Fig. 2

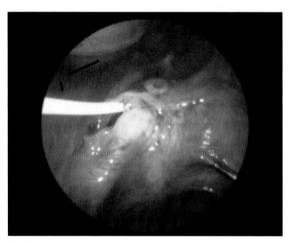

Fig. 3

Suggested Reading

1. Adeloye A. Spontaneous extrusion of the abdominal tube through the umbilicus complicating peritoneal shunt for hydrocephalus. Case report. J Neurosurg 1973; 38:758–760
2. Brunori A, Massari A, Macarone-Palmieri R, Benini B, Chiappetta F. Minimally invasive treatment of giant CSF pseudocyst complicating ventriculoperitoneal shunt. Minim Invasive Neurosurg 1998; 41(1):38–39
3. Esposito C, Porreca A, Gangemi M, Garipoli V, De Pasquale M. The use of laparoscopy in the diagnosis and treatment of abdominal complications of ventriculo-peritoneal shunts in children. Pediatr Surg Int 1998; 13(5–6):352–354
4. Grosfeld JL, Cooney DR, Smith J, Campbell RI. Intra-abdominal complications following ventriculo-peritoneal shunt procedures. Pediatrics 1974; 54:791–796
5. Kim HB, Raghavendran K, Kleinhaus S. Management of an abdominal cerebrospinal fluid pseudocyst using laparoscopic techniques. Surg Laparosc Endosc 1995; 5(2):151–154

Q 96

Christophe Chardot and Sylviane Hanquinet

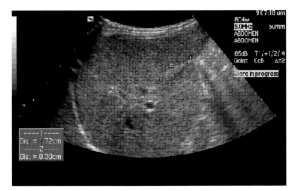

Fig. 1

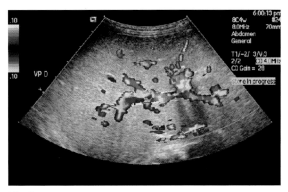

Fig. 2

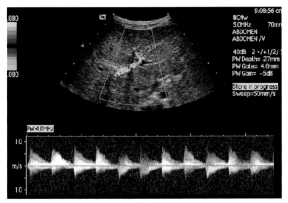

Fig. 3

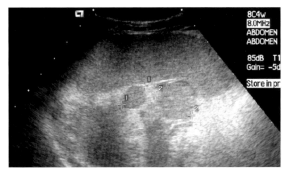

Fig. 4

A 4-week-old boy was taken to a general practitioner for routine examination. He was the third child in a family without any history of congenital disease or malformation. The mother's pregnancy and delivery were uneventful. The boy's birth weight was 3,200 g. He was breastfed, with a normal transit. The mother told the doctor her son's skin and eyes had been slightly yellow since birth, but this had recently become more obvious. He was in good general condition, weighing 3,800 g. His eyes and skin were moderately icteric. On examination, hepatomegaly was found, palpated 4 cm below the costal margin, without splenomegaly. During the examination, the baby passed white stools.

Blood tests confirmed cholestasis. The Quick value was 25%.

- Why is prothrombin time prolonged?
- What severe complication could occur?
- What should be done to avoid this?

Abdominal US was performed to confirm the diagnostic hypothesis.
- In which condition should the child be before the US examination so that adequate information can be obtained?

The US Doppler findings are shown in Figs. 1–4.
- What other US signs may be seen in the syndromic form of the disease?
- Is cholangiography needed in this case? Why?
- What operation is necessary for this disease?
- What are the chances of success of this operation?

A 96

This patient is affected by biliary atresia (BA). The association of neonatal jaundice (lasting after 2 weeks of life), white stools, and hepatomegaly is highly suggestive of this disease.

Prothrombin time is prolonged (Quick value decreased) due to vitamin K deficiency: severe cholestasis induces a lack of bile salts in the intestine, and consequently malabsorption of liposoluble vitamins ADEK. Lack of vitamin K induces deficiency of coagulation factor synthesis. Severe hemorrhage can occur, especially intracranial hemorrhage. Parenteral administration of vitamin K should be carried out urgently.

Before the US examination, the child should be fasting for at least 6 h, and consequently should have an IV line with fluid, glucose, and electrolytes. The aim of fasting is to have a full gallbladder during the US. It is important to check that the child is really nil by mouth when the US is performed, in order to avoid any misinterpretation if a shrunk gallbladder is found.

A shrunk and hyperechogenic gallbladder despite fasting, without intrahepatic bile ducts dilatation, strongly suggests biliary atresia. In the syndromic form of BA (polysplenia syndrome or BA splenic malformation syndrome), the following signs can be seen on US (or CT): multiple spleens; median liver (hypertrophy of the left liver and more or less symmetrical right liver); preduodenal portal vein; absence of retrohepatic vena cava; and situs inversus. Figure 5 shows the operative picture: a cholestatic, fibrotic and enlarged liver and a completely atretic gallbladder, which is characteristic of BA. Complete atresia of the extrahepatic biliary remnant is the most common form of BA.

Since the gallbladder is completely atretic, the diagnosis of BA is certain and cholangiography is not needed (and would be technically unsuccessful).

In other cases of complete neonatal cholestasis (white-gray stools) with a nonatretic gallbladder, cholangiography is mandatory to assess the permeability of the bile ducts and rule out a partial form of BA. This can be done either preoperatively (by interventional radiology or by ERCP) or intraoperatively. It is important to check the color of bile (green or uncolored) before injecting the contrast medium.

The first treatment in patients with BA is to perform hepatoportoenterostomy (Kasai operation), which consists in resection of all the extrahepatic biliary remnant, and anastomosis of a Roux-en-Y jejunal loop at the porta

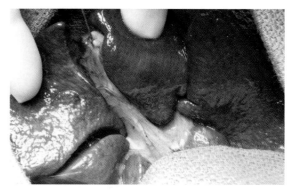

Fig. 5

hepatis. If some intrahepatic bile ducts are still patent, the biliary flow can be restored to the intestine. Yellow liquid is often seen at the porta hepatis after resection of the extrahepatic biliary remnant, and can correspond to either bile or icteric lymph. It is therefore impossible to predict the success of the Kasai operation at this stage.

In Europe and North America, results of the Kasai operation are: clearance of jaundice (normal bilirubin levels) in about one-half of patients; one-third of patients alive with their own liver at the age of 10 years; one-fourth to one-fifth of patients alive with their own liver at the age of 20 years.

When the Kasai operation fails to clear jaundice, biliary cirrhosis progresses and liver transplantation is required, in most cases in the first few years of life. Today, with the sequential treatment of Kasai operation and liver transplantation, if needed, overall survival of BA patients is about 90%.

Suggested Reading

1. Chardot C. Biliary atresia. Orphanet J Rare Dis 2006; 1(1):28
2. Chardot C, Serinet MO. Prognosis of biliary atresia: what can be further improved? J Pediatr 2006; 148(4):432–5
3. Kasai M, Kimura S, Asakura Y, Suzuki Y, Taira Y, Obashi E. Surgical treatment of biliary atresia. J Pediatr Surg 1968; 3(6):665–675
4. Lykavieris P, Chardot C, Sokhn M, Gauthier F, Valayer J, Bernard O. Outcome in adulthood of biliary atresia: a study of 63 patients who survived for over 20 years with their native liver. Hepatology 2005; 41(2):366–71

Q 97

Christophe Chardot and Sylviane Hanquinet

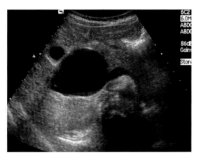
Fig. 1

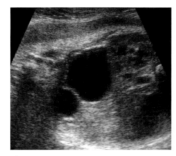
Fig. 2

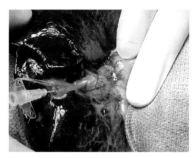
Fig. 4

A 24-year-old woman, without a family history of inherited disease or malformation, was in her second pregnancy. A prenatal ultrasound at 26 weeks' gestation showed a female fetus with normal growth and vitality. A cyst in the liver hilum was discovered (Fig. 1), the liver looked normal, and a small gallbladder was identified. The US was otherwise normal, without any other morphological anomaly.

- What is the suspected diagnosis?
- What can be proposed to the mother?

Prenatal work-up showed no other fetal anomaly, and the pregnancy continued uneventfully. The baby was born after 38 weeks' gestation and after a normal delivery, weighing 3,200 g. The infant's neonatal adaptation was good and clinical examination was normal. Neonatal US confirmed a cystic dilation in the liver hilum (Fig. 2). The gallbladder and the liver looked normal. The rest of the abdominal US was normal.

- What are the possible diagnoses, and how do you manage the infant?

The infant tolerated breast-feeding very well, she passed five to six gold-yellow stools every day, had no jaundice, and her weight progressed normally. Liver test results were normal. An MR image is shown in Fig. 3.

- How do you interpret Fig. 3?
- What is your final diagnosis?
- What anomaly of the common bile duct is usually seen in this condition?
- What are the medium- and long-term risks of this anomaly?
- What surgical treatment is therefore recommended?
- What is the prognosis for this child?

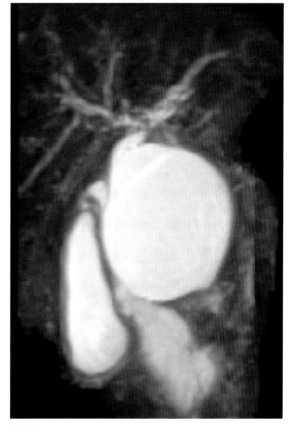
Fig. 3

A 97

A cyst in the liver hilum may correspond to:
- A cystic form of biliary atresia, which requires urgent diagnosis and treatment after birth
- A choledochal cyst
- A duodenal duplication
- An ovarian cyst
- A cystic lymphangioma

The mother needs to be referred to a prenatal diagnosis and counseling center.

Repeated US will follow the evolution of the cyst (size and echogenicity), the liver, and the gallbladder, and will look for other morphological anomalies, especially cardiopathy, situs inversus, and interruption of the inferior vena cava with azygos continuation.

Amniocentesis is not routinely indicated in cases of isolated cyst of the liver hilum. Depending on the associated prenatal findings, it may be advised for:
- Karyotype, although none of the suspected diagnoses is commonly associated with chromosomal anomalies.
- Genetic screening for cystic fibrosis, if indicated.
- Biological screening of digestive enzymes in the amniotic fluid cannot be done in this case. Their level in the amniotic fluid declines between 18 and 24 weeks of gestation, due to closure of the anal sphincter: it is therefore too late to detect a biochemical profile of biliary obstruction (low GGTs and normal intestinal enzymes).

Consultation with a pediatric surgeon is recommended, in order to inform the parents about the postnatal management of the child.

This clinical picture and the US findings (Fig. 2) are highly suggestive of choledochal cyst, although a cystic form of biliary atresia cannot be completely excluded. The child can be fed normally, and must be closely followed up.
- A normal gallbladder does not exclude biliary atresia. Clinical evolution in the first weeks of life will show whether complete cholestasis appears: in the case of biliary atresia, the stools would rapidly become white and jaundice would appear. Blood tests would show cholestasis, and the work-up would confirm obstruction of the bile ducts. Kasai operation should be performed urgently, in the first weeks of life. Figure 4 shows an operative view of another child with a cystic form of biliary atresia, and Fig. 5 is the intraoperative cholangiogram.

In the case of choledochal cyst, the child is likely to have a normal clinical neonatal course, without cholestasis. The surgical treatment can be postponed, and is usually performed after 3 months of life.

Clinical evolution allows one to exclude biliary atresia. MR imaging findings confirm the diagnosis of choledochal cyst, with a major dilation of the common bile duct and hepatic duct, and a mild dilation of the gallbladder and cystic duct. The intrahepatic bile ducts are regular and slightly enlarged.

Choledochal cyst is usually associated with a biliopancreatic common channel: the common bile duct and the Wirsung duct end in a common biliopancreatic duct, which originates above the sphincter of Oddi. This condition causes a reflux of pancreatic juice in the bile ducts, with subsequent biliary epithelium abrasion, inflammation, dysplasia, and finally a risk of cholangiocarcinoma in adulthood. The cystic dilation of bile ducts may also increase in childhood, with chronic cholestasis, liver fibrosis, gallstone formation, and the risk of acute biliary obstruction and/or cholangitis.
- Surgery must:
- Disconnect the pancreatic and biliary ducts, in order to suppress the pancreaticobiliary reflux and subsequent chronic biliary inflammation.
- Resect the diseased extrahepatic bile ducts.

The recommended operation is therefore resection of the extrahepatic biliary tree from the hepatic duct (or extrahepatic biliary bifurcation) to the intrapancreatic termination of the common bile duct, and biliary reconstruction with a hepaticojejunostomy on a Roux-en-Y loop. During the operation, an assay of pancreatic enzymes (amylase, lipase) in bile usually reveals very elevated levels, confirming the reflux of pancreatic juice in the bile ducts. A cholangiogram is recommended (if it has not been done preoperatively) in order to precisely evaluate the intrahepatic extension of the biliary dilations. A liver biopsy is recommended to evaluate potential liver fibrosis.

In this form with limited intrahepatic biliary dilations, the prognosis is good, and the child is likely to have a completely normal life. In cases of large intrahepatic biliary dilations, low-grade cholestasis may persist, with a risk of gallstone formation and cholangitis. Such patients need close follow-up and ursodeoxycholic acid may be necessary to increase the biliary flow, reduce the risk of gallstone formation, and protect the liver against the consequences of chronic cholestasis. Biliopancreatic disconnection and resection of the extrahepatic biliary tree including the intrapancreatic common bile duct are expected to lower the risk of biliary chronic inflammation, dysplasia, and cancer. As with any abdominal surgery, the parents must be informed of the risk of postoperative adhesions and intestinal obstruction. In all cases, a prolonged follow-up is recommended.

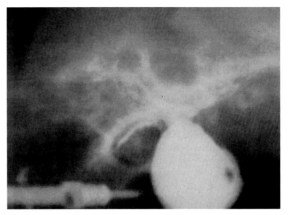

Fig. 5

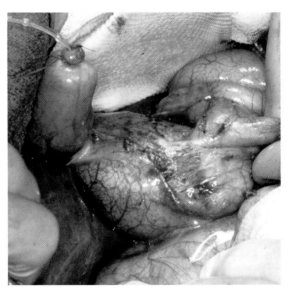

Fig. 6

Suggested Reading

1. Brunero M, De Dreuzy O, Herrera JM, Gauthier F, Valayer L. [Prenatal detection of a cyst in the liver hilum. Interpretation for an adequate treatment]. Minerva Pediatr 1996; 48(11):485–94
2. Muller F, Oury JF, Dumez Y, Boue J, Boue A. Microvillar enzyme assays in amniotic fluid and fetal tissues at different stages of development. Prenat Diagn 1988; 8(3):189–98
3. Todani T, Watanabe Y, Fujii T, Toki A, Uemura S, Koike Y. Congenital choledochal cyst with intrahepatic involvement. Arch Surg 1984; 119(9):1038–43
4. Todani T, Watanabe Y, Fujii T, Toki A, Uemura S, Koike Y. Cylindrical dilatation of the choledochus: a special type of congenital bile duct dilatation. Surgery 1985; 98(5):964–9

Q 98

Christophe Chardot and Sylviane Hanquinet

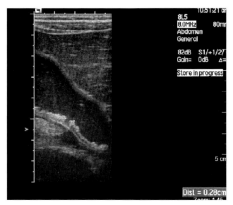

Fig. 1

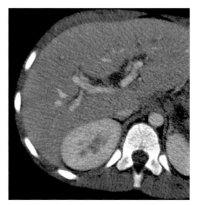

Fig. 2

A 24-month-old girl was referred to the emergency department for episodes of pain and vomiting, which had appeared 3 h previously. She had been in good health until then. During examination, she seemed tired and experienced several episodes of pain. Her temperature was 37°C. She was pale and slightly subicteric. Her abdomen was soft, but palpation of the right upper quadrant was painful. There was no hepatomegaly, no abdominal mass. Splenomegaly was palpated 3 cm below the costal margin. Her nappy contained normal stools, without blood. The rest of the clinical examination was normal.

- What is your first diagnostic hypothesis regarding the current episode?

The abdominal US and CT scan show:
- The absence of intussusception
- A normal liver parenchyma
- A gallbladder containing multiple small stones (Fig. 1)
- A stone in the lower common bile duct
- Dilated bile ducts (Fig. 2).
- An edematous head of the pancreas (Fig. 2)
- A splenomegaly

- What simple US criterion allows you to define splenomegaly, whatever the age of the child?
- How do you interpret the following blood test results?
  Hb 75 g/l; leukocytes 5,600/mm^3; platelets 153,000/mm^3; CRP 15 mg/l; ASAT 245 UI/l; ALAT 234 UI/l; GGT 158 UI/l; total bilirubin 65 μmol/l; direct bilirubin 25 μmol/l; amylase 484 UI/l; lipase 198 UI/l.
- Which relevant clinical information is missing in this observation?

Under painkillers and spasmolytic therapy, the patient's abdominal pain resolved after a few hours. Liver and pancreatic blood values normalized in the following days. Hematological investigations confirmed spherocytosis. Abdominal US confirmed the complete migration of the stone, with regression of the biliary dilation, and normalization of the pancreas. Multiple small stones persisted in the gallbladder.

- What surgical treatment do you propose and why?

A 98

Due to the patient's age and the paroxystic abdominal pain episodes, intussusception has to be ruled out. After this, the suspected diagnosis is biliary stone migration (right upper quadrant abdominal pain, vomiting, and absence of fever), secondary to chronic hemolysis (pale and subicteric, splenomegaly).

If the length of the spleen is more than the length of a normal left kidney, there is a splenomegaly.

These blood tests show an anemia which is probably hemolytic (elevated unconjugated bilirubin), the absence of inflammatory syndrome, mild cholestasis (elevation of liver enzymes with mild elevation of GGTs and of conjugated bilirubin), and mild pancreatic reaction.

These biological findings are consistent with biliary stone migration and chronic hemolysis.

The familial history reveals that the father underwent splenectomy in childhood for hereditary spherocytosis, and the grandfather underwent cholecystectomy in early adulthood for cholelithiasis. Most likely this child also has hereditary spherocytosis.

Biliary lithiasis in childhood can be divided into the following subgroups:

- Asymptomatic biliary lithiasis, without underlying hemolysis: no indication for surgery.
- Symptomatic or complicated biliary lithiasis: indication for surgery (laparoscopic cholecystectomy). It is recommended to search for hemolysis, which may require its own surgical treatment in the same operation.
- Asymptomatic microlithiasis in hemolytic anemias: due to the high risk of severe complications, preventive surgical treatment may be advised, either chole-

cystectomy alone (drepanocytosis) or associated with subtotal splenectomy (spherocytosis).

- Biliary lithiasis in early infancy: it may be related to transient immaturity of bilirubin conjugation in the perinatal period, especially in premature babies. If treatment is needed (due to stone migration) and the bile ducts are presumably normal, a conservative treatment by interventional radiology (percutaneous transhepatic flushing of the stones) without cholecystectomy may be attempted; if successful, biliary lithiasis has a low risk of recurrence.

In the reported case, cholecystectomy is required due to previous stone migration, in order to avoid recurrence of such episodes and potential biliary or pancreatic complications.

Regarding spherocytosis, severe anemia pleads in favor of reducing hemolysis. At this age, the recommended treatment is subtotal (7/8) splenectomy, which allows one to significantly reduce the level of hemolysis and to preserve immunological functions of the splenic remnant.

These two procedures can be combined in the same operation, which can be partly or totally performed by laparoscopy. After subtotal splenectomy, hematological and US Doppler follow-up is needed:

- In the early postoperative period to measure the size and check the blood supply of the splenic remnant (Figs. 3, 4).
- In the follow-up to measure the size of the splenic remnant, since some regrowth is usual and may (rarely) require secondary splenectomy totalization, if significant hemolysis reappears.

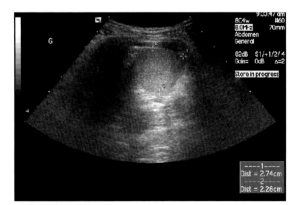

Fig. 3

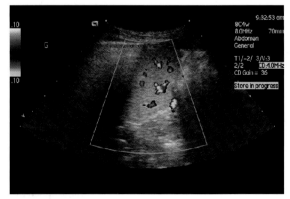

Fig. 4

Q 99

Yves Aigrain and Pascale Philippe-Chomette

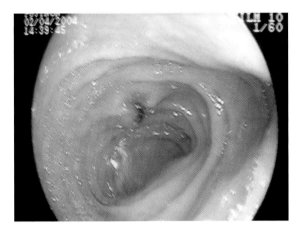

Fig. 1

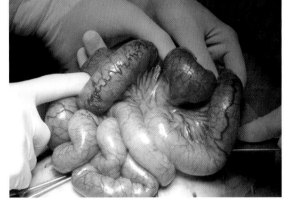

Fig. 2

A 4-year-old girl with Turner syndrome was admitted to hospital for abdominal hemorrhage.

Rectal bleeding and melena were observed.

- What is your strategy and which two examinations do you ask for first?

After these examinations, a US study and CT scan were performed; however, these two examinations were not contributive and laparoscopy was performed. No Meckel diverticulum was observed but intestinal telangiectasias on the small bowel (about 70-cm length) were identified.

A "wait and see" approach was decided on. Two years later, this girl was readmitted for acute gastrointestinal hemorrhage and needed three blood transfusions within 10 days.

A video capsule total intestinal endoscopy was performed and was not contributive, showing only intestinal bleeding without any identifiable lesion.

- What is your hypothesis?

Figures 1 and 2 show the internal and external investigations (endoscopy coupled with laparotomy).

- How do you interpret these images?

A 99

After laboratory tests (patient's blood, platelet count, hemoglobin and hematocrit values), an esophagogastroduodenoscopy and a rectal examination with complete colonoscopy were performed.

Turner's syndrome associated with telangiectasias has been described previously. Telangiectasias are difficult to see at endoscopy and on CT scans. Laparoscopy could be helpful in eliminating Meckel's diverticulum in the case of rapid deglobulization and in establishing the diagnosis of telangiectasia. Hormonal therapy has shown its efficacy in this syndrome but it could not be proposed for this girl before puberty.

Considering that this patient presented with recurrent bleeding, laparotomy was performed with combined upper endoscopy, the bowel was carefully palpated and transilluminated looking for the symptomatic telangiectasias.

Figures 1 and 2 show intra- and extraluminal aspects of telangiectasias. It is rather difficult to localize them with endoscopy alone, and therefore endoscopy should be coupled with laparotomy. After collegial discussion we decided to resect 70 cm of consecutive small bowel. After 5 years of follow-up, there is no recurrent bleeding and no need for hormone therapy.

Suggested Reading

1. Eroglu Y, Emerick KM, Chou PM, Reynolds M. Gastrointestinal bleeding in Turner's syndrome: a case report and literature review. J Pediatr Gastroenterol Nutr 2002 Jul; 35(1):84–7
2. Nudell J, Brady P. A case of GI hemorrhage in a patient with Turner's syndrome: diagnosis by capsule endoscopy. Gastrointest Endosc 2006 Mar; 63(3):514–6
3. Vuillemin E, Rifflet H, Oberti F, Cales P, Wion-Barbot N, Ben Bouali A. Turner syndrome and digestive telangiectasis: an additional value of oestrogen-progestational treatment. Gastroenterol Clin Biol 1996; 20(5):510–1

Q 100

Yves Aigrain and Pascale Philippe-Chomette

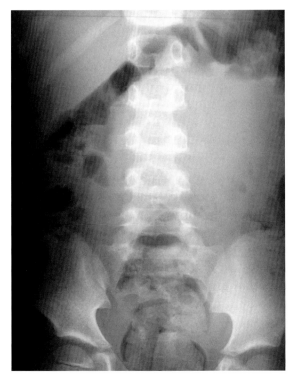

Fig. 1

A healthy 4-year-old boy presented with abdominal obstruction with fever (38.5°C) and pain.

For 2 days the boy had been vomiting and had abdominal distension. The clinical examination revealed a painful medial abdominal mass.

Figure 1 is standard abdominal radiograph and Fig. 2 is a CT scan.

- Can you comment on the case?
- What is your diagnosis?
- As a surgeon, what is your initial approach?
- After a complete recovery, what is your next approach?
- What is the main risk?

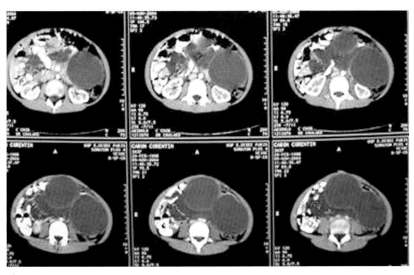

Fig. 2

A 100

The repeat plain abdominal radiographs show a mass effect on the left quadrant of the abdomen with displacement of the viscera.

The CT scan shows a large cystic mass with a hemorrhagic component. The diagnosis is an abdominal cystic lymphangioma with inflammatory and infectious complications.

The initial approach is to treat infection with parenteral antibiotherapy and gastric aspiration.

This benign lesion needs complete excision because of the symptomatic effects and the risk of recurrent intestinal obstruction. This particular lymphangioma developed in the mesenteric area with infiltration of the small bowel and needed small-bowel resection (Fig. 3).

Although cystic lymphangioma is a rare benign lesion, recurrence is the main risk. The resection must be complete and for mesenteric localization bowel resection is often necessary.

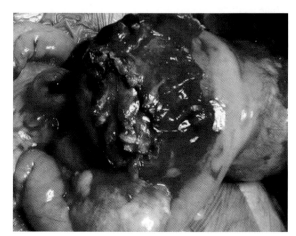

Fig. 3

Suggested Reading

1. Konen O, Rathaus V, Dlugy E, Freud E, Kessler A, Shapiro M, Horev G. Childhood abdominal cystic lymphangioma. Pediatr Radiol 2002 Feb; 32(2):88–94
2. Singh S, Maghrabi M. Small bowel obstruction caused by recurrent cystic lymphangioma. Br J Surg 1993 Aug; 80(8):1012

Q 101

Yves Aigrain and Pascale Philippe-Chomette

A premature twin (30 weeks), weighing 900 g, with a dilated jejunum detected at 20 weeks' gestation was referred to our department.

At birth, the boy was clinically healthy and needed no respiratory assistance.

A standard radiograph was obtained (Fig. 1).

- Can you comment on this examination?
- Before birth, what sort of examinations would you request if intestinal obstruction is suspected?
- Considering the prematurity, what is your initial approach as a surgeon?

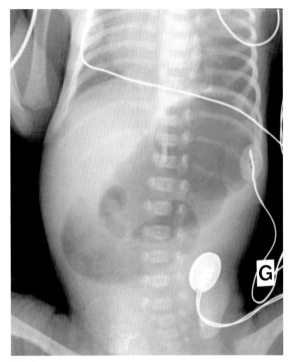

Fig. 1

A 101

A gastric and duodenal distension with "double bubble sign" and a gasless abdomen were identified.

These findings could fit the description of a proximal intestinal atresia or the description of a midgut volvulus. In view of the enlarged jejunum described at 20 weeks, we diagnosed proximal jejunal atresia, with uncertainty about the rest of the small bowel (multiple atresias, antenatal volvulus, apple peel syndrome).

Prenatal ultrasound examinations detect some anomalies evoking proximal intestinal obstruction:

- Isolated enlarged stomach and duodenum ("double bubble sign") associated with polyhydramnios are suggestive of duodenal junction obstruction, while calcifications or hyperechogenicity of the loops may indicate meconium peritonitis.

As we detected these anomalies, MR imaging was performed within 2 weeks of the US examination. Obstruction is considered proximal when the dilated loops are hypointense on T1-weighted images and distal when they are hyperintense on T1-weighted images with normal loops visible below the stomach.

Amniocentesis is proposed for amniotic fluid assays for karyotyping, cystic fibrosis screening, and digestive enzyme assays.

This boy did not undergo MR imaging considering his prematurity; however, amniocentesis was carried out

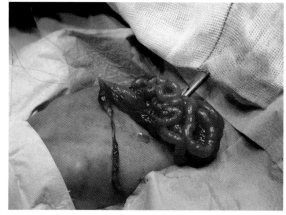

Fig. 2

with a digestive enzyme assay which suggested proximal obstruction with no detection of cystic fibrosis.

This premature twin had jejunal atresia, and an intestinal permeability test revealed an associated jejunal diaphragm 3 cm below. We performed a "onetime" reparation without stoma (Fig. 2) and with duodenal caliber reduction; at the same time a CVC was inserted. Three weeks after reparation, intestinal transit started and enteral feeding could be initiated. We recommend "onetime" reparation when there is proximal atresia without involvement of the distal bowel.

Suggested Reading

1. Besner GE, Bates GD, Boesel CP, Singh V, Welty SE, Corpron CA. Total absence of the small bowel in a premature neonate. Pediatr Surg Int 2005 May; 21(5):396–9
2. Escobar MA, Ladd AP, Grosfeld JL, West KW, Rescorla FJ, Sherer LR, Engum SA, Rouse TM, Billmire DF. Duodenal atresia and stenosis. J Pediatr Surg 2004 Jun; 39(6):867–71: long term follow up over 30 years.
3. Garel C, Dreux S, Philippe-Chomette P, Vuillard E, Oury JF, Muller F. Contribution of fetal magnetic resonance imaging and amniotic fluid digestive enzyme assays to the evaluation of gastrointestinal tract abnormalities. Ultrasound Obstet Gynecol 2006; 28:282–291

Q 102

Felix Schier

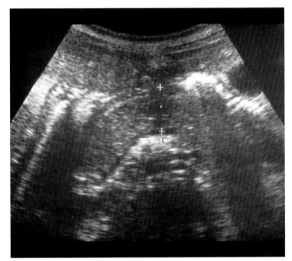

Fig. 1

Fig. 2

A 6-year-old girl presented with acute, persistent upper abdominal tenderness and distension. There was no trauma or sepsis, and she was not taking any medication. The girl had nausea and vomiting.

Serum and urinary amylase and lipase levels were elevated.

An ultrasound examination was performed, shown in Figs. 1 and 2.

Puncture and aspiration yielded hemorrhagic ascites.
- What does Fig. 1 show?
- What does Fig. 2 show?
- What is the most likely diagnosis?
- What may be the cause?
- What is the most adequate therapy?

A 102

Figure 1 shows a transverse ultrasonographic section of the upper abdomen at the level of the pancreas.

The pancreas is markedly enlarged in all segments and is of reduced echogenicity.

Figure 2 shows a longitudinal cross-section at the level of the left anterior axillary line. The *black area* is a broad fluid collection with fine internal echoes caudally to the inferior spleen pole, also cranially and ventrally to the left kidney.

The most likely diagnosis is hemorrhagic pancreatitis.

The pathophysiology of acute pancreatitis is unclear in most cases. The most frequent causes in children are idiopathic, cystic fibrosis or diabetes, biliary tract disease, and trauma with ductal lesions. Also, systematic diseases such as lupus erythematosus, sepsis, or shock have been described as possible causes.

Clinically, more than 90% of the children will have pain, more than 60% will vomit, and more than 30% will have fever.

Bowel rest, nasogastric tube, intravenous support, and the correction of electrolytes, glucose, and calcium are the main aspects of therapy for acute pancreatitis. The basic idea is to reduce pancreatic activity by stopping enteral feedings. The efficacy of the nasogastric tube is controversial. In parallel, a search for a possible anatomical, chemical, or metabolic cause should be conducted, leading to a specific therapy when identified.

More than 75% of patients will recover without needing surgery.

Despite the figures shown above, the sensitivity of ultrasonography in detecting acute pancreatitis is inferior to the sensitivity of CT.

Suggested Reading

1. Akel S, Khalifeh M, Makhlouf Akel M. Gallstone pancreatitis in children: atypical presentation and review. Eur J Pediatr 2005; 164:482–485, Review
2. Benifla M, Weizman Z. Acute pancreatitis in childhood: analysis of literature data. J Clin Gastroenterol 2003; 37:169–172, Review
3. Nydegger A, Couper RT, Oliver MR. Childhood pancreatitis. J Gastroenterol Hepatol 2006; 21:499–509, Review
4. Stringer MD. Pancreatitis and pancreatic trauma. Semin Pediatr Surg 2005; 14:239–246, Review

Q 103

Felix Schier

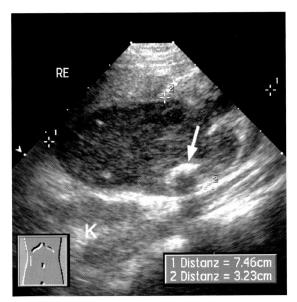

Fig. 1

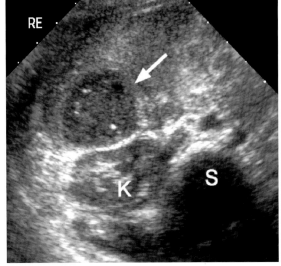

Fig. 2

A 4-year-old boy presented with right-sided lower abdominal pain that had started 4 days earlier. The pain increased over the last 2 days, reached a peak on the 2nd day, and decreased slightly over the next 2 days. Initially there was vomiting; his fever persisted.

There was marked tenderness on palpation of the right lower abdomen. The remaining abdomen was tender.

Both Rovsing and Blumberg signs were positive. The child avoided walking, had to be carried, and especially avoided moving the right psoas muscle. However, the child had a good appetite and wished to eat and drink.

Laboratory tests demonstrated an elevated leukocyte count and C-reactive protein level.

Ultrasound studies yielded the images shown in Figs. 1 and 2.
- What is the most likely diagnosis?
- What is the therapy?

A 103

Figure 1 is a longitudinal section of the right lower abdomen. There is a fluid collection of 7-cm diameter caudally to the right kidney (*K*) with marked internal echoes. Most conspicuous is a semilunar hyperechoic structure with a dorsal acoustic shadow (*arrow*). This is a fecalith within an abscess (*RE*, patient's right side).

Figure 2 shows a transversal section of the right middle abdomen. Just ventrally to the kidney (*K*), again, the fluid-containing structure is seen with marked internal echoes (*arrow*). The abscess is almost the size of the kidney (*K*). "*S*" marks the vertebral column.

The diagnosis is perityphlitic abscess with a fecalith inside the abscess cavity.

CT is not very good in detecting perforation in appendicitis.

The best treatment of appendiceal masses is controversial at present. It would appear that evacuation of the abscess, for example, by ultrasonographic guidance, is indicated as soon as the diagnosis is established. Several studies support this approach. An appendectomy will follow later.

Suggested Reading

1. Bixby SD, Lucey BC, Soto JA, Theyson JM, Ozonoff A, Varghese JC. Perforated versus nonperforated acute appendicitis: accuracy of multidetector CT detection. Radiology 2006; 241:780–786
2. Brown CV, Abrishami M, Muller M, Velmahos GC. Appendiceal abscess: immediate operation or percutaneous drainage? Am Surg 2003; 69:829–832
3. Lasson A, Lundagards J, Loren I, Nilsson PE. Appendiceal abscesses: primary percutaneous drainage and selective interval appendicectomy. Eur J Surg 2002; 168:264–269
4. Samuel M, Hosie G, Holmes K. Prospective evaluation of nonsurgical versus surgical management of appendiceal mass. J Pediatr Surg 2002; 37:882–886
5. Wootton-Gorges SL, Thomas KB, Harned RK, Wu SR, Stein-Wexler R, Strain JD. Giant cystic abdominal masses in children. Pediatr Radiol 2005; 35:1277–1288

Q 104

Felix Schier

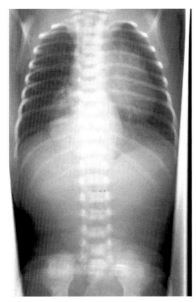

Fig. 1

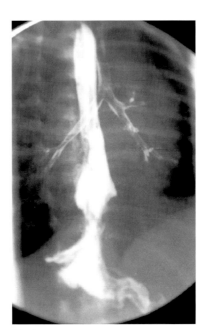

Fig. 2

In a newborn boy, all attempts at feeding resulted in immediate vomiting. Prenatal ultrasound examinations were normal. The abdomen was not distended and the vomit did not smell sour.

On examination, the child appeared otherwise normal. No malformations were known and all laboratory values were normal. Radiological studies yielded the images shown in Figs. 1 and 2.

- What is the most likely diagnosis?

A 104

Figure 1 shows a large, oval epiphrenic mass, shifting the heart to the left. The abdomen is gasless. Figure 2 is a contrast study of the esophagus and the stomach. The stomach is small and located mostly intrathoracically. The esophagus is unusually short. The contrast medium is promptly regurgitated and even aspirated, additionally contrasting the trachea and bronchi.

The diagnosis is brachyesophagus and microgastria.

Congenital microgastria has been postulated to be the result of impaired normal foregut development. Apparently, only 39 cases have been described in the literature. Clinically, reflux signs, failure to thrive, and growth retardation are the consequences.

Preliminary jejunostomy feeding has been suggested as a primary treatment modality. Subsequently, gastric augmentation (Hunt-Lawrence pouch) is performed. From the few cases described so far, it seems that even the gastroesophageal sphincter may regain its competence once the reservoir capacity of the small stomach is restored.

An initial diagnosis of gastroesophageal reflux is not unusual in children with microgastria. The child may be referred to the surgeon for fundoplication or placement of a gastrostomy with the referring physician not being aware of the presence of microgastria. For the same reasons, surgical correction may be delayed. The youngest child to have undergone gastric augmentation was 3 months old. As a consequence, in children with severe reflux symptoms since birth, radiographic contrast studies should be evaluated carefully for reduced gastric reservoir capacity. Prolonged medical management is not beneficial in congenital microgastria, because the stomach size does not increase significantly with the passage of time.

After gastric augmentation the gastroesophageal reflux will cease.

Microgastria is seldom an isolated symptom. In most children there are associated congenital malformations. They include asplenia, intestinal malrotation, cardiopulmonary anomalies, central nervous system and renal anomalies, laryngotracheobronchial clefts, and limb-reduction defects including total amelia. Prenatal ultrasonographic demonstration of these anomalies should alert the surgeon.

Suggested Reading

1. Hoehner JC, Kimura K, Soper RT. Congenital microgastria. J Pediatr Surg 1994; 29:1591–1593
2. Kroes EJ, Festen C. Congenital microgastria: a case report and review of literature. Pediatr Surg Int 1998; 13:416–418
3. Menon P, Rao KL, Cutinha HP, Thapa BR, Nagi B. Gastric augmentation in isolated congenital microgastria. J Pediatr Surg 2003; 38:E4–6
4. Murray KF, Lillehei CW, Duggan C. Congenital microgastria: treatment with transient jejunal feedings. J Pediatr Gastroenterol Nutr 1999; 28:343–345
5. Ramos, CT, Moss RL, Musemeche CA. Microgastria as an isolated anomaly. J Pediatr Surg 1996; 31:1445–1447

Q 105

Felix Schier

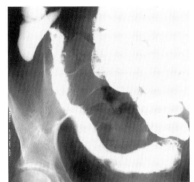

Fig. 1

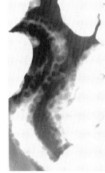

Fig. 2

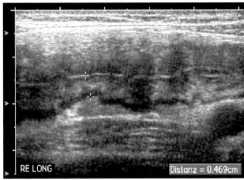

Fig. 3

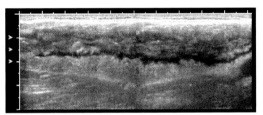

Fig. 4

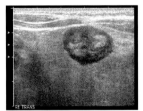

Fig. 5

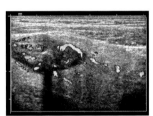

Fig. 6

A 12-year-old boy presented with right-sided lower abdominal pain that had started 4 days earlier. The pain decreased over the last 2 days. His aunt suffered from ulcerative colitis.

Initially there was vomiting, and bloody diarrhea had set in during the last 2 days. He had a moderate fever.

There was tenderness and possibly a mass on palpation of the right lower abdomen.

Laboratory tests showed a slightly elevated leukocyte count and a markedly elevated C-reactive protein level. The erythrocyte sedimentation rate was markedly elevated and the hemoglobin value decreased.

Ultrasound examinations yielded the images shown in Figs. 1–6.

- What is the most likely diagnosis?

A 105

Figure 1 shows the terminal ileum, which is stenotic and displays an increased distance to the adjacent small bowel loops. The cecum is compressed. Multiple spiculae are identified (a source of fistulae).

In Fig. 2, in addition to the stenosis of the terminal ileum, a cobblestone mucosa is seen. The bowel wall is thickened.

Figure 3 is a longitudinal section of the terminal ileum. Again, there is marked thickening of the bowel wall, especially at the level of the submucosa. The muscularis propria is also thickened and demonstrates irregular interphases with the broadened mesenterial fat.

In Fig. 4, as before, there is wall thickening of the terminal ileum, especially of the submucosa. The muscularis propria shows infiltrations of the massively thickened mesenterial fatty tissue.

Figure 5 is a cross-section of the terminal ileum. The bowel wall is thickened and contains an enlarged hyperechoic submucosa. There is massive enlargement of the hyperechoic mesenterial fatty tissue, almost completely encircling the bowel loops ("creeping fat"). A few spiculae are cross sectioned from the muscularis propria into the mesenterial fat.

On color-coded Doppler images (Fig. 6) a hypervascularity of the mesenterial fat and especially of the thickened ileum is noticeable, a sign of acute inflammation.

The diagnosis is Crohn's disease.

There are only few data on inflammatory bowel disease in young children. It seems that these children often present with rectal bleeding and primarily colonic involvement. Furthermore, it has been observed that half of the children had a positive history of neonatal or early-onset bacterial infection with the use of antibiotics before the onset of inflammatory bowel disease. Some patients were even still being breastfed, others were just weaned when GI symptoms started. Most children eventually needed bowel rest, parenteral nutrition, and steroid, azathioprine, or cyclosporine medication. One-third of patients required surgery. Neonatal inflammatory bowel disease seems to be more severe in presentation and evolution.

Crohn's disease patients often have a positive family history of the disease.

It is not unusual for primary manifestations of Crohn's disease to be misinterpreted as acute appendicitis or gastrointestinal infection.

Ultrasonographic diagnosis of Crohn's disease in such a small child is unusual. Usually contrast studies are undertaken in order to search for stenosis, mucosal disease, and skip lesions. Bowel wall thickening is better seen with CT. Recently, 18F-FDG-PET has been attributed with a high diagnostic value in pediatric patients with chronic inflammatory bowel disease. In addition, CE-mannitol-MR imaging has been described to contribute significantly to the identification of disease extension, severity, and intestinal complications with adequate diagnostic accuracy. This technique has been suggested for diagnostic exploration in young patients with suspected Crohn's disease.

Wireless video capsule endoscopy (VCE) is increasingly described, possibly also used, in children with a diagnosis of functional abdominal pain. Even children can swallow the capsules without major problems. VCE has also been used to detect Crohn's disease. VCE is more sensitive than endoscopy for detection of macroscopic gastric and small-bowel pathologies.

Laparoscopy has been used for early detection of Crohn's disease, also in combination with endoscopy. It provides an early macroscopic impression of Crohn's disease in children, a picture not obtained previously. However, since primary treatment of Crohn's disease is usually nonsurgical, and is directed by the "activity" of the disease process, the significance of the macroscopic picture is relatively unimportant.

The most efficient screening strategy for Crohn's disease in children seems to be measurement of the erythrocyte sedimentation rate and hemoglobin. This combination appears to have a higher positive predictive value and is more sensitive, more specific, and less costly than commercial serologic testing.

Q 106

Felix Schier

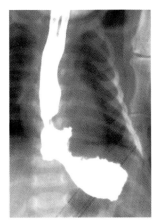

Fig. 1

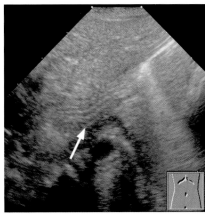

Fig. 2

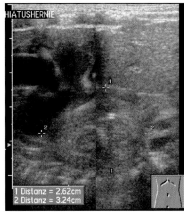

Fig. 3

A 9-month-old child presented with intermittent vomiting since birth. There had been several previous episodes of pneumonia.

On auscultation there were normal breath sounds. Laboratory values were normal except for signs of anemia. Imaging studies yielded the pictures shown in Figs. 1–3.

- What is the most likely diagnosis?

A 106

Figure 1 is an esophagogram demonstrating parts of the fundus within the thorax.

On the ultrasound image in Fig. 2, a layered, longitudinal, tubular structure is seen at the hiatus (*arrow*).

In Fig. 3 the structure can be followed cranially to an epiphrenic parenchymal mass.

The diagnosis is paraesophageal hiatal hernia.

Paraesophageal hernias are uncommon in children and are different from the more common sliding hiatus hernias. They may be combined with a sliding hernia. Most often they are found on the right side. They also occur as a complication after a previous antireflux operation, especially if there was no crural plication. Children with preoperative gagging or slow corrected gastric emptying seem to be at higher risk of developing a paraesophageal hernia postoperatively.

The most common symptoms in children with paraesophageal hernias are chest infections, vomiting, anemia, failure to thrive, and dysphagia. In some children, the diagnosis is established incidentally. Strangulation, in contrast to what one would expect, virtually does not exist. Mechanical obstruction owing to organoaxial volvulus requiring emergency surgery does occur, however. Some children will also have malrotation.

Radiologically, a cystic or opaque mass is seen in the posterior mediastinum in the right lower chest, occasionally an air–fluid level in the cystic mass or a dilated esophagus is also noted. In most cases, the gastroesophageal junction is displaced into the stomach. Some have the gastroesophageal junction within the abdomen.

Ultrasonographically obvious pictures, as demonstrated here, are usually not obtained.

The principles of surgery are the reduction of the contents, partial excision of the sac, crural approximation, and a fundoplication. Omission of a fundoplication is likely to result in reflux.

The laparoscopic treatment of large paraesophageal and mixed hiatal hernias is feasible and safe. The long-term results, however, are less favorable. The anatomical and functional recurrence rate is around 40%. It is unknown at present which patients are at risk of failure and which technical modifications need to be made in order to prevent recurrences.

Suggested Reading

1. Avansino JR, Lornez ML, Hendrickson M, Jolley SG. Characterization and management of paraesophageal hernias in children after antireflux operation. J Pediatr Surg 1999; 34:1610–1614

2. Imamoglu M, Cay A, Kosucu P, Ozdemir O, Orhan F, Sapan L, Sarihan H. Congenital paraesophageal hiatal hernia: pitfalls in the diagnosis and treatment. J Pediatr Surg 2005; 40:1128–1133

3. Karpelowsky JS, Wieselthaler N, Rode H. Primary paraesophageal hernia in children. J Pediatr Surg 2006; 41:1588–1593

4. Schier F. Indications for laparoscopic antireflux procedures in children. Indications for laparoscopic antireflux procedures in children. Semin Laparosc Surg 2002; 9:139–45

5. Targarona EM, Novell J, Vela S, Cerdan G, Bendahan G, Torrubia S, Kobus C, Rebasa P, Balague C, Garriga J, Trias M. Mid term analysis of safety and quality of life after the laparoscopic repair of paraesophageal hiatal hernia. Surg Endosc 2004; 18:1045–1050

Q 107

Felix Schier

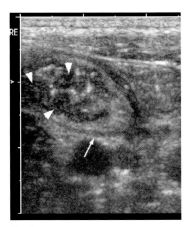

Fig. 1

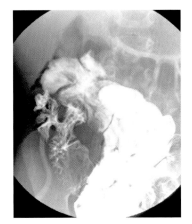

Fig. 2

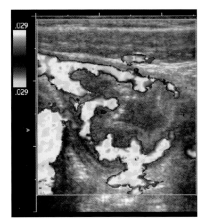

Fig. 4

A 7-year-old boy presented with right lower quadrant mass and pain, fever, vomiting, and leukocytosis. The leukocyte and C-reactive protein levels were moderately elevated.

Imaging studies yielded the pictures shown in Figs. 1–4.

- What is the most likely diagnosis?

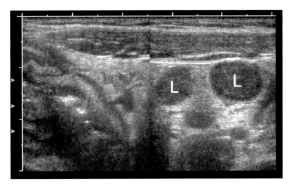

Fig. 3

A 107

Figure 1 is a cross-section of the terminal ileum. The wall is thickened. Hyperechoic structures are identified within the submucosa (*arrowheads*), representing lymphofollicular hypertrophy. There is slight thickening of the submucosa. The muscularis propria is unchanged (*arrow*).

In Fig. 2, there is normal haustration near the cecum. Several enlarged lymph follicles make the shape of the lumen irregular.

Figure 3 is an ultrasonogram of the right lower abdomen. There are enlarged lymph nodes within the mesentery (*L*).

Figure 4 is a color-coded Doppler cross-sectional sonogram of the terminal ileum. The bowel wall is enlarged and displays increased vascularity. The mesenteric fat is not involved. The lymph follicles are hyperplastic.

The diagnosis is ileitis terminalis (yersiniosis). The differential diagnosis to Crohn's disease includes no spiculae and no or only little broadening of the mesenterial fat.

The clinical symptoms are very similar to classic appendicitis: lower abdominal pain, fever, vomiting, and a right lower quadrant mass associated with leukocytosis. Upon surgery, terminal ileitis is found, and eventually cultures of peritoneal fluid and of mesenteric lymph nodes will grow *Yersinia enterocolitica*.

There is no consistently reliable nonoperative way to separate a sporadic case of appendicitis from one whose appendicitis-like symptoms are due to *Yersinia*. In addition, a small percentage of *Yersinia* patients will present with true appendicitis as a complication of their disease.

In a study of 352 patients who were hospitalized with symptoms of an acute appendicitis, *Yersinia* infections were determined in almost 20% of patients by cultural and serological methods. Infections due to *Y. enterocolitica* serovar 0:3 were approximately six times more frequent than those due to *Y. enterocolitica* serovar 0:9. *Yersinia pseudotuberculosis* could only be isolated in one patient from a mesenterial lymph node. The majority of the infections were found in the age group of 9–12 years. The incidence was highest in the summer months, June–August.

Other studies have found lower rates of yersiniosis in "appendicitis," especially in the United States.

Numerous publications discuss the advantages and disadvantages of preoperative ultrasonography and CT in the diagnosis of appendicitis. This case demonstrates that ultrasonography, when performed by an expert, may be helpful in establishing the correct diagnosis.

Suggested Reading

1. Baier R, Puppel H, Zelder O, Heiming E, Bauer E, Syring J. Frequency and significance of infections due to Yersinia enterocolitica in "acute appendicitis". Z Gastroenterol 1982; 20:78–83
2. Bennion RS, Thompson JE Jr, Gil J, Schmit PJ. The role of Yersinia enterocolitica in appendicitis in the southwestern United States. Am Surg 1991; 57:766–768
3. Shorter NA, Thompson MD, Mooney DP, Modlin JF. Surgical aspects of an outbreak of Yersinia enterocolitis. Pediatr Surg Int 1998; 13:2–5
4. York D, Smith A, Phillips JD, von Allmen D. The influence of advanced radiographic imaging on the treatment of pediatric appendicitis. J Pediatr Surg 2005; 40:1908–1911

Q 108

Felix Schier

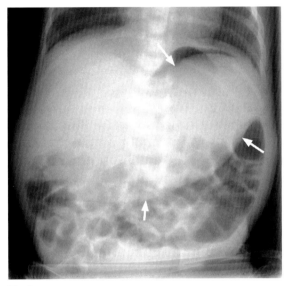

Fig. 1

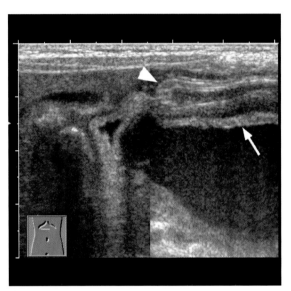

Fig. 2

A newborn presented with vomiting immediately after any feeding attempt. No mass or olive was palpated. The shape of the abdomen looked normal and peristalsis was not seen.

Laboratory values were also normal. Imaging studies yielded the pictures shown in Figs. 1 and 2.

- What is the most likely diagnosis?

A 108

Figure 1 is a plain view radiograph. There is a mass at the greater curvature (*arrows*). The gastric air is dislocated cranially and the transverse colon is pushed caudally.

Figure 2 is a sonogram of the antrum. The *arrowhead* points to the compressed antrum. Caudally to the compressed antrum, a large fluid-containing structure is identified with the characteristic layers of the gastrointestinal wall, typical for these kinds of lesions. To the left, the compressed bulbus duodeni is seen, also containing some fluid.

The diagnosis is gastric duplication.

Gastric duplications represent only 5% of all alimentary tract duplications. Most become symptomatic before the age of 2 years. A duplication of the size presented here will become symptomatic from shear mass effect, other duplications may bleed or cause peptic ulceration, depending on location, size, presence of gastric mucosa, and whether there is a communication with the lumen of the stomach (in the majority there is none).

This patient was a newborn. The diagnosis, however, was not known prenatally, despite several sonographic evaluations of the pregnancy. Antenatal ultrasound diagnosis has become the rule for larger gastric duplications.

Symptoms of children with gastric duplication cysts vary widely. There are asymptomatic duplication cysts. Pain, bleeding, obstruction, palpable mass, failure to thrive, perforation, and recurrent pancreatitis have been described in children with gastric duplication, and some have even eroded up into the chest.

Diagnostically, ultrasound and CT will establish the diagnosis, perhaps aided by an upper GI study.

Surgical excision is the therapy of choice. Complete excision is usually feasible.

Laparoscopic resection of gastric duplication cysts has been described. Some cysts, however, are difficult to localize laparoscopically, even when aided by intraoperative gastroscopy.

Suggested Reading

1. Carachi R, Azmy A. Foregut duplications. Pediatr Surg Int 2002; 18:371–374
2. Ford WD, Guelfand M, Lopez PJ, Furness ME. Laparoscopic excision of a gastric duplication cyst detected on antenatal ultrasound scan. J Pediatr Surg 2004; 39:e8–e10
3. Master V, Woods RH, Morris LL, Freeman J. Gastric duplication cyst causing gastric outlet obstruction. Pediatr Radiol 2004; 34:574–576
4. Nakazawa N, Okazaki T, Miyano T. Prenatal detection of isolated gastric duplication cyst. Pediatr Surg Int 2005; 21:831–834
5. Rodriguez CR, Eire PF, Lopez GA, Alvarez EM, Sanchez FM. Asymptomatic gastric duplication in a child: report of a new case and review of the literature. Pediatr Surg Int 2005; 21:421–422

Q 109

Felix Schier

A mature newborn had a distended abdomen, bilious vomiting, and failed to pass meconium for 3 days. There were no associated anomalies and all laboratory values were normal.

An imaging study yielded the picture in Fig. 1.

- What is the most likely diagnosis?

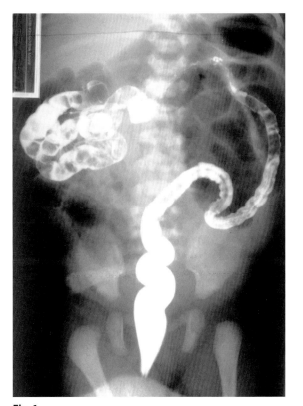

Fig. 1

A 109

Figure 1 is a contrast study of the colon. A microcolon extends over the whole colon length, containing numerous small meconium globules. The small bowel in the left upper abdomen is distended secondary to the distal obstruction.

The diagnosis is meconium ileus from cystic fibrosis (as diagnosed subsequently).

As newborns, children with cystic fibrosis usually present with gastrointestinal or pancreaticobiliary symptoms. Meconium ileus is the typical first manifestation. These symptoms persist throughout childhood. Only later do pulmonary complications become more prominent.

Radiologically, the colon is of normal length but has a decreased caliber. If there is reflux into the terminal ileum, the site of obstruction will be identified. A barium enema also serves to differentiate an uncomplicated meconium ileus from an intestinal atresia or volvulus.

Later in life, the combination of fat deposition and pancreatic fibrosis leads to varying CT and MR appearances. A higher than normal incidence of pancreatic cysts and calcification is also seen. Decreased transport of water and chloride increases the viscosity of bile, with subsequent obstruction of the biliary ductules. If extensive, this can progress to obstructive cirrhosis, portal hypertension, and esophageal varices. Diffuse fatty infiltration, hypersplenism, and gallstones are also commonly seen in these patients.

There is a risk to confuse meconium ileus radiologically with Hirschsprung's disease. It has been stated that the presence of right lower quadrant intraluminal calcifications should raise the suspicion of long-segment intestinal aganglionosis even if the operative findings are typical of meconium ileus and a biopsy should be performed.

Later in life, a neonate with meconium ileus will not have a poorer nutritional status or poorer lung function tests than a cystic fibrosis patient without meconium ileus.

Up to one-third of children with meconium ileus may be treated nonsurgically with hypertonic enemas. Children with small-bowel atresias may constitute up to 20% of cases with meconium ileus.

Approximately 60% of children with meconium ileus have uncomplicated disease. Uncomplicated cases are those with simple obstruction of the terminal ileum. One-third has complications such as perforation, volvulus, atresia, or meconium peritonitis.

In this case, there is meconium obstruction without cystic fibrosis.

If surgery is required, up to 60% of the children with uncomplicated disease will need bowel resection and enterostomy. Of the complicated cases, about half may be managed by bowel resection and anastomosis, the other half of patients will require an enterostomy.

Suggested Reading

1. Chaudry G, Navarro OM, Levine DS, Oudjhane K. Abdominal manifestations of cystic fibrosis in children. Pediatr Radiol 2006; 36:233–240
2. Cowles RA, Berdon WE, Holt PD, Buonomo C, Stolar CJ. Neonatal intestinal obstruction simulating meconium ileus in infants with long-segment intestinal aganglionosis: radiographic findings that prompt the need for rectal biopsy. Pediatr Radiol 2006; 36:133–137
3. Escobar MA, Grosfeld JL, Burdick JJ, Powell RL, Jay CL, Wait AD, West KW, Billmire DF, Scherer LR 3rd, Engum SA, Rouse TM, Ladd AP, Rescorla FJ. Surgical considerations in cystic fibrosis: a 32-year evaluation of outcomes. Surgery 2005; 138:560–571
4. Munck A, Gerardin M, Alberti C, Eizenman C, Lebourgeois M, Aigrain Y, Navarro J. Clinical outcome of cystic fibrosis presenting with or without meconium ileus: a matched cohort study. J Pediatr Surg 2006; 41:1556–1560
5. Rescorla FJ, Grosfeld JL. Contemporary management of meconium ileus. World J Surg 1993; 17:318–325

Q 110

Felix Schier

The radiograph is of a 6-month-old boy with coughing after feedings. Asthma was suspected and treated earlier. Quite often, the child choked and coughed during feedings.

A physical examination was normal, and all laboratory values were normal. An imaging study yielded the picture in Fig. 1.

- What is the most likely diagnosis?

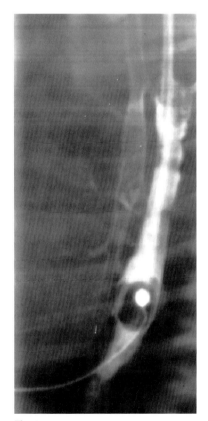

Fig. 1

A 110

Figure 1 is an esophagogram, obtained by advancing a balloon catheter into the distal esophagus, followed by a second catheter ending more proximally. This avoids aspiration during swallowing. Contrast medium is injected into the proximal catheter, resulting in contrasting the esophagus and subsequently the fistula in a retrograde manner from distally to cranially.

The diagnosis is tracheoesophageal H-fistula

H-type tracheoesophageal fistulae are rare. Although most cases are diagnosed in the neonatal period because of choking and cyanosis during feeding, there are rather frequent reports of older children and even adults with H-type fistulae. The reason is that the diagnosis is difficult and elusive, with a high percentage of false-negative findings.

Several radiologic techniques have been described on how to identify an H-type fistula. The technique demonstrated in Fig. 1 is simple and efficient.

Closure of H-fistulae is attempted in three different approaches: (a) the conventional "open" approach if the fistula is high up in the neck, (b) the thoracoscopic approach if the fistula is within the thorax, and (c) the endoscopic approach using electrocautery and histoacryl glue or fibrin glue. Success with the third technique is variable. It has been stated that a fistula that has not closed after two endoscopic attempts is not suitable for further endoscopic treatment and therefore an external approach should be recommended.

Although cine-esophagography is described to be highly effective in demonstrating H-type tracheoesophageal fistulae, bronchoscopy should be used in every patient suspected of having a fistula, especially when radiological methods fail. Bronchoscopy is helpful in diagnosis, in evaluation of associated respiratory tract anomalies, and in treatment.

Preoperative placement of a catheter in order to facilitate identification of the cyst has repeatedly been suggested. Identification of the fistula, however, is not that difficult in typical cases.

Suggested Reading

1. Aziz GA, Schier F. Thoracoscopic ligation of a tracheoesophageal H-type fistula in a newborn. J Pediatr Surg 2005; 40:35–36
2. Blanco-Rodriguez G, Penchyna-Grub J, Trujillo-Ponce A, Nava-Ocampo AA. Preoperative catheterization of H-type tracheoesophageal fistula to facilitate its localization and surgical correction. Eur J Pediatr Surg 2006; 16:14–17
3. De Schutter I, Vermeulen F, De Wachter E, Ernst C, Malfroot A. Isolated tracheoesophageal fistula in a 10-year-old girl. Eur J Pediatr 2006; 21:2006
4. García NM, Thompson JW, Shaul DB. Definitive localization of isolated tracheoesophageal fistula using bronchoscopy and esophagoscopy for guide wire placement. J Pediatr Surg 1998; 33:1645–1647
5. Karnak I, Senocak ME, Hicsonmez A, Buyukpamukcu N. The diagnosis and treatment of H-type tracheoesophageal fistula. J Pediatr Surg 1997; 32:1670–1674
6. Tzifa KT, Maxwell EL, Chait P, James AL, Forte V, Ein SH, Friedburg J. Endoscopic treatment of congenital H-Type and recurrent tracheoesophageal fistula with electrocautery and histoacryl glue.Int J Pediatr Otorhinolaryngol 2006; 70:925–930

Q 111

Felix Schier

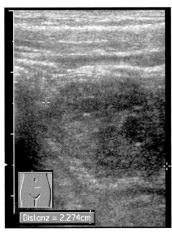

Fig. 1

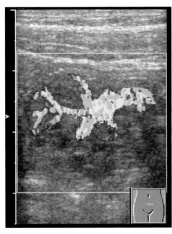

Fig. 2

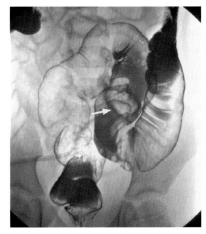

Fig. 3

A 7-year-old boy passed a moderate amount of fresh blood perianally. The child was otherwise healthy and had no abdominal pain. All laboratory values were normal.

Imaging studies yield the pictures shown in Figs. 1–3.

• What is the most likely diagnosis?

A 111

Figure 1 is a sonogram of the lower abdomen. A circular mass of 2.3-cm diameter and of mean echogenicity is identified, interspersed with hypoechoic areas.

As seen in the color-coded Doppler sonogram (Fig. 2), the structure has a central vessel, branching into several smaller vessels.

The double contrast study of the colon (Fig. 3) demonstrates a round mass in the descending part of the sigmoid (*arrow*).

The diagnosis is juvenile polyp of the sigmoid.

Juvenile polyps are the most common cause of rectal bleeding in children above the age of 1 year. In this age, they are the most common polypoid lesion of the colon. They are usually relatively large.

Clinically, the children present with mild, asymptomatic perianal bleeding. Profuse bleeding, however, has repeatedly been reported. Some children also have diarrhea, in others the polyp prolapses.

The origin and the natural history are unknown. Earlier it was believed that they were solitary. Colonoscopy has demonstrated, however, that more than half of the patients have additional polyps further up.

There seems to be a potential risk of developing carcinoma because of the presence of adenomatous changes in some juvenile polyps, warranting colonoscopic removal.

The patient presented here is a typical case. The mean presenting age of juvenile polyps is around 6 years, and boys are mostly affected.

It has been found that roughly 50% of the polyps are in the rectosigmoid, 15% in the descending colon, and another 30% near the splenic flexure. Overall, proximal polyps were seen in 37% of pancolonoscopies. The conclusion of these observations was that although most juvenile polyps are located in the left colon, a pancolonoscopy should be the initial procedure because: (a) 37% of pancolonoscopies revealed proximal polyps, (b) 32% of polyps were located proximal to the splenic flexure, (c) persistence of symptoms from missed proximal polyp(s) necessitates a repeat study with attendant risks, and (d) there is a possibility of malignant transformation in an unidentified juvenile polyp.

Suggested Reading

1. Gupta SK, Fitzgerald JF, Croffie JM, Chong SK, Pfefferkorn MC, Davis MM, Faught PR. Experience with juvenile polyps in North American children: the need for pancolonoscopy. Am J Gastroenterol 2001; 96:1696–1697
2. Katz AL. Juvenile polyps and poyposis syndromes. In: Surgery of Infants and Children: Scientific principles and practice. Keith T. Oldham, Paul M. Colombani, and Robert P. Foglia (eds). Lippincott-Raven Publishers, Philadelphia, p 1313–1314, 1997
3. Pratap A, Tiwari A, Sinha AK, Kumar A, Khaniya S, Agarwal RK, Shakya VC. Nonfamilial juvenile polyposis coli manifesting as massive lower gastrointestinal hemorrhage: report of two cases. Surg Today 2007; 37:46–49
4. Ukarapol N, Singhavejakul J, Lertprasertsuk N, Wongsawasdi L. Juvenile polyp in Thai children-clinical and colonoscopic presentation. World J Surg 31 2007; 395–398

Q 112

Felix Schier

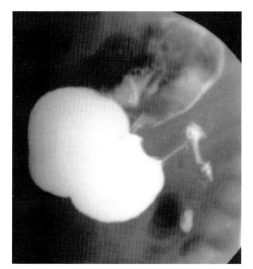

Fig. 2

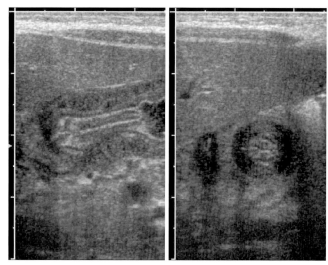

Fig. 3

A 5-week-old boy presented with projectile vomiting that had set in from one day to another. An "olive" could not be palpated.

Laboratory values showed hypochloremia and alkalosis.

Imaging studies yielded the findings shown in Figs. 2 and 3.

- What is the most likely diagnosis?

A 112

Figure 1 serves only for comparison. It is a normal, longitudinal sonogram of the pylorus and the bulbus duodeni.

To the extreme right the antrum is seen, entering into the pyloric channel. All five layers of the intestinal wall are easily distinguishable: mucosa, muscularis mucosae, submucosa, and muscularis propria including the serosa. This is a normal picture.

Figure 2 shows an abnormal sonogram. The plane is almost identical to Fig. 1. The pyloric channel is markedly elongated. The sphincter musculature is thickened, hypoechoic, and less structured. The pyloric region is enlarged to 14 mm. On the right, a transsection of the stenotic and "multiluminal" channel is seen.

Figure 3 is a gastric contrast study and shows the characteristic "string sign." The pyloric channel is highly stenosed and markedly elongated. The gastric antrum is impressed by the hypertrophic pyloric musculature. The diagnosis is pyloric hypertrophy.

Years ago, the diagnosis of pyloric hypertrophy was established by palpating the enlarged muscle as an "olive." The advent of ultrasonography has replaced palpation. However, surgeons have never trusted palpation of an olive more than ultrasonography. It has been shown that introducing a guideline to require palpation by a surgeon first and ultrasonographic imaging second did not reduce the total amount of ultrasonography. The final diagnosis is eventually based on ultrasonography exclusively.

Radiologists have established criteria for the ultrasonographic diagnosis of hypertrophic pyloric stenosis: A pyloric canal length of 18–20 mm (normal 11 mm), a diameter of 13–14 mm, and a muscle thickness of 4–5 mm (normal <2 mm) have been stated to be diagnostic for hypertrophic pyloric stenosis; 4.8 ± 0.6 mm, muscle length 2.1 ± 0.3 cm, and channel length 1.8 ± 0.3 cm were measured in this case. Thickness of the pyloric muscle is the most discriminating and accurate criterion for hypertrophic pyloric stenosis.

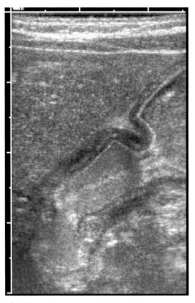

Fig. 1

As in a number of pediatric surgical diseases, the etiology of pyloric hypertrophy is still unknown. Numerous theories are still being proposed. If some day the etiology is identified, the role of surgery, namely, a destructive intervention, will consequently be revisited.

Today, the role of laparoscopic surgery in hypertrophic pyloric stenosis is not yet well established. The conventional, open approach has passed the test of time and naturally has fewer complications. It has been stated that it also has a higher efficacy. On the other hand, recovery time appears to be shorter following the laparoscopic approach.

An indication that surgeons no longer feel comfortable with the conventional transverse upper abdomen incision is the fact that, in addition, a transumbilical approach has been introduced, for cosmetic reasons.

Q 113

Giuseppe Ascione

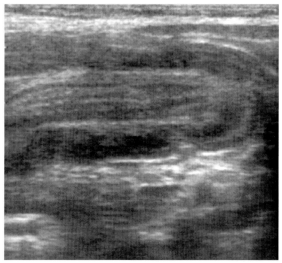

Fig. 1

A 7-month-old infant presented with vomiting, abdominal pain, and lethargy. The parents reported an attack of intermittent abdominal pain on the previous day.

On physical examination, the child was chubby and in good health. Because of abdominal distension, no abdominal mass was palpable. An examining finger passed into the anus revealed blood in the stools.

- What does the examination in Fig. 1 show?
- What is the most likely diagnosis?
- What is the best treatment?

A 113

Figure 1 is an abdominal ultrasonography scan and it reveals the classic target sign.

The diagnosis is idiopathic intussusception (in older patients intussusception can be associated with others medical conditions such as Henoch–Schönlein purpura, hemophilia, Peutz–Jeghers syndrome, cystic fibrosis etc.).

Ultrasonography and barium enema are the imaging studies to be conducted for confirmation of the diagnosis.

The barium enema (Fig. 2) shows intussusception in the ascending colon.

The treatment of intestinal intussusception is hydrostatic reduction or surgical reduction that can be performed via an open or laparoscopic approach.

Hydrostatic reduction (air insufflation or barium or water-soluble contrast) is conditioned by the patient's age, duration of symptoms, and presence of lead points.

The recommended pressure of air insufflation for therapeutic enema should not exceed 120 cm of H_2O. Operative reduction (Fig. 3) is indicated if hydrostatic reduction is unsuccessful or if perforation exists.

Suggested Reading

1. Di Fiore JW. Intussusception: Semin Pediatr Surg 1999 Nov; 8 (4):214–220
2. Eklof OA, Johanson L, Lohr G. Childhood intussusception: hydrostatic reducibility and incidence of leading points in different age groups. Pediatr Radiol 1980 Nov; 10(2):83–86
3. Kirks DR. Air intussusception reduction: "the wind of change" Pediatr Radiol 1995; 25(2)89–91

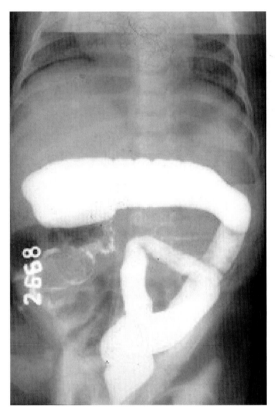

Fig. 2

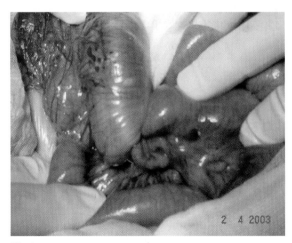

Fig. 3

Q 114

Giuseppe Ascione

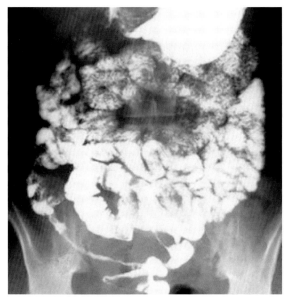

Fig. 1

A 9-year-old boy had a history of fatigue, anorexia, abdominal pain, diarrhea, and weight loss.

Several types of medical therapies did not improve the symptoms. The boy presented to the emergency department after a severe episode of rectal bleeding and abdominal distension.

The patient had a recent appendectomy scar; in the right lower quadrant there was a palpable abdominal mass.

There was bilateral joint swelling at the knees. Examination of the anus was normal.

Laboratory values revealed an iron-deficiency anemia, an erythrocyte sedimentation rate of 50 mm in 1 h, and a low concentration of serum albumin.

An upper gastrointestinal series is shown in Fig. 1.
- What does Fig. 1 show?
- What pathological condition is affecting this child?
- How do you confirm the diagnosis in this case?
- What medical or surgical option is better for resolving this problem?

A 114

The barium meal shown in Fig. 1 demonstrates a "string sign" leading to obstruction.

This child has a Crohn's disease with terminal ileum involvement.

Endoscopy (Fig. 2) with biopsies of the mucosa (Fig. 3) confirm the diagnosis.

Figure 3 is a histologic specimen showing a granuloma.

Fibroendoscopy is quite accurate when ileocolic or colonic Crohn's disease is present.

Other noninvasive tests are sucralfate scan to detect the presence of active disease and radio-labeled leukocyte scan to determine progressive disease.

Remission can be achieved by dietary manipulations (elemental or semielemental diet) or intestinal rest.

If symptoms are severe, the mainstay therapy is steroids (5 mg. m^2). In intractable disease with steroids, 5-ASA preparations and immunosuppressants such as azathioprine, methotrexate, and cyclosporin A have been used.

Indications for surgery are:
a) In emergency, massive hemorrhage, perforation or intestinal obstruction
b) Growth and sexual development failure
c) Fistulas or persistent inflammatory mass
d) Perianal lesions that may precede intestinal problems

Complete eradication is unnecessary because of the multifocality of the disease (risk of short bowel syndrome). In all, 85% of children with Crohn's disease will have had surgery within 15 years after presentation of the disease.

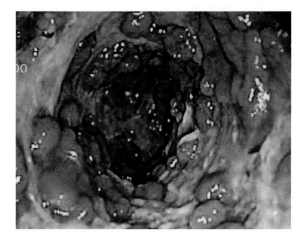

Fig. 2

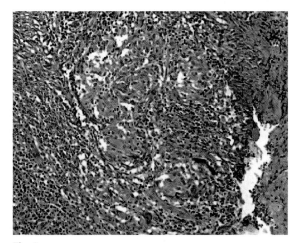

Fig. 3

Suggested Reading

1. Ruemmele FM, Roy CC. Nutrition as primary therapy in pediatric Crohn disease: fact or fantasy? J Pediatr 2000 Mar; 136(3):285–91
2. Sawczenco A, Sandu BK. Presenting features of inflammatory bowel disease. Arch Dis Child Nov 88(11):995–1000
3. Zholudef A, Zurakoswsky D. Serologic testing with ANCA, ASCA and anti-Ompc In children. Am J Gastroenterol 2004 Nov 99(11):2235–41

Q 115

Craig T. Albanese

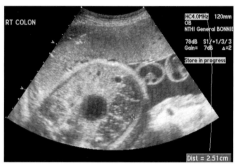

Fig. 1

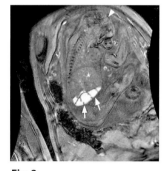

Fig. 2

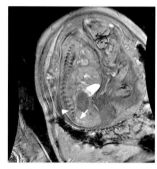

Fig. 3

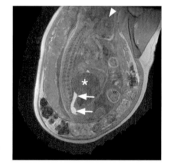

Fig. 4

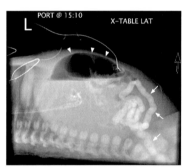

Fig. 5

A routine screening ultrasound at 22 weeks' gestation was obtained. An ultrasound of the fetal abdomen revealed a dilated portion of bowel, most likely of the proximal colon (Fig. 1, calipers).

- What is the differential diagnosis?

Prenatal MR imaging (Fig. 2) was performed, which also suggested an obstruction of the proximal colon (*arrows*). The liver (*asterisk*), fetal head (*arrowhead*), and the more distal microcolon (Fig. 3, *arrow*) can be seen. For comparison, Fig. 4 shows the spine (*arrowhead*), liver (*asterisk*), normal fetal colon (*arrows*), bladder (*asterisk*), and fetal head (*arrowhead*).

The baby was uneventfully delivered at term. Polyhydramnios was never present.

A postnatal contrast enema was performed (Fig. 5).

- What are the findings and what is your diagnosis?

A 115

There is a dilated, meconium-filled segment of bowel. It appears to be the proximal colon, although the distal ileum cannot be ruled out.

The differential diagnosis is colon atresia, ileal atresia, and meconium ileus.

The MR image shows meconium (bright signal) in the dilated right colon with virtually no fluid/meconium entering a small distal colon.

The postnatal contrast enema demonstrates a microcolon (*arrows*) and obstruction of the dilated proximal colon (*arrowheads;* stomach, *asterisk*). This is most consistent with a right colon atresia. A type IIIb atresia was noted at operation. This accounts for less than 1% of all intestinal atresias. Intestinal continuity was established and the baby recovered uneventfully.

Suggested Reading

1. Blair GK, Jamieson DH. Colon atresia—type III. J Pediatr Surg 2001 Mar; 36(3):530–1
2. Etensel B, Temir G, Karkiner A, Melek M, Edirne Y, Karaca I, Mir E. Atresia of the colon. J Pediatr Surg 2005 Aug; 40(8):1258–68
3. Karnak I, Ciftci AO, Senocak ME, Tanyel FC, Buyukpamukcu N. Colonic atresia: surgical management and outcome. Pediatr Surg Int 2001 Nov; 17(8):631–5

Q 116

Francois Becmeur

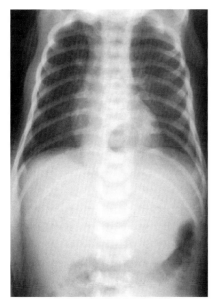

Fig. 1

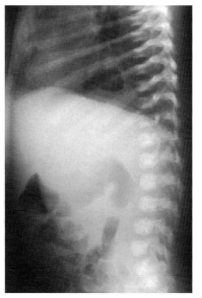

Fig. 2

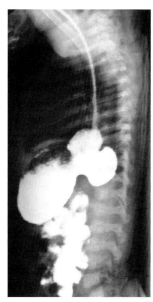

Fig. 4

The patient in this case was born at full term weighing 3,550 g. The mother consulted the pediatric emergency department when the infant was 13 days old because of tears, weight loss, and frequent regurgitations. On admission, the infant weighed 3,200 g, he had a temperature of 37°C, and seemed well. The clinical examination did not show any possible anomalies.

Plain radiographs of the abdomen and thorax were acquired in two planes: anteroposterior and lateral (Figs. 1, 2).

• Can you comment on the radiographs?

An esophagogastroduodenal transit study was requested, which is shown in Figs. 3 and 4.
• What do you make of this study?
• What is your diagnosis and what are the possible treatments?

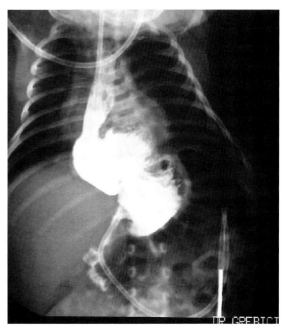

Fig. 3

A 116

An air bubble in the base of the thorax is seen on the radiographs, evoking the presence of part of the stomach in the posterior mediastinum.

It is a large right hernia which does not allow enteral feeding (Figs. 3, 4).

Postural treatment may be attempted, with the child in vertical position and placement of a nasogastric probe. The hernia can thus be reduced gradually while the child grows in weight. In this case, as often occurs in this situation, this medical treatment failed. We decided to perform a laparoscopy to reduce the hernia, to close the diaphragmatic opening, and to create an antireflux gastroesophageal valve (Nissen–Rossetti type of fundoplication). The postoperative course was uneventful and at 3 years the child was perfectly normal.

Suggested Reading

1. Fasching G, Huber A, Uray E, Sorantin E, Lindbichler F, Mayr J. Gastroesophageal reflux and diaphragmatic motility after repair of congenital diaphragmatic hernia. Eur J Pediatr Surg 2000 Dec; 10(6):360–4

2. Gorenstein A, Cohen AJ, Cordova Z, Witzling M, Krutman B, Serour F. Hiatal hernia in pediatric gastroesophageal reflux. J Pediatr Gastroenterol Nutr 2001 Nov; 33(5):554–7

3. Mayr J, Sauer H, Huber A, Pilhatsch A, Ratschek M. Modified Toupet wrap for gastroesophageal reflux in childhood. Eur J Pediatr Surg 1998 Apr; 8(2):75–80

4. Samujh R, Kumar D, Rao KL. Paraesophageal hernia in the neonatal period: suspicion on chest X-ray. Indian Pediatr 2004 Feb; 41(2):189–91

Q 117

Ciro Esposito and Giovanni Esposito

An 8-year-old boy had undergone surgery at the age of 2 years for subocclusive abdominal pains that were thought to be due to a defect of fixation and rotation of the midgut; the surgery was complicated by a postoperative occlusion due to adherence that required another operation.

Since that time the child had not fed correctly with scarce growth and he had recurrent episodes of upper abdominal distension. At 7 years of age, vomiting appeared. Therefore, the child was taken to hospital where a plain abdominal radiograph was acquired, followed by a contrast meal. After these studies, he was transferred to our department for surgery. On physical examination the child had a distended and tympanic abdomen, overall in the epigastrium and left hypochondrium. Before surgery, other examinations were performed.

- What does the contrast meal show (Fig. 1)?
- Which other examinations should be performed?
- What is the diagnosis?
- What was the treatment?
- What was the follow-up?

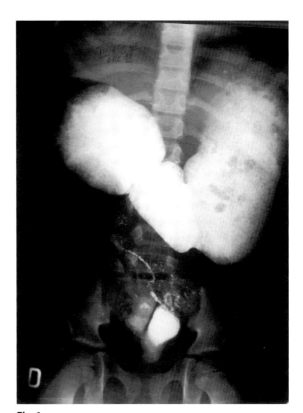

Fig. 1

A 117

The abdominal radiograph shows the presence of a double bubble, due to a dilated, gas-filled stomach and duodenum. The contrast meal (Fig. 1) reveals a large dilatation of the first part of the duodenum.

Gastroduodenoscopy was performed revealing a stenosis in the second part of the duodenum due to the diaphragm with a very small hole.

The delayed diagnosis is a diaphragmatic duodenal stenosis.

The operation consisted in a duodenotomy and a complete web excision, coupled with a tapering duodenoplasty. Postoperative nasogastric decompression with a tube is necessary. Postoperative imaging through the nasogastric tube showed a regular gastroduodenal transit (Fig. 2).

The postoperative course was uneventful and hospitalization lasted 10 days. At the 5-year follow-up, the child was growing well without any intestinal problems.

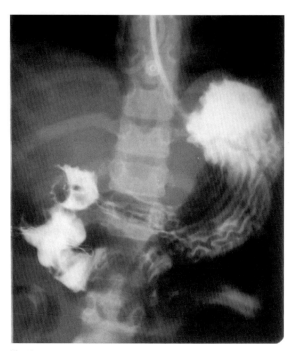

Fig. 2

Suggested Reading

1. Diamond IR, Hayes-Jordan A, Chait P, Temple M, Kim PC. A novel treatment of congenital duodenal stenosis: image-guided treatment of congenital and acquired bowel strictures in children. J Laparoendosc Adv Surg Tech A 2006 Jun; 16(3):317–20
2. Escobar MA, Ladd AP, Grosfeld JL, West KW, Rescorla FJ, Scherer LR 3rd, Engum SA, Rouse TM, Billmire DF. Duodenal atresia and stenosis: long-term follow-up over 30 years. J Pediatr Surg 2004 Jun; 39(6):867–71
3. McCollum MO, Jamieson DH, Webber EM. Annular pancreas and duodenal stenosis. J Pediatr Surg 2002 Dec; 37(12):1776–7
4. van Rijn RR, van Lienden KP, Fortuna TL, D'Alessandro LC, Connolly B, Chait PG. Membranous duodenal stenosis: initial experience with balloon dilatation in four children. Eur J Radiol 2006 Jul; 59(1):29–32

Q 118

Alessandro Settimi and Ciro Esposito

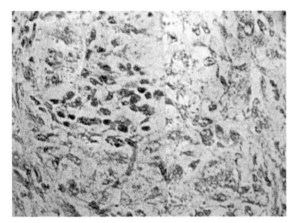

Fig. 1

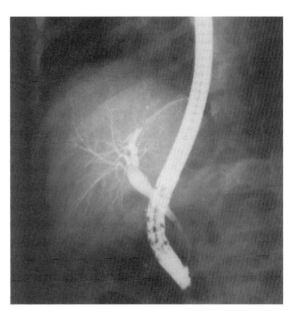

Fig. 2

A 5-year-old girl, born at term after an uncomplicated pregnancy and delivery, had developed normally without any disease until the age of 5 months, when, during hospitalization for gastroenteritis with episodes of biliary vomiting, high levels of transaminases were found. After discharge, the hypertransaminasemia persisted and the child was hospitalized again. A hepatic biopsy was performed that showed mild inflammatory fibrosis of the liver (Fig. 1). The child was transferred to a gastroenterology department where US, photoscintigraphy with 99mTc-dimethyl-iminodiacetic acid scintigraphy (HIDA), and intravenous cholangiography were performed, which revealed nonvisualization of the gallbladder with a dilatation of the choledochus and a slow elimination of the HIDA.

In order to define the disease and to establish a therapeutic plan, the child was sent to our surgical department. On admission, the physical examination revealed no pathology except for a mild increase in the size of the liver, which was palpated at 1 cm to the costal margin with a normal surface. Laboratory test results were normal except for glutamyl oxaloacetic transaminase (GOT) and glutamyl pyruvic transaminase (GPT) levels with values of 134 U/l and 394 U/l, respectively. Endoscopic retrograde cholangiopancreatography (ERCP) was scheduled to define the exact diagnosis and to provide a therapeutic indication (Fig. 2).

- What does Fig. 1 show?
- What was the diagnosis?
- What was the therapeutic indication?
- What was the follow-up?

A 118

On the ERCP scan, the papilla of Vater was found in a normal localization but it was difficult to cannulate.

Injection of radiopaque contrast medium into the papilla demonstrated a duplication of the hepatic left duct, absence of the gallbladder, and hypoplasia of the distal choledochus with dilatation of its proximal portion (Fig. 2).

The diagnosis is a complex congenital malformation of the biliary tree, consisting in anomaly of the biliary tract, agenesis of the gallbladder, and hypoplasia of the distal choledochus.

The therapeutic indication is a biliodigestive diversion, which the child's parents refused.

Follow-up until the age of 7 years did not show any aggravation of the disease. Subsequently, the child was lost to follow-up.

Suggested Reading

1. Kabiri H, Domingo OH, Tzarnas CD. Agenesis of the gallbladder. Curr Surg 2006 Mar–Apr; 63(2):104–6
2. Peloponissios N, Gillet M, Cavin R, Halkic N. Agenesis of the gallbladder: a dangerously misdiagnosed malformation. World J Gastroenterol 2005 Oct 21; 11(39):6228–31
3. Wazz G, Branicki F, Chishti I, Taji H. Role of intraoperative cholangiography in detecting rare bile duct anomalies. JSLS 2002 Oct–Dec; 6(4):393–5s
4. Okada T, Sasaki F, Honda S, Naitou S, Onodera Y, Todo S. sefulness of axial planes of helical computed tomography for diagnosis of pancreaticobiliary maljunction in early infants with negative findings on magnetic resonance cholangiopancreatography. Pediatr Surg 2008 Mar;43(3):579-82.
5. Fitoz S, Erden A, Boruban S. Magnetic resonance cholangiopancreatography of biliary system abnormalities in children. Clin Imaging. 2007 Mar-Apr;31(2):93-101.
6. Ishida M, Egawa S, Takahashi Y, Kohari M, Ohwada Y, Unno M. Gallbladder agenesis with a stone in the cystic duct bud. J Hepatobiliary Pancreat Surg. 2008;15(2):220-3.

Q 119

Giovanni Esposito and Ciro Esposito

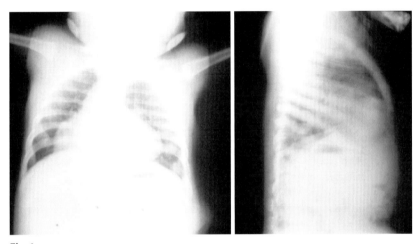

Fig. 1

A 3-year-old child without any previous serious disease came to our attention because of the incidental detection of a thoracic opacity. On admission, physical examination of the child did not reveal any anomaly. After other examinations, surgery was scheduled.

- What does Fig. 1 show?
- Which other examinations were performed and what were their results?
- What was the diagnostic suspicion?
- What was found during the intervention and what was the treatment?
- What was the definitive diagnosis?
- What was the follow-up?

A 119

The radiograph of the thorax (Fig. 1) shows the presence of an opacity the size of a small mandarin in the right phrenopericardial angle.

CT was performed (Fig. 2) that demonstrated the presence of a round mass occupying the left phrenopericardial angle. The diagnostic suspicion was a pericardial cyst.

At operation, a Morgagni–Larrey hernia with hepatic contents (Fig. 3) was found.

After incision of the hernial sac, the liver was replaced in the abdomen, the sac was excised, and the margins of the Morgagni–Larrey hole were sutured.

The postoperative course was uneventful and at 2 years' follow-up the child is doing well.

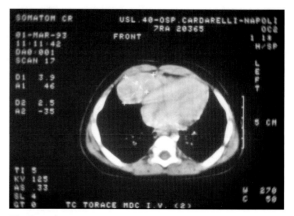

Fig. 2

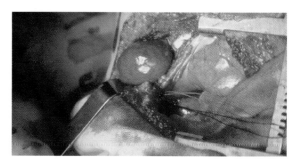

Fig. 3

Suggested Reading

1. Laparoscopic treatment of Morgagni-Larrey hernia: technical details and report of a series. J Laparoendosc Adv Surg Tech A 2005 Jun; 15(3):303–7
2. Huttl TP, Meyer G, Geiger TK, Schildberg FW. Indications, techniques and results of laparoscopic surgery for diaphragmatic diseases. Surg Tod 2002 Jul; 127(7):598–603
3. Ipek T, Altinli E, Yuceyar S, Erturk S, Eyuboglu E, Akcal T. Laparoscopic repair of a Morgagni-Larrey hernia: report of three cases. Surg Today 2002; 32(10):902–5
4. Lima M, Lauro V, Domini M, Libri M, Bertozzi M, Pigna A, Domini R. Laparoscopic surgery of diaphragmatic diseases in children: our experience with five cases. Eur J Pediatr Surg 2001 Dec; 11(6):377–81
5. Ridai M, Boubia S, Kafih M, Zerouali ON. Morgagni-Larrey hernias treated by laparoscopy. Presse Med 2002 Sep 14; 31(29):1364–5

Q 120

Ciro Esposito and Giovanni Esposito

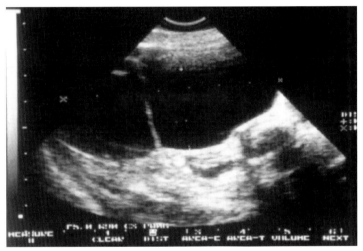

Fig. 1

A 10-year-old girl without any significant disease presented with abdominal colic accompanied by bile-stained vomiting.

On physical examination, a mobile, aching mass was revealed in the upper region of her abdomen.

US was performed (Fig. 1), which confirmed the presence of the mass. Other procedures were subsequently required to make a precise diagnosis and establish the treatment.

- What did the US show?
- Which other procedures were performed and what was their result?
- What was the diagnosis?
- What was the treatment?
- What was the follow-up?

A 120

The US (Fig. 1) image shows a large cystic mass that is surrounded by some dilated intestinal loops.

To define its nature, laparoscopy was performed that revealed an intestinal lymphangioma.

Laparotomy was subsequently performed.

The diagnosis was confirmed.

The treatment consisted in the simple excision of the lymphangioma (Fig. 3).

The postoperative course was uneventful and the girl was discharged 7 days after the intervention. At the 1-year follow-up, she was doing well.

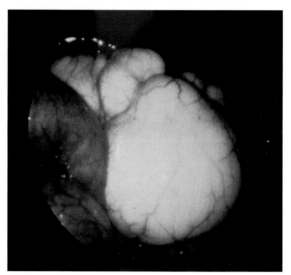

Fig. 2

Suggested Reading

1. Menon P, Rao KL, Vaiphei K. Isolated enteric duplication cysts. J Pediatr Surg 2004 Aug; 39(8):67–69
2. Morgan K, Ricketts RR. Lymphangioma of the falciform ligament—a case report. J Pediatr Surg 2004 Aug; 39(8):1276–9
3. Ng WT. Mesenteric lymphangioma infected with non-typhoidal Salmonella: the first case. Pediatr Surg Int 2005 Jun; 21(6):504–5. Epub 2005 May 19
4. Ratan SK, Ratan KN, Kapoor S, Sehgal T. Giant chylolymphatic cyst of the jejunal mesentry in a child: report of a case. Surg Today 2003; 33(2):120–2
5. Takeuchi K, Takaya Y, Maeda K, Maruo T. Peritonitis caused by a ruptured, infected mesenteric cyst initially interpreted as an ovarian cyst. A case report. J Reprod Med 2004 Jan; 49(1):65–7

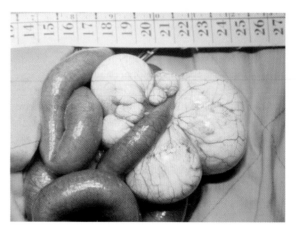

Fig. 3

Q 121

Vincenzo Di Benedetto and Ciro Esposito

A neonate, born at 34°weeks' gestation because of maternal gestosis, and delivered by cesarean section, at birth presented with respiratory distress with intense dyspnea and ingravescent cyanosis that required immediate respiratory assistance with intubation and a ventilator at high frequencies and low pressures. After acquiring a standard thoraco-abdominal radiograph, an intervention was scheduled. This was performed after stabilization of the infant's respiratory function and normalization of laboratory values, which were considerably altered, showing hypoxia and acidosis.

- What does Fig. 1 show?
- What was the diagnosis?
- When was the intervention performed?
- What was found during the intervention?
- What was the follow-up?

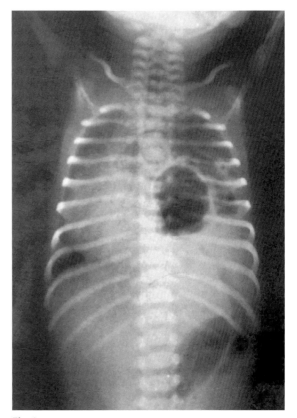

Fig. 1

A 121

The radiograph shows the presence of a large gaseous area inferiorly and medially in the left hemithorax and the presence of other translucent areas laterally, with a complete shift of the mediastinum and dextrocardia.

The diagnosis was of congenital diaphragmatic hernia (Bochdalek hernia) with transposition of the stomach and of some intestinal loops in the thorax.

Two days after birth, once stabilization of the respiratory function was obtained and the oxygenation and acid-base balance were normalized, the neonate was operated on.

The intervention consisted in a subcostal left laparotomy that showed a large posterior diaphragmatic defect through which the stomach and left colon were migrated in the thorax (Fig. 2). After repositioning these organs in the abdomen, the diaphragmatic defect was closed with interrupted sutures, without leaving a drain in the thorax according to the suggestions of Cloutier.

After a radiographic check-up of the chest 8 days after operation, which was normal with a good expansion of the lung, the neonate was discharged on the 10th postoperative day. After 1 year, the child was in good condition.

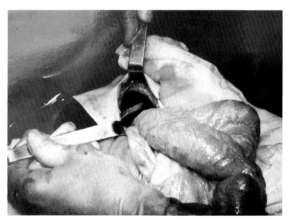

Fig. 2

Suggested Reading

1. Crankson SJ, Al Jadaan SA, Namshan MA, Al-Rabeeah AA, Oda O. The immediate and long-term outcomes of newborns with congenital diaphragmatic hernia. Pediatr Surg Int 2006 Apr; 22(4):335–40

2. Kamata S, Usui N, Kamiyama M, Tazuke Y, Nose K, Sawai T, Fukuzawa M. Long-term follow-up of patients with high-risk congenital diaphragmatic hernia. J Pediatr Surg 2005 Dec; 40(12):1833–8

3. Koumbourlis AC, Wung JT, Stolar CJ. Lung function in infants after repair of congenital diaphragmatic hernia. J Pediatr Surg 2006 Oct; 41(10):1716–21

4. Luis AL, Avila LF, Encinas JL, Andres AM, Suarez O, Elorza D, Rodriguez I, Martinez L, Murcia J, Lassaletta L, Tovar JA. Results of the treatment of congenital diaphragmatic hernia with conventional therapeutics modalities. Cir Pediatr 2006 Jul; 19(3):167–72

5. Rygl M, Pycha K, Stranak Z, Melichar J, Krofta L, Tomasek L, Snajdauf J. Congenital diaphragmatic hernia: onset of respiratory distress and size of the defect: Analysis of the outcome in 104 neonates. Pediatr Surg Int 2007 Jan; 23(1):27–31

Q 122

Francois Becmeur

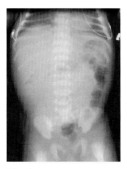 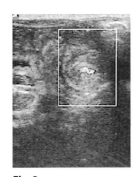 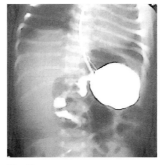 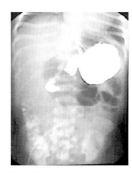

Fig. 1 **Fig. 2** **Fig. 3** **Fig. 4**

A 6-month-old infant, born at 37 weeks and weighing 3,090 g, presented with greenish vomiting, diarrhea, refusal of bottle-feeding, no tears, and no painful crises, which had started when he was 2 months old. These episodes appeared regularly.

- What are the plausible diagnoses?

The pediatrician diagnosed an allergy to cow's milk proteins, and thus performed the Diallertest® (patch test), which was positive. A dietetic treatment was started, substituting the usual milk by Peptijunior®. The greenish vomiting continued and the doctor suggested complementary examinations. An abdominal ultrasound was performed to search for an obstruction. The radiologist was satisfied with the sonogram of the cardia and did not perform supplementary examinations or radiography of the abdomen, although the symptoms had been persisting for 1 month.

A diagnosis of gastroesophageal reflux (GER) was made.

- Which treatment would you have proposed for the GER?

The medical therapy was with anti-acid drugs and a stimulant of intestinal motility.

However, the symptoms continued, and the child vomited all the time, although the amount of procinetic was increased. Moreover, abdominal pain appeared, with increasingly long crises until the pain became continuous.

The baby was taken to hospital again. On clinical examination, a flexible, distended, and swollen abdomen was found with no signs of defense.

- Which diagnoses do you eliminate and which do you consider further?
- How did the doctor in the emergency department proceed?
- Which examinations were requested?

A plain anteroposterior abdominal radiograph and an ultrasound scan were acquired (Figs. 1, 2). Subsequently an esophagogastric-duodenal transit was carried out (Figs. 3, 4)

- What do you observe?
- Which treatment do you propose?

A few hours after treatment, abdominal meteorism and pain appeared.

- What went wrong?

A 122

The GER is due to bad gastroduodenal voiding. Any bile-stained vomiting should suggest an occlusion caused by a vaterian obstruction (bulb of Vater: bile duct).

Volvulus around the base of the narrow midgut common mesentery can provoke recurrent episodes of subacute intestinal obstruction.

Laparoscopic surgery is the right treatment. The last radiograph showed a gastric probe not in place: it is at the bottom of the esophagus. It is enough to descend it in the stomach.

Suggested Reading

1. Boyle JT. Gastroesophageal reflux disease in 2006: The imperfect diagnosis. Pediatr Radiol 2006 Sep; 36(Supplement 14):192–195
2. Gold BD. Review article: epidemiology and management of gastro-oesophageal reflux in children. Aliment Pharmacol Ther 2004 Feb; 19 Suppl 1:22–7
3. Ida S. Evaluation and treatment of gastroesophageal reflux in infants and children. Nippon Rinsho 2004 Aug; 62(8):1553–8
4. Ostlie DJ, Holcomb GW 3rd. Laparoscopic fundoplication and gastrostomy. Semin Pediatr Surg 2002 Nov; 11(4):196–204
5. Suwandhi E, Ton MN, Schwarz SM. Gastroesophageal reflux in infancy and childhood. Pediatr Ann 2006 Apr; 35(4):259–66

4

Genitourinary Disorders

Introduction

Clinical history and physical examination represent an important aspect in the management of infants and children with urological diseases.

However, the role of instrumental and in particular of radiological examinations is fundamental for making a certain and correct diagnosis in all clinical cases.

In the last 20 years, there has been a considerable improvement in the diagnosis of children with urological problems. The most important reason for this is the advent of ultrasonography as a prenatal and postnatal screening tool.

Nowadays, this examination allows a complete and accurate study of the upper urinary tract.

Obviously, a good knowledge of the most common congenital urinary malformations is essential for the correct interpretation of the ultrasonographic findings.

Two other examinations that are frequently adopted to confirm the diagnosis are voiding cystography and isotopic renography.

Ultrasound, voiding cystography, and renal scanning together allow one to study the majority of obstructive congenital uropathies in pediatric patients.

Urography on its own is rarely performed on children, even if it is indicated in some cases of obstructive uropathies to obtain more anatomo-functional data.

MR imaging and MR urography require anesthesia in the pediatric age and they are mainly adopted to study renal masses or in cases of ureteral duplications with a nonfunctioning upper or lower renal pole.

Urodynamic studies always complete the diagnostic work-up in patients with neurological or functional vesical dysfunctions.

Obviously, the diagnostic work-up can change case per case and it is related to the clinical experience of the pediatric urologist and is generally focused on obtaining a correct diagnosis, avoiding certain invasive diagnostic examinations without benefit to the child.

The therapeutic procedures described in the clinical cases presented in this section are: endoscopic, laparoscopic, video-assisted, and open surgical techniques. Frequently, these procedures are complementary, allowing resolution of the majority of cases with very good results and guarantying young patients not only resolution of their disease but a good quality of life too.

Q 123

Jean Stephane Valla

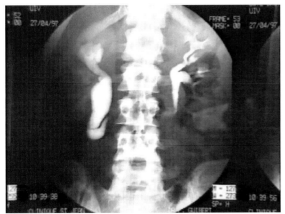

Fig. 1

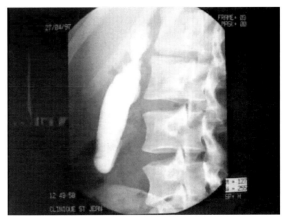

Fig. 2

A 14-year-old boy presented with a 1-year history of intermittent right flank pain radiating from the loin to the groin. He had also had two episodes of hematuria. The physical examination was normal.

Ultrasonography showed mild dilatation of the upper urinary tract on the right side. Excretory urography was performed.

- What do Figs. 1 and 2 show?
- What pathological condition is affecting this adolescent?
- Which other diagnostic examinations are necessary in this case?
- How do you manage this condition?

A 123

The IV urogram shows a right-sided hydronephrosis and dilatation of the proximal ureter up to the level of the transverse process of L3 (Fig. 1, frontal view; Fig. 2, lateral view). In addition there is a medial deviation of the ureter at this level, usually described as an "S" or "fish hook" deformity at the point of obstruction.

This adolescent has a retrocaval ureter. Retrocaval (circumcaval) ureter is an uncommon anomaly. It originates form a developmental error in the formation of the vena cava and not of the ureter; this can cause varying degrees of ureteral obstruction. Retrocaval ureter should be suspected in any case of pyelectasis and ureterectasis of the upper third ureter on the right side.

In order to reduce irradiation, the MAG-3 scan (technetium-99m mercaptoacetyltriglycine) is likely to replace IV urography, CT, and diuretic renography. This examination allows one to confirm the diagnosis, to underline other associated malformations, and to assess the function of the right kidney.

Surgical repair is indicated only when symptoms develop or functionally significant obstruction exists. In our opinion, minimally invasive repair, by a trans- or retroperitoneal approach, should be considered before open surgery, provided the surgeon is comfortable with advanced laparoscopic techniques. During the procedure the patency of the ureter must be verified to determine whether it is necessary or not to excise the retrocaval segment and to avoid any residual ureteral stenosis.

Figure 3 is an intraoperative uretero-pyelograph. In Fig. 4, the intraoperative view is shown (retroperitoneoscopic approach) after dissection. Figure 5 shows the final result after division of the pelvis, uncrossing of the ureter, and ureteropelvic reanastomosis.

Suggested Reading

1. Simforoosh N et al. Laparoscopic pyelostomy for retrocaval ureter without excision of the retrocaval segment: first report of 6 cases. J Urol Vol 175 2006; p 2166–2169
2. Uthappa MC et al. Retrocaval ureter: MR appearances. Br J Radiol 2002; Vol 75 p 177–179

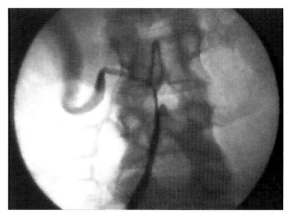

Fig. 3

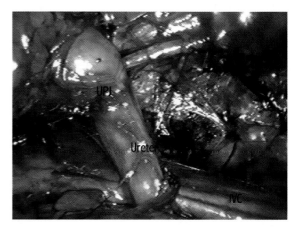

Fig. 4

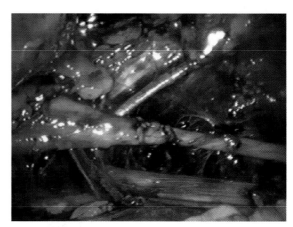

Fig. 5

Q 124

Jean Stephane Valla

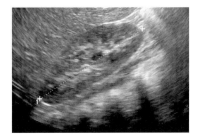

Fig. 1

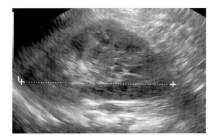

Fig. 2

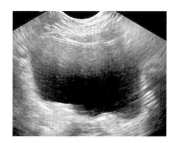

Fig. 3

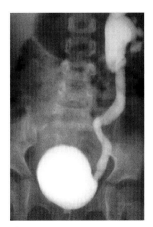

Fig. 4

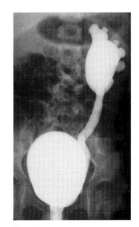

Fig. 5

A 4-year-old girl presented with a recurrent upper urinary tract infection with fever up to 40°C, irritability, and left flank pain. The antenatal ultrasound examination of her kidney was normal. She had been hospitalized 6 months earlier for 1 week because of an initial episode of pyelonephritis due to *Escherichia coli*. At that time, ultrasonography (Figs. 1–3) and retrograde cystography (Figs. 4, 5) were performed; the girl was discharged with continuous antibiotic prophylaxis.

- How would you interpret the radiographic studies in Figs. 1–5?
- Which other examinations are needed in this case?
- On the basis of which arguments could you distinguish a primary vesicoureteral reflux (VUR), referred to as a congenitally deficient ureterovesical junction, from a secondary VUR due to bladder or sphincter disease?
- How do you manage this case?

A 124

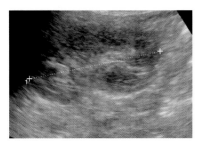

Fig. 6

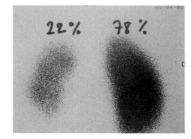

Fig. 7

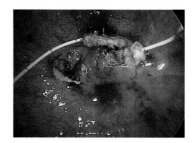

Fig. 8

The first ultrasonography was judged as normal: normal echostructure and renal growth (Fig. 1, right kidney: 71 mm; Fig. 2, left kidney: 75 mm) no visible ureter, normal bladder (Fig. 3, capacity, thickness). The retrograde cystogram confirmed a normal bladder and unilateral left high-grade reflux (Figs. 4, 5). Follow-up with antibiotic prophylaxis was appropriate at that time.

The present recurrent pyelonephritis needs rapid intravenous antibiotherapy for at least 10 days after collection of urine samples for bacteria identification (*E. coli*) and blood samples for infection and renal function evaluation. A more complete investigation is then necessary.

A careful history and physical examination revealed: no voiding symptom, no incontinence, no constipation, normal neuro-urological test results.

A new renal ultrasound found asymmetric renal growth (left side 66 mm, right side 75 mm; Fig. 6) which was not present 6 months earlier.

A new retrograde cystogram revealed persistence of the high-grade left VUR. Urodynamics testing yielded normal results. A radioisotope renal scan (dimercaptosuccinic acid, DMSA) confirmed the loss of left renal function (Fig. 7).

All these arguments point to renal scarring due to primary VUR: unilateral VUR, normal bladder and sphincter, and recent unilateral renal loss of growth and function.

Because of the patient's age, the nature of the VUR, the recurrent urinary tract infection in spite of antibiotic prophylaxis, medical management should be given up. Correction of the VUR by classical surgery or submucosal endoscopic injection was suggested to the parents, some weeks after the latest episode. In this case, ureteral reimplantation was performed using a minimally invasive technique (Fig. 8).

Suggested Reading

1.   Demede D et al. Evidence-based medicine and vesico ureteral reflux. Ann Urol (Paris) Vol 43 2006; p 161–74
2.   Greenbaum LA, Mesrobian HG. Vesico ureteral reflux. Pediatr Chir North Ann Vol 53 2006; p 413–427
3.   Steyaert H, Valla JS. Minimally invasive urologic surgery in children: an overview of what can be done. Eur J Pediatr Surg Vol 15 2005; p 307–13

Q 125

Jean Stephane Valla

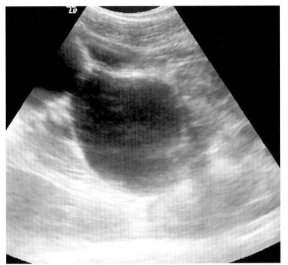

Fig. 1

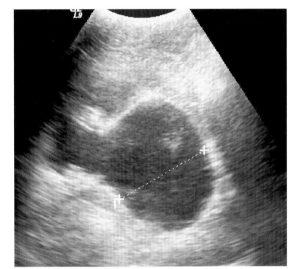

Fig. 2

A 15-year-old boy presented with recurrent left flank pain with hematuria, but without dysuria and no fever. Urinary culture did not demonstrate urinary tract infection. After questioning, the mother told us that during pregnancy a left renal pelvis dilatation was noted; this dilatation was controlled after birth, and had regressed at 1 year of age. No ultrasonographic follow-up was made after 2 years of age.

- What are the first diagnostic hypotheses to explain pain with hematuria in an adolescent?
- How do you interpret the renal sonography study (Figs. 1–3)?
- What is the suspected pathological condition?
- How do you complete the diagnostic work-up?
- How do you manage this case?

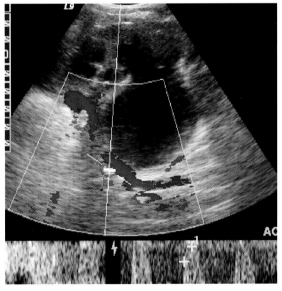

Fig. 3

A 125

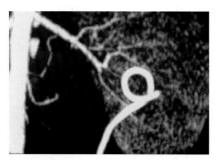

Fig. 4

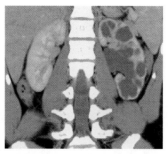

Fig. 5

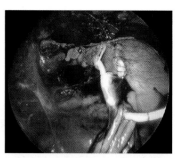

Fig. 6

The two most frequent etiologies to explain flank pain with hematuria are lithiasis and obstructive uropathy, in particular ureteropelvic junction obstruction (UPJO). These two causes could be associated.

The ultrasonography shows:

a. Sagittal US (Fig. 1), pelvis and calices are largely dilated, renal parenchyma is thin.

b. Transversal US (Fig. 2), anteroposterior diameter of the pelvis is up to 40 mm.

c. Doppler US (Fig. 3), no lower pole crossing vessel is clearly visible.

The suspected pathological condition is pyeloureteral junction obstruction because no lithiasis is visible and the ureter is not distended.

A radionuclide renal study using Tec-99 MAG 3 is mandatory to calculate the relative renal function of each kidney (in this case, left kidney 17%, right kidney 83%) and the degree of obstruction (in this case major obstruction on the left side). Angiography (Figs. 4, 5) could be useful in detecting crossing vessels (extrinsic cause of UPJO).

Surgery is needed in this case; because the left renal function was down to 15%, pyeloplasty must be preferred to nephrectomy and if possible by using a minimally invasive approach (Fig. 6). Nevertheless, the patient and parents must be informed of a possible failure of this reconstructive surgery (10% of cases) in such a distended and poorly functioning kidney. This case demonstrates that it would have been better to make an earlier diagnosis by performing annual ultrasound examinations and not to stop the surveillance after 1 year.

Suggested Reading

1. Balster S, Schiborr M, Brinkmann OA, Hertle L. Obstructive uropathy in childhood. Aktuelle Urol 2005 Aug; 36(4):317–28

2. Kaselas C, Papouis G, Grigoriadis G, Klokkaris A, Kaselas V. Pattern of renal Function Deterioration as a predictive factor of unilateral ureteropelvic junction obstruction treatment. Eur Urol 2006 Jun 15

3. McDaniel BB, Jones RA, Scherz H, Kirsch AJ, Little SB, Grattan-Smith JD. Dynamic contrast enhanced MR urography in the evaluation of pediatric hydronephrosis: Part 2, anatomic and functional assessment of ureteropelvic junction obstruction. AJR Am J Roentgenol 2005 Dec; 185(6):1608–14

4. McMann LP, Kirsch AJ, Scherz HC, Smith EA, Jones RA, Shehata BM, Kozielski R, Grattan-Smith JD. Magnetic resonance urography in the evaluation of prenatally diagnosed hydronephrosis and renal dysgenesis. J Urol 2006 Oct; 176(4 Pt 2):1786–92

5. Sheu JC, Koh CC, Chang PY, Wang NL, Tsai JD, Tsai TC. Ureteropelvic junction obstruction in children: 10 years' experience in one institution. Pediatr Surg Int 2006 Jun; 226:519–23

Q 126

Jean Stephane Valla

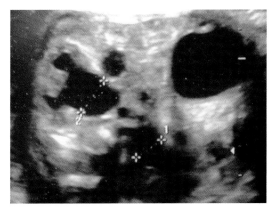

Fig. 1

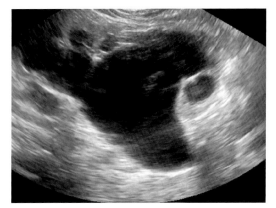

Fig. 2

A full-term normal-weight baby was supervised before birth because an ultrasound examination at 22 weeks of pregnancy had revealed a dilatation of the left pelvis. This dilatation increased at 32 weeks, reaching 22 mm in diameter (Figs. 1). At 4 days of life, ultrasonography confirmed the dilatation of the left upper urinary tract (Fig. 2). A urine sample was sterile.

- How do you interpret Fig. 2?
- What is the suspected diagnosis?
- How do you complete the diagnostic work-up?
- How do you manage this case?

A 126

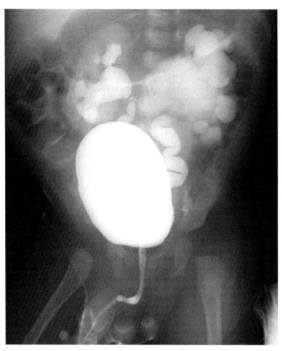

Fig. 3

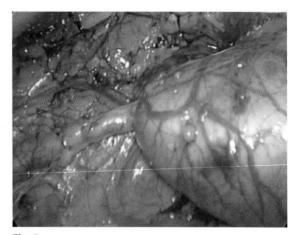

Fig. 4

Figure 2 shows a typical aspect of ureteropelvic junction obstruction (UPJO): a central cystic structure with connecting peripheral cysts representing the dilated calyces. The renal parenchyma is thin but its echogenicity looks normal.

Hydronephrosis on a prenatal examination is today the most common mode of presentation of UPJO.

Two examinations are mandatory before making a therapeutic decision: first a retrograde cystogram (Fig. 3), which shows a normal urethra, normal bladder, and bilateral stage III vesicoureteral reflux with diluted contrast liquid in the left pelvis. Second, a MAG-3 renal scan (Fig. 4) allows one to measure the value of the left kidney (34%), to confirm the obstruction.

Management can be debatable; in this case antibiotic prophylaxis was given. A clinical, bacteriological, and radiological follow-up was performed each month. At 3 months, ultrasonography and MR imaging demonstrated no improvement of the left pelvic dilatation; the left ureter was not visible. At 4 months, this infant was sent to hospital because of febrile urinary tract infection. An Anderson–Hynes dismembered pyeloplasty (excision of the abnormal segment as well as redundant renal

Fig. 5

pelvis) was performed at 6 months (Fig. 5, on the right, dilated pelvis, on the left, normal ureter, in the middle, stenotic segment). Preoperative cystoscopy allowed assessment of the two ureteral orifices to be made (mild malformation) and catheterization of the left side to be carried out.

Q 127

Sabine Sarnacki

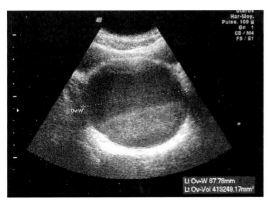

Fig. 1

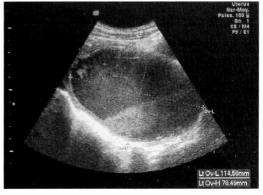

Fig. 2

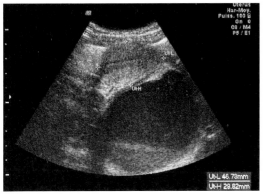

Fig. 3

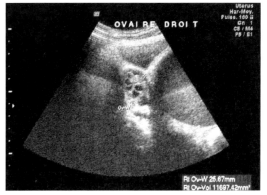

Fig. 4

A 12.5-year-old girl presented with a 3-week history of abdominal pain. Clinical examination showed a healthy girl with patent signs of puberty (Tanner stage IV) and an abdominopelvic mass, which was not mobile. A pelvic ultrasound examination was performed *before* the consultation (Figs. 1–4).

Laboratory tests were also performed on the basis of the first US examination, yielding the following results:
- ACE: 8 ng/ml (normal <5 ng/ml)
- CA 19-9: 2,252 U/ml (normal <39 U/ml)
- CA 125: 1,129 U/ml (normal <35 U/ml)
- β-HCG: <1 UI/l (normal <5 UI/L)
- Alpha-fetoprotein (AFP): 2 ng/ml (normal <15 ng/ml)

Questioning of the patient and the clinical examination finally allowed the correct diagnosis to be made.
- How do you interpret the US images (Figs. 1–4)?
- How do you interpret the results of the laboratory tests?
- What are the main questions and the principal features of the clinical examination that make the US examination useless, and in this case confusing?
- What is the main diagnosis that leads to a very simple operation and a complete relief of the symptoms?

A 127

The discovery of an abdominopelvic mass in a girl of 12–13 years with patent signs of puberty raises several diagnoses that could be explored through clinical, radiological, and biological examinations. The presence of the symptoms for several weeks is not common in adnexal torsion, but this diagnosis must be considered. The mobility of the mass may clearly point to an ovarian nature, but the immobility cannot eliminate this hypothesis. In contrast, the fact that the mass is painful does not favor the diagnosis of an ovarian tumor but rather the diagnosis of an obstruction of the genital tract with retention of menstruation.

In the presence of an abdominopelvic mass, laboratory tests are required only when there is a suspicion of ovarian tumor to detect the presence of a malignant component (alpha-fetoprotein for the yolk sac tumor component and HCG for the choriocarcinoma component), which may require preoperative chemotherapy. Measurements of CA 19-9, CA 125, and ACE levels are useless in a pubertal girl, since adult-type ovarian carcinoma is exceptional in this age group.

Questioning the patient and a complete clinical examination in this case would have avoided a misinterpretation of the US and laboratory tests.

Figures 1 and 2 show a hypoechogenic mass that was interpreted as an ovarian cyst. There is, however, a clear line of sedimentation that could not be present in an ovarian cyst. Figure 3 shows an adult-type uterus with signs of hormonal impregnation, and Fig. 4 a normal right ovary with multiple follicles.

The markers for malignant germinal tumors are negative (alpha-fetoprotein and HCG). The elevation of ACE, CA 19-9, and CA 125 levels is nonspecific, due to the inflammatory context.

The main question to ask is whether this girl with patent signs of puberty has already started having her periods, and the sign to search for during the clinical examination is the presence of a hymenal swelling.

The diagnosis was hematocolpos due to imperforate hymen.

Suggested Reading

1. Nazir Z, Rizvi RM, Qureshi RN, Khan ZS, Khan Z. Congenital vaginal obstructions: varied presentation and outcome. Pediatr Surg Int 2006; 22:749–753
2. Posner JC, Spandorfer PR. Early detection of imperforate hymen prevents morbidity from delays in diagnosis. Pediatrics 2005; 115:1008–1012
3. Stone SM, Alexander JL. Images in clinical medicine. Imperforate hymen with hematocolpometra. N Engl J Med 2004; 351:e6
4. Wall EM, Stone B, Klein BL. Imperforate hymen: a not-so-hidden diagnosis. Am J Emerg Med 2003; 21:249–250

Q 128

Sabine Sarnacki

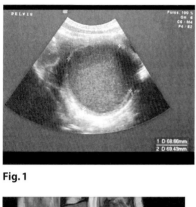

Fig. 1

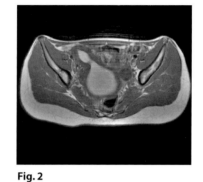

Fig. 2

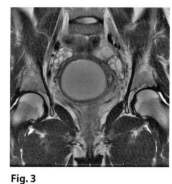

Fig. 3

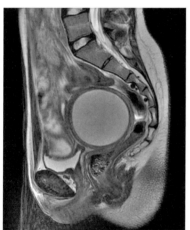

Fig. 4

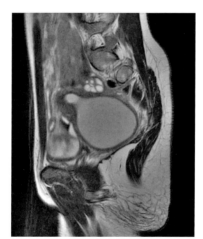

Fig. 5

A 12-year-old girl presented with a 2–3-month history of coccygeal pain. Clinical examination showed a healthy girl with patent signs of puberty (Tanner stage IV) and a normal aspect of the sacrococcygeal region.

- Which important question should be asked?

A US examination was performed and showed normal ovaries with peripheral follicles and a mass in the pelvis (Fig. 1).

- What is the other region that is important to analyze on this examination?
- What is the first diagnosis to be proposed?

An MR imaging study was requested by the surgeon.

- How do you interpret Figs. 2–5?
- What are the important points to assess on these images?
- How do you manage this situation?

A 128

The most important question to ask this girl who had reached puberty is about the date of onset of her period. The pain related to a hematocolpos typically has a coccygeal projection, and this diagnosis should be considered in this pubertal girl. If periods had already occurred, the notion of a two-step menstruation with two different colors (one red and one brown) is important to consider and gives information about the anatomical type of the potential malformation (incomplete septum, see below).

The US examination shows a hypoechogenic mass with a well-defined wall and a line of sedimentation within. The presence of two normal ovaries (Fig. 3) with signs of hormonal activity eliminates an ovarian origin. The retroperitoneal region has to be analyzed for the presence of both kidneys. Müllerian duplication is usually associated with a renal agenesis on the side of the interrupted genital tract. This malformation proceeds from mesonephric anomalies with absence of the wolffian duct opening to the urogenital sinus and of the ureteral bud sprouting (and, therefore, renal agenesis). The 'inductor' function of the wolffian duct on the müllerian duct is also failing and there is usually a uterovaginal duplicity plus ipsilateral blind hemivagina with the renal agenesis. This malformation is thus associated with a large unilateral hematocolpos with a partial resorption of the intervaginal septum. These types can be associated with a vaginal ectopic ureter and interseptal or interuterine communication. Vaginal or complete cervicovaginal unilateral agenesis, ipsilateral with the renal agenesis, with or without communication between both hemiuteri, is less common.

Figures 2–5 are fat-saturated T2-weigthed sequences which demonstrate the fluid nature of the collection. Figure 2 shows the hematocolpos in the blind hemivagina on a transversal section of the pelvis. A hematometra is visible in the right hemiuterus. Figure 3 is an axial section where both ovaries with multiple follicles can be seen from one part of the fluid collection to another in the blind hemivagina. The ipsilateral hemiuterus is anteverted and is not seen on this section. Figures 4 and 5 show sagittal sections of the pelvis, where the mucosal line of the open hemivagina reaching the perineum can be followed.

The diagnosis of müllerian duplication could be made on the basis of a simple US. This examination allows one to determine the uterine didelphys, the blind hemivagina, and the location of the cervix. MR imaging is, however, interesting for the precise study of the level of the vaginal partition. Retention of blood often gives an ovoid or round shape to the filled hemivagina, such that the vaginal partition is not sagittal, but transversal, as in the present case. Axial and sagittal MR imaging representations give a more precise evaluation of the distance of the septum from the perineal level, which is helpful in anticipating the difficulties of the intervention.

The degree of emergency for curing the malformation depends on the symptoms. The intervaginal septum may be seen as a 'buttonhole' on the anterolateral wall of the normal vagina when the septum is incomplete but is difficult to locate when the septum is complete. A true collection swelling in the vagina is mandatory in this case to determine precisely the site of incision of the septum. If the girl is symptom-free, the distension of the hemivagina can be followed with a US examination and the intervention planned when it is filled. In the present case, the intervention can be planned at once. Some authors recommend preoperative hormonal treatment to block ovary functions, with the aim of preventing later onset of endometriosis. Resection of the vaginal septum is performed via the normal vagina. Preoperative cystoscopy could attest to the expected trigonal agenesis, and laparoscopy may provide additional information on the pelvic and urological anatomy beyond radiologic tests.

Suggested Reading

1. Acien P, Acien M, Sanchez-Ferrer M. Complex malformations of the female genital tract. New types and revision of classification. Hum Reprod 2004; 19:2377–2384
2. Acién P. Incidence of Müllerian defects in fertile and infertile women. Hum Reprod 1997; 12:1372–1376
3. The American Fertility Society. Classification of adnexal adhesions, distal tubal occlusion, tubal occlusion secondary to tubal ligation, tubal preganancies, müllerian anomalies and intrauterine adhesions. Fertil Steril 1988; 49:944–955
4. Zurawin RK, Dietrich JE, Heard MJ, Edwards CL. Didelphic uterus and obstructed hemivagina with renal agenesis: case report and review of the literature. J Pediatr Adolesc Gynecol 2004; 17:137–141

Q 129

Antonio Savanelli, Marianna De Marco, and Hana Dolezalova

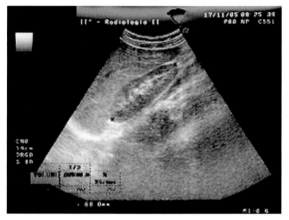

Fig. 1

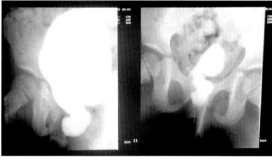

Fig. 2

A child who was affected by urinary tract infections (UTIs) since birth had been diagnosed with right urethral duplication and bilateral vesicourethral reflux, which was treated in another hospital first with endoscopic injection and then with a right ureteral implantation using the Cohen technique.

Recurrent UTIs persisted after surgery and a serious urinary incontinence appeared.

Because of the complaint of urinary incontinence, the child was admitted to our hospital at the age of 5 years. Firstly, ultrasound and voiding cystography studies were performed, which are shown in Figs. 1 and 2.

- What does the renal ultrasound show (Fig. 1)?
- What does the second examination (Fig. 2) show?

Following these studies, another examination was necessary so as to examine the urinary continence.

- Which study was performed?
- What does the urodynamic study show (Fig. 3)?
- Which malformation is causing persistence of the symptoms in this girl?
- Why did she develop urinary incontinence?
- What is the optimal treatment for this condition?

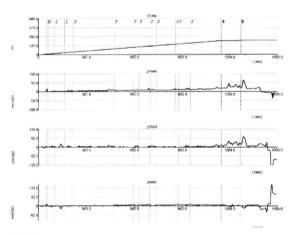

Fig. 3

A 129

The girl had a duplicated right kidney, bilateral vesico-urethral reflux, and *ipsilateral blind ectopic ureterocele*, misdiagnosed during the first operation. Cystoscopic detection of ureteroceles can be quite variable and frequently confused. A compressible ureterocele may come to resemble only a minor mucosal fold with bladder filling; even when the ureterocele has poor detrusor support and prolapses, at cystoscopy it may be misdiagnosed as a bladder diverticulum. In the other hospital the child also underwent intravenous pyelography that was negative for ureterocele. Most ectopic ureteroceles are associated with the upper pole of a duplex kidney that shows minimal or no function, as in our case, and in these cases the radiographic signs of ureterocele are primarily negative. Ureteroceles are described as blind when no kidney or upper pole associated with ureterocele can be demonstrated. Despite thorough radiological investigation in all patients, a correct assessment of the anatomic defect can be achieved only by surgical exploration. If preoperative radiological evaluation is equivocal, a high index of suspicion after cystography and intraoperative recognition of an unusual anatomic presentation of the ectopic ureterocele are essential for appropriate management and a successful outcome.

The first examination (Fig. 1) in this case is an ultrasound and shows no pelvic dilatation and a normal renal structure.

The second study (Fig. 2) is a cystogram showing a large and irregular bladder neck and a dilated urethra, with an image resembling a urethral diverticulum.

In order to evaluate urinary incontinence it is useful to perform a urodynamic study. In our case the study

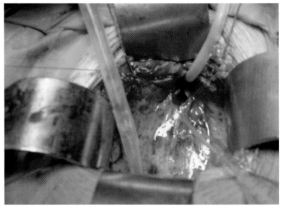

Fig. 4

(Fig. 3) shows a good *detrusor* contraction with urinary leakage at the end of filling.

Persistent urinary incontinence was due to the flow of urine from the bladder directly into the postsphinteric urethra. It was attributed to failure to resect the misdiagnosed ureterocele.

Finally, we performed cystoscopy, which revealed the real malformation. The urethral diverticulum is actually the distal part of the ureterocele that comes out in the urethra. Ureterocelectomy and neck bladder reconstruction were performed (Fig. 4).

In Fig. 4 it is possible to see the intravesical hole responsible for the urinary incontinence.

The child remains continent 1 year after the surgical treatment.

Suggested Reading

1. Byun E, Merguerian PA. A meta-analysis of surgical practice patterns in the endoscopic management of ureteroceles. J Urol 2006; 176(4 Pt2):1871–7
2. Castagnetti M, Cimador M, Sergio M de Grazia E. Transureteral incision of duplex system ureteroceles in neonates: does increase the need for secondary surgery in intravesical and ectopic cases? BJU Int 2004; 93(9):1313–7
3. Chertin B, Rabinowitz R, Pollack A, Koulikov D, Fridmans A, Hadas-Halpern I, Farkas. Does prenatal diagnosis influence the morbidity associated with left in situ non-functioning or poorly functioning renal moiety after endoscopic puncture of ureterocele? J Urol 2005; 173(4):1349–52
4. Hoebeke P, De Kuyper P, Goeminne H, Van Laecke E, Everaert K. Bladder neck closure for treating pediatric incontinence. Eur Urol 2000 Oct; 38(4):453–65
5. Shekarriz B, Upadhyay J, Fleming P, Gonzales R, Barthold JS. Long-term outcome based on the initial surgical approach to ureterocele. J Urol 1999; 162(3Pt2):1072–6

Q 130

Antonio Savanelli, Flavio Perricone, Gianfranco Vallone,
and Pier Francesco Rambaldi

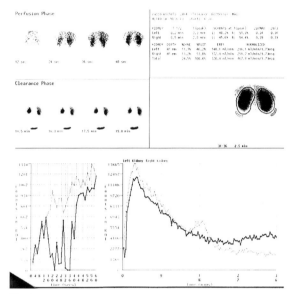

Fig. 1

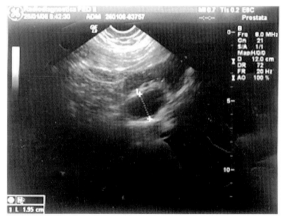

Fig. 2

A 10-year-girl with abdominal pain and pelvic and caliceal dilatation diagnosed on ultrasound was admitted to
our unit.

During a previous hospitalization 4 years earlier, the
patient, after an episode of abdominal pain, underwent
ultrasonography. A caliceal and pelvic dilatation was
detected with an anteroposterior (AP) diameter of the
renal pelvis of 34×27 mm.

At the same time, the girl also underwent cystography, which was normal, and Tc-99 MAG-3 dynamic renal scintigraphy (Fig. 1).

• What does Fig. 1 show?

The girl underwent annual ultrasonographic follow-ups
that showed an unchanging condition.

The patient returned to hospital at the age of 10 years,
after another ultrasound study for a renal colic episode
(Fig. 2).

After analgesic treatment and when the symptoms
disappeared, the girl underwent an ultrasound examination after 12 h (Fig. 3).

• What does Fig. 3 show?

Fig. 3

Another investigation was then performed.
• What is the diagnosis?
• What is the preferred therapeutic approach?
• Which preoperative investigation would have al-
  lowed an etiologic diagnosis to be made?
• What is the follow-up?

A 130

Figure 1 shows a renal scintigraphy study with normal relative renal function and adequate elimination after furosemide (80%). It shows a urinary dilatation without obstruction.

The ultrasound image (Fig. 2) shows a caliceal and pelvic dilatation with AP diameter of 66 mm and a thinning cortical parenchyma.

The ultrasound after 12 h (Fig. 3) shows an improvement with AP diameter of 20 mm.

The intravenous urogram (IVU), necessary to improve the diagnosis and to provide other anatomo-functional details, shows a reduced and delayed elimination of contrast media and hydronephrosis signs. Since the marked improvements in the quality of ultrasound examinations, the indications to perform an IVU have been more restricted, but there is still a role for this modality in some patients before surgical intervention.

The improved dilatation and pain lead to the diagnosis of intermittent hydronephrosis, which in patients of this age is typically produced by a crossing renal vessel.

Indications for surgery in children with unilateral hydronephrosis are the presence of symptoms, failure to improve the dilatation over time, and poor relative renal function.

The girl underwent surgery with Anderson–Hynes dismembered pyeloplasty.

A dynamic MR image should permit a more specific preoperative diagnosis to be made, by depicting the anomalous vessel; however, the etiologic diagnosis should not change the therapeutic planning.

Follow-up entails 6-month ultrasound and scintigraphy evaluations.

The MAG-3 scintigraphy (Fig. 4) provides evidence of worsening renal function despite a good excretion phase, and the ultrasound shows a small left kidney without dilatation.

The delay in the diagnosis and the treatment of hydronephrosis as an anomalous vessel probably caused the renal damage. The presence of pelvic–caliceal system dilatation associated with renal colic in childhood should always suggest an anomalous vessel and indicate the surgical treatment.

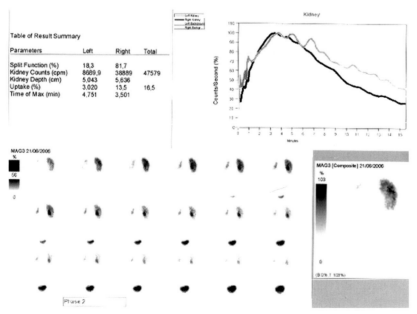

Fig. 4

Q 131

Antonio Savanelli, Francesca Alicchio, and Luigi Mansi

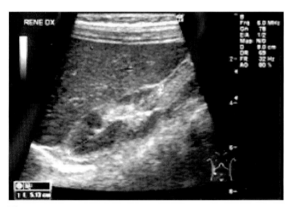

Fig. 1

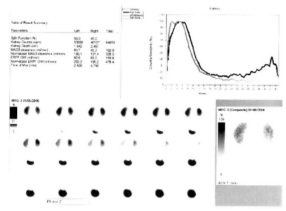

Fig. 3

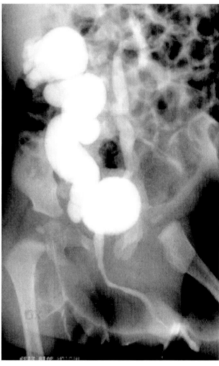

Fig. 2

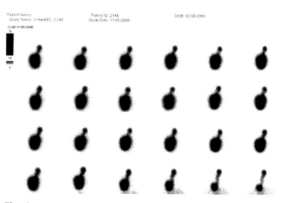

Fig. 4

A newborn boy had an antenatal ultrasound diagnosis of dilatation of the upper urinary tracts. Urinary tract infections (UTIs) were not reported.

- Which examinations do you perform?

The examinations shown in Figs. 1 and 2 were performed.

- What does Fig. 1 show? What does Fig. 2 show?
- Why are other examinations necessary?
- What does Fig. 3 show?
- What is the diagnosis?
- What is the treatment of this malformation in the newborn?

- What is the follow-up?
- What does Fig. 4 show?
- What is the final treatment?

A 131

The newborn could have a congenital bilateral vesico-ureteral reflux (VUR) and he needs to undergo an ultrasound examination and voiding cystourethrography.

The ultrasound (Fig. 1) allows the diagnosis of a left pyeloureteral duplication to be made. Figure 2 shows a cystography. You can see a huge left refluxing megaureter corresponding to the inferior renal segment and a moderate right VUR. The urethral profile is normal.

To complete the diagnostic approach, a Tc-99m DMSA static renal scan is necessary, so as to estimate the renal function and the presence of reflux nephropathy, or dynamic renography. The Tc-99m DMSA isotopic scan is the gold standard for evaluating the function of the involved renal tissue, but the differential renal function is more reliably assessed with Tc-99m MAG-3 dynamic renography.

In Fig. 3 you can see a MAG-3 dynamic renogram showing a normal renal function and a good washout.

The diagnosis is VUR of severe grade at the left side of the lower renal segment and of moderate grade at the right.

Preventing urinary infections by using prophylactic antimicrobials is generally the first treatment step.

Children with high-grade reflux have a spontaneous resolution rate of about 30%.

Indications for surgical treatment are recurrent symptomatic urinary infections, despite prophylactic antimicrobials, failure to improve the grade of reflux over time, new scars and compliance problems. A nonfunctioning lower renal segment can be removed. At follow-up, radioisotope cystography (Fig. 4) shows persistent VUR after 1 year of prophylactic treatment.

The principles of management of VUR associated with complete ureteral duplication do not differ substantially from those for management of reflux into a single ureteral system. The most common surgical treatment is intravesical repair described by Cohen, where the ureters are placed in a common transtrigonal submucosal tunnel in their common sheath without changing the ureteral hiatus. In order to obtain such a ratio, when the ureter caliber is wider than 10 mm, the last 10 cm of the ureter needs to be tapered.

Endoscopic subureteric injection of bulking agents is another modern approach. Proposals for a randomized clinical trial of immediate endoscopic treatment versus conservative management are pending at this time.

Suggested Reading

1. Badwan KH, Diamond DA. Vesicoureteral reflux: diagnosis and management. J Med Liban 2005 Apr–Jun; 53(2):61–5
2. Bhide A, Sairam S, Farrugia MK, Boddy SA, Thilaganathan B. The sensitivity of antenatal ultrasound for predicting renal tract surgery in early childhood. Ultrasound Obstet Gynecol 2005 May; 25(5):489–92
3. Cohen AL, Rivara FP, Davis R, Christakis DA. Compliance with guidelines for the medical care of first urinary tract infections in infants: a population-based study. Pediatrics 2005 Jun; 115(6):1474–8
4. Dillon MJ, Goonasekera CD. Reflux nephropathy. J Am Soc Nephrol 1998 Dec; 9(12):2377–83
5. Smellie JM, Barratt TM, Chantler C, Gordon I, Prescod NP, Ransley PG, Woolf AS. Medical versus surgical treatment in children with severe bilateral vesicoureteric reflux and bilateral nephropathy: a randomised trial. Lancet 2001 Apr 28; 357(9265):1329–33

Q 132

Antonio Savanelli, Pier Francesco Rambaldi, Gianfranco Vallone, and Barbara Greco

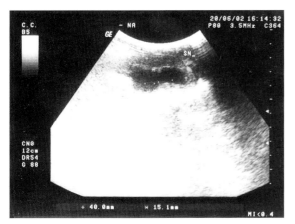

Fig. 1

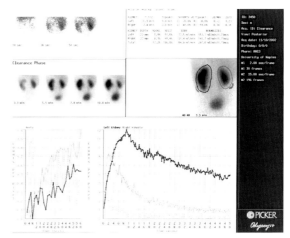

Fig. 2

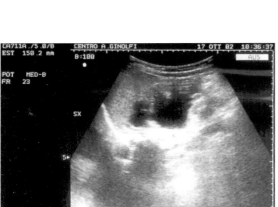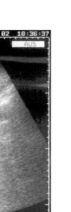

Fig. 3

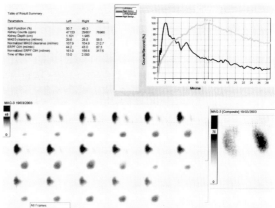

Fig. 4

A newborn was affected by monolateral left hydronephrosis identified on antenatal ultrasound (Fig. 1).
- What does the antenatal ultrasound show?
- What other examinations do you perform in this case?
- What does Fig. 2 show?

- What is the diagnosis?
- What is the therapeutic planning?
- What do the examinations in Figs. 3 and 4 show (performed when the boy was 3 and 6 months old, respectively)?
- What is the follow-up?

A 132

The antenatal ultrasound (Fig. 1) allows one to see a thinner renal parenchyma and a monolateral severe dilatation of the calyx and pelvis without ureteral dilatation.

We performed a new ultrasound at 5 days of life confirming a severe dilatation with an AP diameter of the pelvis of 34 mm. A MAG-3 renogram was planned after the first month of life, maintaining prophylactic therapy until the diagnosis of obstruction is excluded.

Figure 2 shows a renogram with a good renal relative function and late washout.

The diagnosis is monolateral dilatation of the upper urinary tract without obstruction.

In this case, there are no indications to surgical treatment. An ultrasound and another MAG-3 renogram were repeated after 3–6 months.

The ultrasound (Fig. 3) shows an improved dilatation of the upper urinary tract with an AP diameter of the pelvis of 19 mm and the MAG-3 (Fig. 4) shows an improved washout too.

Follow-up studies using a MAG-3 renal scan and an ultrasound should be performed at 12 and 24 months. In this case, at follow-up the AP diameter of the pelvis improved reaching 14 mm (Fig. 5), and the MAG-3 renogram showed a good washout after furosemide administration.

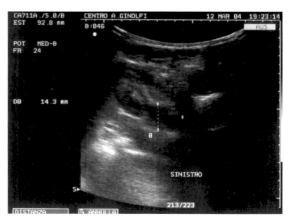

Fig. 5

Suggested Reading

1. Bhide A, Sairam S, Farrugia MK, Boddy SA, Thilaganathan B. The sensitivity of antenatal ultrasound for predicting renal tract surgery in early childhood. Ultrasound Obstet Gynecol 2005 May; 25(5):489–92

2. Chandrasekharam VV, Shah MA. Outcome of patients with antenatally detected pelviureteric junction obstruction. Pediatr Nephrol 2005; 20:547

3. Riccabona M. Assessment and management of newborn hydronephrosis. World J Urol 2004; 22:73

Q 133

Antonio Savanelli, Gianfranco Vallone, Barbara Greco, and Luigi Mansi

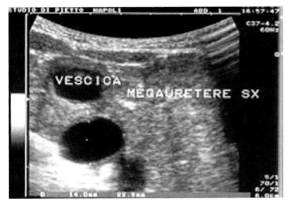

Fig. 1a

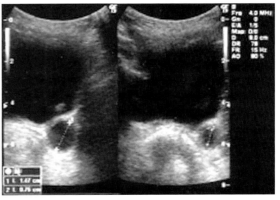

Fig. 1b

A 9-month-old child with an antenatal diagnosis of left hydronephrosis was admitted to our unit. The patient had a history of a urinary tract infection (UTI) occurring postnatally. In order to exclude vesicoureteral reflux (VUR), voiding cystourethrography was performed. The cystography was normal. Antibiotic prophylaxis for the UTI was begun soon after cystography. Two months later renal ultrasonography (Fig. 1a, b) was performed.

- What does Fig. 1 show?

After admission in our unit, the diagnostic examinations were completed with excretory urography and a MAG-3 renal scan (Fig. 2).

- What do you see in Fig. 2?
- What is the diagnosis?
- What is the therapeutic approach?
- What is the follow-up for this malformation?

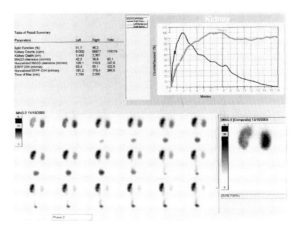

Fig. 2

A 133

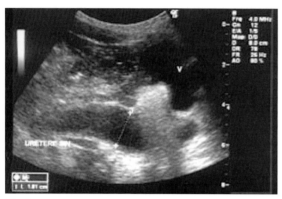

Fig. 3

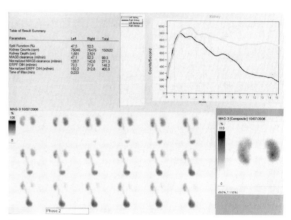

Fig. 4

UTIs are the most common cause of fever due to bacterial infection in the neonatal age. The causes of UTI can be VUR, obstructive uropathies like posterior urethral valves (PUV), megaureter etc.

Figure 1 (a, b) shows severe hydronephrosis of the left kidney with renal parenchymal thickness.

An intravenous urography study showed delayed contrast excretion with dilution of material contrast within the calices and pelvis, with a late image of hydroureteronephrosis. A diuretic radionuclide urography with MAG-3 (Fig. 2) confirmed the delayed elimination of the tracer without obstruction and a normal renal function.

The diagnosis was of a partially obstructive megaureter.

Spontaneous resolution or improvement of many cases of urinary tract dilatation is becoming more common. Many asymptomatic primary megaureters in infancy improve spontaneously and do not require surgical treatment. When the upper urinary tract is dilated, patients may need antibiotic prophylaxis, because the dilatation of the upper urinary tract increases the risk of

UTIs. Surgical treatment is indicated in the event of deteriorating renal function with permanent obstruction.

These patients are followed up with ultrasonography and nuclear renography until stable improvement or complete resolution of hydroureteronephrosis is noted. An excretory urogram should be limited to cases in which anatomical details are required before surgical treatment. In our case the last echogram repeated after 2 years showed remarkable improvement (Fig. 3). The MAG-3 scan that showed a conserved parenchymal function remained unmodified in spite of the persistence of incomplete washout (Fig. 4).

Comment: The diagnosis and the treatment of a not refluxing obstructive megaureter still represent one of the most challenging dilemmas in pediatric urology today. The indication to treatment is the presence of clinical symptoms, decrease of renal function, and dilatation. The aims of diagnosis, treatment, and long-term follow-up are the preservation of renal function and the prevention of UTIs.

Q 134

Alfonso Papparella, Mercedes Romano, and Pio Parmeggiani

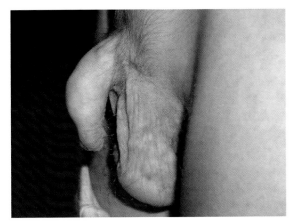

Fig. 1

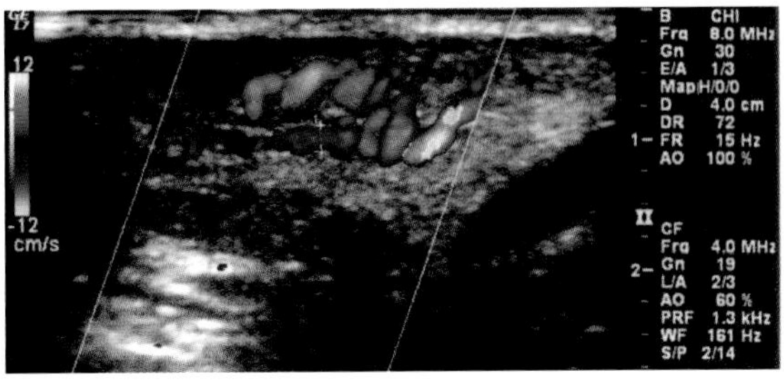

Fig. 2

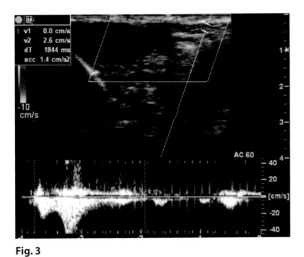

Fig. 3

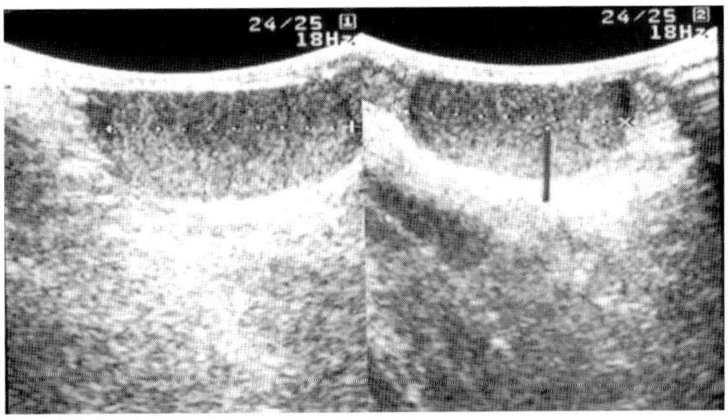

Fig. 4

An 11-year-old patient presented with a soft mass in the upper part of the left scrotal region. The lesion was painless and was associated with ipsilateral testicular hypotrophy.

- What is the most likely diagnosis? (See Fig. 1)
- What should the clinical examination evaluate?

An echo color Doppler of the spermatic vessels was requested.

- What does the test show (Figs. 2, 3)?
- What does Fig. 4 show?
- What are the most likely grade and classification of this pathological condition?
- Would you suggest further diagnostic investigations?
- What is the surgical treatment for this condition?

A 134

The diagnosis is varicocele. Palpation should evaluate the size of the testis, the condition of the pampiniform plexus and the spermatic cord, in addition to the patency of the vaginal peritoneal duct. Palpation highlights a dilation of the pampiniform plexus that is evident even with the patient in the standing position; it resembles the typical "bag of worms" and is associated with ipsilateral testicular hypotrophy. In the clinostatic position, the varicose swelling decreases, and it increases after the Valsalva maneuver. Examination of the contralateral region is normal.

The power color Doppler shows a 2.8-s reflux on the left side after the Valsalva maneuver (normal range: 0.8 s).

The comparative testicular ultrasound shows a reduced size in the left testis compared with the right testis (Fig. 4)

The classification is grade II varicocele with type I reflux (renospermatic) and testicular hypotrophy.

Instrumental tests to be performed include: abdominal–scrotal ultrasound (symptomatic, bilateral varicocele), scrotal echo color Doppler, retrograde phlebography of the internal spermatic vein that could be useful in recurrences, and CT scan in the case of obstructive varicocele.

The therapeutic approach in this patient can be ligation of the spermatic vessels, either using the retroperitoneal approach according to Palomo with ligation of the spermatic artery or the inguinal approach according to Ivanissevich (ligation of the spermatic, cremasteric, and deferential veins); the subinguinal microsurgical approach (ligation of the spermatic and cremasteric veins, external spermatic vein and gubernaculums); derivative microsurgical anastomosis;or sclerotizing treatment. More recent approaches use transperitoneal videosurgery, where the spermatic vein and artery are isolated several centimeters away from the internal inguinal ring,

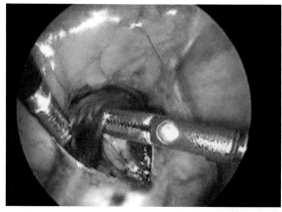

Fig. 5

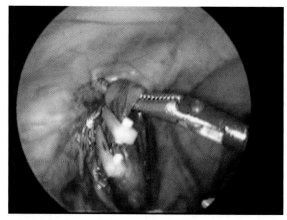

Fig. 6

clipped (Figs. 5, 6), and then sectioned (Palomo procedure). A retroperitoneoscopic technique could also be applied for varicocele.

Complications include hydrocele, testicular atrophy, recurrence, and persistence.

Suggested Reading

1. Esposito C, Monguzzi GL, Gonzalez-Sabin MA, Rubino R, Montinaro L, Papparella A, Amici G. Laparoscopic treatment of pediatric varicocele: a multicenter study of the Italian society of video surgery in infancy *J Urol* 2000; 163(6):1944–1946

2. Esposito C, Monguzzi G, Gonzalez-Sabin MA, Rubino R, Montinaro L, Papparella A et al. Results and complications of laparoscopic surgery for pediatric varicocele. *J Pediatr Surg* 2001; 36(5):767–9

3. Koyle MA et al. Laparoscopic Palomo varicocele ligation in children and adolescents: results of 103 cases. *J Urol* 2004; 172:1749–52

Q 135

Alfonso Papparella, Mercedes Romano, and Pio Parmeggiani

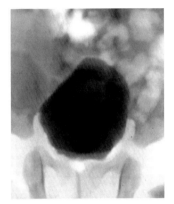

Fig. 1

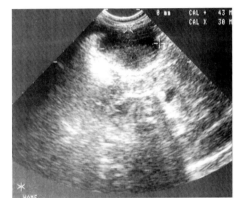

Fig. 2

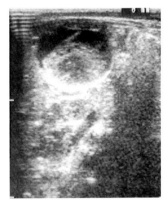

Fig. 3

A 1-month-old girl was hospitalized following the prenatal diagnosis of an abdominal mass.

The general objective examination was normal; laboratory test results (alpha-fetoprotein and CA 125) were within normal ranges. Results from the urinalysis showed small amounts of blood with leukocyturia, whereas the urine culture was positive for *Escherichia coli* (10^5). A micturitional cystourethrography and a complete abdominal ultrasound were performed.

- What does Fig. 1 (micturitional cystourethrography) show?
- What do Figs. 2 and 3 show?
- What additional diagnostic tests would you suggest?
- What is the most likely diagnosis?
- Which is the most appropriate surgical management in this case?
- What other conditions can we suspect?

A 135

The diagnosis in this girl is self-amputated ovarian cysts.

Ovarian cysts are generally rare in the pediatric age. They represent a heterogeneous group of conditions that range from functional (nonneoplastic) ovarian cysts, to ovarian torsion, benign tumors, or even malignant and extremely aggressive neoplasm.

The micturitional cystourethrography shows a normal-sized and normally localized bladder, with a lateral deflection of vesical imaging probably due to mass compression (Fig. 1). The course and caliber of the urethral duct are regular and there is no vesicoureteral reflux.

The abdominal ultrasound shows a roundish mass with linear and exogenous margins, located in an anteromedian position compared to both the lower pole of the right kidney and the subhepatic region; the mass is about $4 \times 3 \times 3$ cm, and has a mixed solid–liquid echostructure (Figs. 2, 3).

CT and MR imaging should be performed to better understand the origin and the localization of the cyst; as a matter of fact, the former confirmed the presence of the lesion in the subhepatic regions, whereas the latter located it in the right iliac fossa, and ruled out the involvement of other organs or apparatuses.

In such cases, the value of a diagnostic laparoscopy is beyond doubt, as it is able to evaluate the anatomical relationships of the mass, verifying its nature and the organ of origin through video-guided biopsies. Moreover, it can also be surgical or can help choose the most suitable surgical strategy. Laparoscopy is essential for the management of pediatric pathologies involving the annexes.

In this specific case, laparoscopy was able to detect a 4-cm cystic formation in the subhepatic region. The mass was mobile, well delimited by the surrounding organs, filled with blood, and attached by a thin long vessel (Figs. 4, 5).

Although the diagnostic test results were normal, to completely rule out a neoplastic formation the mass was totally removed through a right pararectal laparotomic incision, to avoid disseminating the fluid within the abdominal cavity in case of cyst rupture.

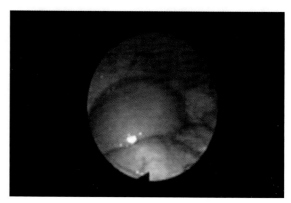

Fig. 4

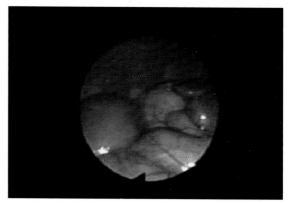

Fig. 5

Histological examination indicated a self-amputated ovarian cyst, morphologically devoid of malignant features. A self-amputated ovarian cyst results from a prenatal or neonatal torsion, followed by necrosis and calcification.

The differential diagnosis of ovarian cysts includes lymphangiomas and intestinal duplications, hepatic tumors, hypersplenism, neuroblastoma, and renal masses.

Q 136

Antonio Marte, Maria Domenica Sabatino, and Pio Parmeggiani

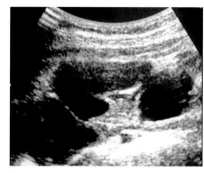

Fig. 1

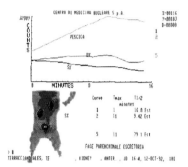

Fig. 2

A 14-year-old boy presented with recurrent lower abdominal pain. His mother told the doctor that her child
had been diagnosed with a kidney anomaly at birth.
When he was 1 year old he underwent the examinations
shown in Figs. 1 and 2.

- What does Fig. 1 show?
- What does Fig. 2 show?
- What pathological condition is affecting this child?
- What is the way to manage this condition?

A 136

This patient has an ectopic right pelvic kidney, an abnormality of renal migration with an incidence of 1 in 5,000. The ectopic kidney can be asymptomatic or associated with vesicoureteral reflux (VUR) 26%, ureteropelvic junction (UPJ) obstruction 37%, and functional ureterovesical junction (UVJ) 15%.

Figure 1 shows the ectopic pelvic kidney (note the proximity of the bladder) with a mild dilation of the pelvis.

The DTPA nuclear scintigram (Fig. 2) shows a bilateral good function of both kidneys with a mild delay of the tracer washout on the right side—split function: right kidney, glomerular filtration rate (GFR) 32.7 ml/m², relative function 41.7%; left kidney, GFR 37.7 ml/m², relative function 58.3%.

On admission we planned MAG-3 nuclear scintigraphy with indirect voiding cystourethrography (VCG) and MR urography.

Another important aspect the surgeon must consider is that the ectopic kidney is quite often associated with other malformations such as skeletal, cardiovascular, pulmonary, and genital system malformations. In girls, Rokitansky-Mayer-Kuster-Hauser syndrome is frequent.

In this case, echocardiography showed a mild mitral insufficiency.

The URO-MR study (Figs. 3, 4) confirms the position of the kidney, the iliac pelvic blood supply, the abnormal pelvicaliceal rotation, and the dilation.

The anterior view of the MAG-3 nuclear scintigraphy shows a reduction of right renal function (split right function (%), 39.1%) and confirms the obstruction (Fig. 5).

The nuclear VCG shows no VUR.

Because of the reduction of the right renal function (<40%) and the abdominal symptoms, the patient underwent laparoscopic-assisted pyeloplasty according to Anderson-Hynes.

After the 1-year follow-up, the child was well and free of symptoms.

Suggested Reading

1. Allen D, Bultitude MF, Nunan T, Glass JM. Misinterpretation of radioisotope imaging in pelvic kidneys. Int J Clin Pract Suppl 2005; 147:111–2

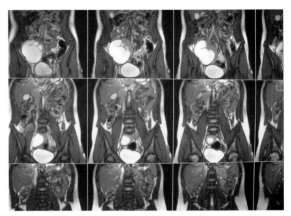

Fig. 3

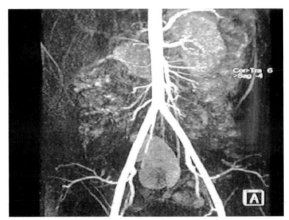

Fig. 4

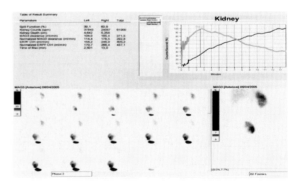

Fig. 5

Q 137

Antonio Marte, Maria Domenica Sabatino, and Pio Parmeggiani

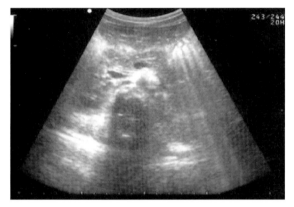

Fig. 1

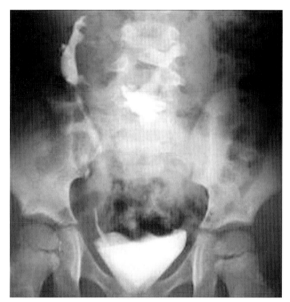

Fig. 2

A 5-year-old boy presented with an 8-month history of a febrile *Escherichia coli* urinary tract infection (UTI) with abdominal pain. The patient was referred to us by his pediatrician for other diagnostic investigations.

The patient was on antibiotic prophylaxis with co-trimoxazole and intermittently took spasmolytic drugs.

The mother showed us the examinations performed during a previous hospitalization (Figs. 1, 2).

- What do Figs. 1 and 2 show?
- Is there a need for other examinations?
- What pathological condition is affecting this child?
- What is the best way to manage this condition?

A 137

This child has a horseshoe kidney. Figure 1 shows an ultrasound scan demonstrating the abnormality of position as well as the connecting isthmus.

Figure 2 shows a typical appearance of a horseshoe kidney on an excretory urogram with a mild hydronephrosis of the left segment. The renal pelvis remains anterior with the ureter crossing the isthmus. The renal axis appears to be vertical with the lower poles lying closer than the upper pole. A frequent urographic finding is a low-lying kidney and the lower outer border of the kidney appears to continue across the midline (*arrow*), in this case the right kidney.

Associated urological anomalies (52%) are frequently identified in patients with horseshoe kidney, including primary vesicoureteral reflux (VUR), ureteropelvic junction obstruction, and ectopic ureter.

Figure 3 is a MAG-3 renal scan that shows the two kidneys fused through their lower poles. The left kidney and the isthmus show minimal function, elimination of tracer after IV furosemide; and after micturition it does not show elimination of tracer material from the pelvis. Split function percentage is: effective renal plasma flow (ERPF) left kidney 8.3%; ERPF right kidney 91.7%. The right kidney has a normal function.

Most horseshoe kidneys are asymptomatic throughout the patient's life. However, segmental hydronephrosis, reflux, lithiasis, or malignancy may lead to surgical intervention because of UTI, abdominal pain, or hematuria. Because of the recurrent UTI, the abdominal pain, and the poor function of the left kidney, the patient underwent left segment nephrectomy.

The intraoperative view shows a large parenchymatous renal isthmus that made the dissection difficult.

After a 10-month follow-up, the patient was well and free of symptoms.

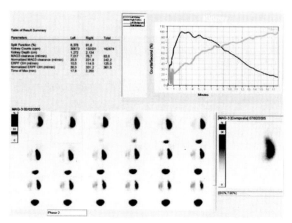

Fig. 3

Suggested Reading

1. Cascio S, Sweeney B, Granata C, Piaggio G, Jasonni V, Puri P. Vesicoureteral reflux and ureteropelvic junction in children with horseshoe kidney. Treatment and outcome. J Urol 2002; 167:2566–8

2. Pitts WR jr, Muecke EC. Horseshoe kidneys: a 40 years experience. J Urol 1975; 113:743–6

3. Yoannes P, Smith AD. the endourological management of complications associated with horseshoe kidney. J Urol 2002; 168:5–8

Q 138

Antonio Marte, Maria Domenica Sabatino, and Pio Parmeggiani

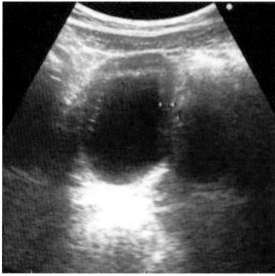

Fig. 1

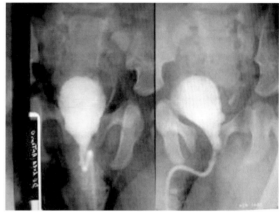

Fig. 2

A 3-month-old boy with a history of a febrile urinary tract *Escherichia coli* infection underwent urologic evaluation. The boy was on antibiotic prophylaxis.

The boy had been operated on at birth for myelomeningocele (MMC) prenatally detected with US. He did not need a ventricular shunt. The physical examination and blood test results were all normal. The child seemed to be leaking urine constantly. The motility of the lower limbs was intact. We performed the examinations shown in Figs. 1–3.

- What does Fig. 1 show?
- What does Fig. 2 show?
- What does Fig. 3 show?
- How should we manage this case?

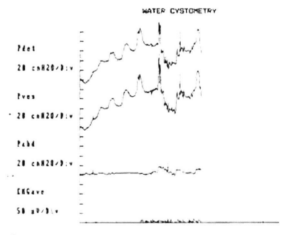

Fig. 3

A 138

The patient has a neuropathic bladder without urinary retention.

Figure 1 is a US study of the bladder showing a thickened bladder. The renal US is normal.

Figure 2 is a voiding cystourethrography (VCG) that shows a typical neuropathic bladder with trabeculation and anomalies of the bladder profile. There is a left grade-1 (according to international classification: grade 1–5) vesicoureteral reflux (VUR).

The urodynamics shows a hyperactive bladder with high pressures and detrusor-sphincter dyssynergia. The leak point pressure (LPP) is 50 cm of water and the leak point volume (LPV) 30 cc. Pressures over 40 cm H_2O pose a risk for the upper urinary tract.

The patient was treated with oral oxybutynin, CIC, and antibiotic prophylaxis.

Despite the treatment, he developed a bilateral VUR at the age of 3 years (Fig. 4). The MAG-3 nuclear scintigraphy showed a relative function of 55.5% on the left and of 44.5% on the right side. There was no evidence of obstruction or scars.

The patient continued with antibiotic prophylaxis and CIC and when he was 6 years old underwent endoscopic correction of the VUR with a subureteral Deflux injection.

In order to increase the patient's bladder capacity, at the age of 11 years he underwent intradetrusor botulin A toxin injection of 200 UI. The injection was repeated 8 months later. At the time of writing, the patient is 14 years old, infection-free, and dry between the CIC without oxybutynin; moreover, his bladder capacity has increased from 180 cc to about 400 cc. A follow-up VCUG was normal, and the urodynamics study yielded the following results: LPP 54 cm H_2O, LPV 411 c.

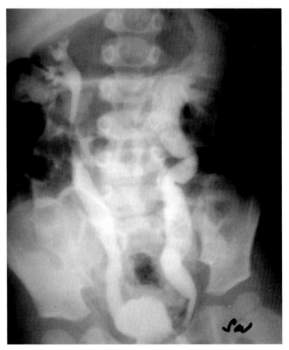

Fig. 4

The stool incontinence is treated with a continent enema device two times a week and occasionally the boy takes loperamide.

In some cases, neuropathic bladder secondary to MMC has an unfavorable evolution which requires bladder augmentation and/or an increase of the bladder outlet resistance in order to prevent urinary tract infections, intractable VUR, and continuous incontinence.

Suggested Reading

1. Bauer SB. Evaluation and management of the newborn with myelomeningocele. In Gonzales ET, Roth D (eds) Common Problems in Pediatric Urology. Mosby-Year Book Inc 1991; pp 169–80

2. Marte, A Vessella, P Cautiero, M Romano, M Borrelli, C Noviello, R Del Gado, P Parmeggiani. Efficacy of toxin-A Botulinum for treating intractable bladder hyperactivity in children affected by neuropathic bladder secondary to myelomeningocele: an alternative to enterocystoplasty. Minerva Pediatrica 2005; 57(1):35–40

Q 139

Antonio Marte, Maria Domenica Sabatino, and Pio Parmeggiani

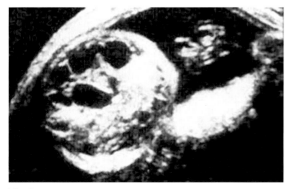

Fig. 1

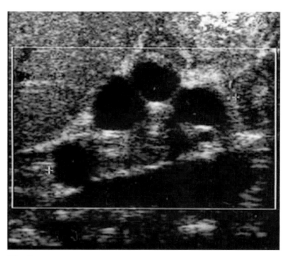

Fig. 2

We were asked to see a full-term newborn female. During the mother's pregnancy, a prenatal ultrasound performed at 32 weeks showed a cystic mass in the retroperitoneum on the left side (Fig. 1).

The baby appeared to be healthy. Physical examination confirmed a left upper quadrant mass which was hard and with an irregular surface. Otherwise, the child was normal.

A US study was performed (Fig. 2).
- What does Fig. 1 show?
- What does Fig. 2 show?
- What pathological condition is affecting this baby?
- Does she need to undergo other examinations?
- What is the best way to manage this condition?

A 139

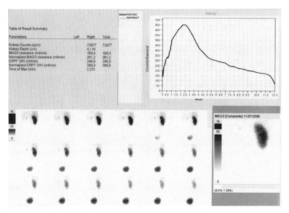

Fig. 3

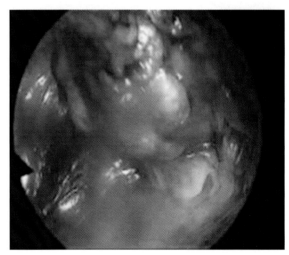

Fig. 4

This girl has a left multicystic dysplastic kidney (MCDK) presenting with an abdominal mass on the upper left quadrant (Fig. 1).

The lesion feels hard and has a knobbly surface, while the hydronephrotic kidney has a smooth surface (other postnatal presentations are: flank pain, urinary tract infection, or hypertension).

The postnatal US examination (Fig. 2) shows: randomly arranged and varied-sized cysts, the presence of interfaces between the cysts, a nonmedial location of the largest cyst, a lack of an identifiable renal sinus, and an absence of renal parenchyma. The right kidney shows compensatory hypertrophy. MCDK is found commonly in children with other major anomalies such as those of the respiratory, cardiac, gastrointestinal, and musculoskeletal system.

A nuclear renogram is the best imaging study with which to differentiate MCDK from hydronephrotic kidney and to detect a contralateral ureteropelvic junction (UPJ) obstruction. A CT scan would require sedation, it exposes the child to more radiation, and it is more expensive. Multicystic kidneys do not function. The MAG-3 nuclear scintigraphy shows that there is no

tracer in the left retroperitoneum. Only the right well-functioning kidney is seen (Fig. 3).

VCUG can detect associated vesicoureteral reflux.

The management of this case was conservative with periodic ultrasonographic checkups every 6 months until the patient was 3 years of age, and yearly until she was 6 years old.

MCDK might persist without any change, increase in size, or undergo spontaneous involution. Most cases of unilateral MCDK undergo spontaneous involution.

Complications of multicystic kidney disease include hypertension and infection. The danger of malignancy in this lesion is considered remote.

The surgical treatment of MCDK should be considered in only few selected conditions: with a very large MCK (>6 cm), when the retained mass appears to be growing or not involuting, when adequate follow-up cannot be assured, when the diagnosis is in question, and if hypertension or symptoms develop.

At the age of 6 years the patient presented with hypertension and left flank pain. The mass appeared nearly unchanged on US. Therefore, the girl underwent retroperitoneoscopic nephrectomy (Fig. 4).

Q 140

Antonio Marte

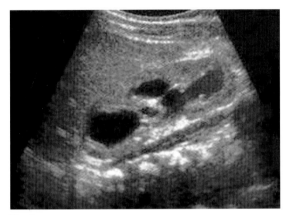

Fig. 1

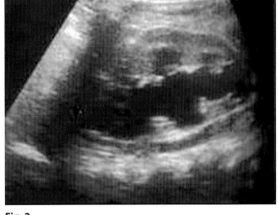

Fig. 2

A 6-year-old girl presented with a history of secondary nocturnal enuresis, urinary urgency associated with recurrent flank pain and febrile urinary tract infections (UTIs). The patient was on antibiotic prophylaxis with cotrimoxazole. The mother showed us previous examinations (Figs. 1–3).

- What do Figs. 1 and 2 show?
- What does Fig. 3 show?
- Which pathological condition is affecting this girl?
- Are other examinations necessary?
- What is the best way to manage this condition?

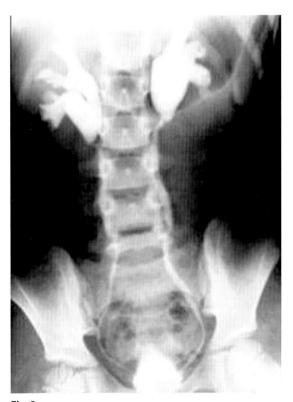

Fig. 3

A 140

This girl has a bilateral vesicoureteral reflux (VUR).

The renal sonograms (left–right) in Figs. 1, 2 show a dilatation of both pelvises.

Figure 3 is a voiding cystourethrography (VCUG) scan during the voiding stage and shows a grade-III bilateral VUR, dilation of both pelvises, and trabeculation of the bladder wall.

Because the patient has a history of recurrent UTI and urinary urgency, a DMSA nuclear scan and urodynamics were requested.

The DMSA scan (Fig. 4) shows both the kidneys scarred with central and peripheral scars.

The urodynamics demonstrates a hyperactive bladder with high waves of detrusor contraction during the bladder filling.

The girl was kept on antibiotic prophylaxis with amoxicillin-clavulanic acid and oxybutynin 0.3 mg/kg/die.

After 1 year of therapy the urinary symptoms resolved but a nuclear cystogram (Fig. 5) revealed the persistence of bilateral VUR.

The parents were offered three options: (a) to go on with continuous antibiotic therapy, (b) open bilateral reimplantation, (c) endoscopic correction of the VUR.

The parents chose the third option and the girl underwent endoscopic correction of the VUR with a bulking agent (Deflux).

Eight months later the nuclear voiding cystogram showed no reflux. The girl's nocturnal enuresis resolved but she is still taking oxybutynin for sporadic urgency.

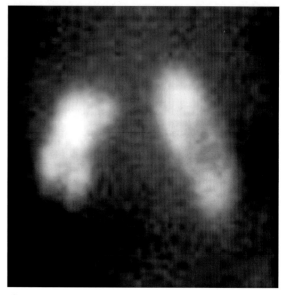

Fig. 4

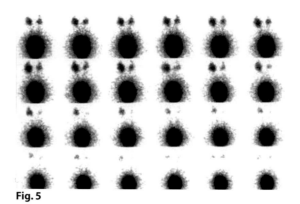

Fig. 5

Suggested Reading

1. Elder JS, Diaz M, Caldamone A, Cendron M, Greenfield S, Hurwitz R, Kirsch A, Koyle MA, Pope J, Shapiro E. Endoscopic therapy for vesicoureteral reflux: a meta-analysis. I. Reflux resolution and urinary tract infection. J Urol 2006; 175:716–22

2. Stenberg A, Hensle TW and Lackgren G. Vesicoureteral reflux: a new treatment algorithm. Curr Urol Rep 2002; 3:107–14

3. Unver T, Alpay H, Bivikli NK, Ones T. Comparison of direct radionuclide cystography and voiding cystourethrography in detecting vesicoureteral reflux. Pediatr Int 2006; 48:287–91

Q 141

Marcelo Martinez-Ferro

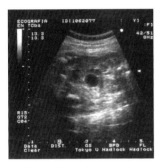

Fig. 1

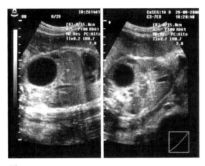

Fig. 2

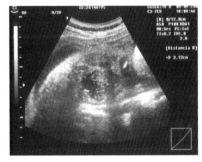

Fig. 3

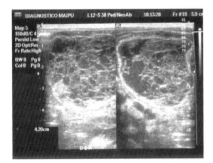

Fig. 4

On a routine prenatal ultrasound scan (Fig. 1), performed at 32 weeks, a 21-mm cystic mass lying over the urinary bladder was observed in the fetal abdomen. The rest of the fetal anatomy was normal for a female fetus and the amniotic fluid volume was also normal.

At 34 weeks (Fig. 2) the mass had doubled in volume and now measured 43 mm. Its content was liquid and completely anechogenic with thin walls. It occupied a big portion of the abdominal cavity.

At 36 weeks (Fig. 3) the mass reduced in size measuring 33 mm, but its content had turned echogenic with a fluid/debris pattern. The walls of the mass were thick and crumpled.

An immediate postnatal ultrasound revealed a 5-cm echogenic mass with multiple internal septa (Fig. 4).

- What are the possible differential diagnoses for a fetal abdominal cystic mass?

On an ultrasound scan performed at 20 weeks, the cystic mass was not seen.

- Is this possible or could it be a misdiagnosis?
- How can you explain the fact that after presenting a considerable growth, by the end of pregnancy this mass diminished in size?
- What could be the reason for the ultrasonographic (from anechogenic to echogenic with septa) changes that this mass showed?
- Would you expect to palpate this mass after birth? If so, what clinical characteristics would you expect to find during palpation?
- What is the most probable diagnostic condition?
- Would you ask for further postnatal imaging studies?
- What is the best way to manage this condition?

A 141

This patient has a prenatally diagnosed ovarian cyst.

The differential diagnoses for fetal cystic abdominal masses are: choledochal cyst, intestinal duplications, mesenteric cysts, hydronephrosis, urachal cyst, and omphalomesenteric cysts among others.

It has been proposed that placental hormone stimulation is the trigger factor that provokes follicular stimulation and growth.

There are no reports of fetal ovarian cysts before 27 gestational weeks, probably because the ovarian tissue requires some degree of maturity in order to respond to hormonal stimulation. These data together with the determination of fetal sex are important diagnostic tools that help in the differential diagnosis.

The diagnostic criteria are: (1) female fetus (2) older than 37 weeks (3) absence of urogenital and gastrointestinal anomalies, (4) presence of a cystic mass in the fetal abdominal cavity.

Depending on their ultrasound pattern, the cysts are called simple (completely anechogenic with thin walls) and complex or complicated (presence of septa, fluid/debris, calcification).

The morphological changes shown by the mass are due to its complication with torsion of the vascular pedicle and internal hemorrhage followed by necrosis. Torsion may occur in up to 50% of cases in cysts larger than 5 cm.

Figure 5 shows the size of the mass as palpated after birth. The mass could be moved all around the abdomen without resistance.

Laparoscopy is the treatment of choice for complicated cysts, as it provides diagnosis and treatment. No further imaging studies are required in this case.

Figure 6 shows the necrotic aspect of the left ovary (*Ov*) during laparoscopy. The vascular pedicle (*Ped*) was completely torted and the left tube was amputated up to the left uterine horn. In addition, the torted vascular pedicle partially occluded the sigmoid colon. The cyst was resected and excised through the umbilicus.

One-week postoperative cosmetic results were optimal after laparoscopy (Fig. 7).

Suggested Reading

1. Brandt ML, Helmrath MA. Ovarian cysts in infants and children. Semin Pediatr Surg 2005; 14:78–85

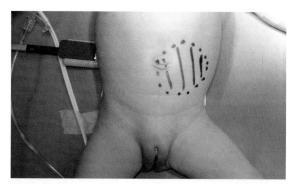

Fig. 5

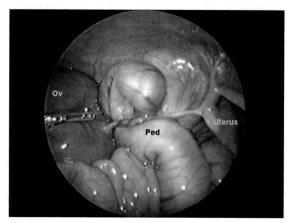

Fig. 6

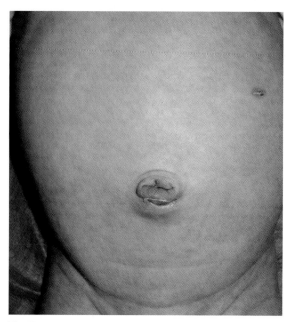

Fig. 7

Q 142

Antonio Savanelli, Salvatore Iacobelli, and Hana Dolezalova

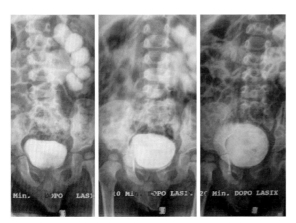

Fig. 1

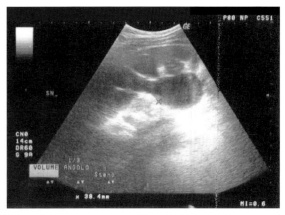

Fig. 2

A 26-month-old child presented with a 5-month history of urinary tract infections (UTIs). A US scan and a urography study were performed, shown in Figs. 1 and 2.

- What do you see in Figs. 1 and 2?
- Which procedures do you need so as to complete the diagnosis?
- What does Fig. 3 show?
- What is the differential diagnosis?
- What is your diagnosis?
- Which treatment do you prefer in this case?
- What is the follow-up?
- What does Fig. 4 show?

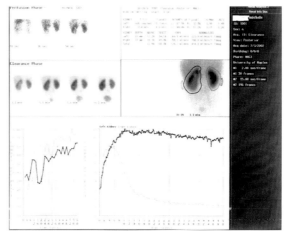

Fig. 3

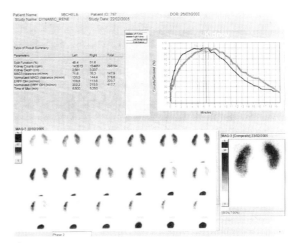

Fig.4

A 142

The diuretic urography shows, on the right, regular elimination of the contrast medium with a normal-looking pyelocaliceal system and ureter. On the left side we can see a delayed washout with hydronephrosis and no visualized ureter. After 12 h, there is persistence of contrast medium on the left side. The US scan shows a high degree of hydronephrosis on the left. The anteroposterior diameter of the pelvis measures 38 mm.

In order to complete the diagnosis, MAG-3 scintigraphy was indicated. We can see a dishomogeneous left renal perfusion and capitation with poor washout after the diuretic test. Effective renal plasma flow (ERPF) in the left kidney was 54.1%; ERPF in the right kidney was 45.9% (Fig. 3).

Unilateral hydronephrosis can be found in the following pathologies: vesicoureteral reflux, obstructive megaureter, ureterocele and ectopic ureter, and ureteropelvic junction obstruction (UPJO).

As there is no dilated ureter, the most probable diagnosis is UPJO.

The UPJO can be treated medically or surgically. Surgical indications are: symptomatic patient, UTI with fever and failure of growth, and poor renal function. Open pyeloplasty using the Anderson–Hynes dismembered pyeloplasty is still the most widely used method.

At the 6-month follow-up, we performed a US scan and dynamic scintigraphy. The last US scan shows a small hydronephrosis on the left with a normal ureter. The renal scintigram (Fig. 4) shows a renogram with a good washout after the diuretic test.

Comment: Stenosis of the pyeloureteral junction represents the most common malformation of the upper urinary tract. US scans and renal scintigraphy concur in most cases in providing a definitive diagnosis. Diuretic urography has been supplanted by scintigraphy, but is still occasionally used in the preoperative phase for a better diagnostic definition.

Suggested Reading

1. Ismail A, Elkholy A, Zaghmout O, Alkadhi A, Elnaggar O, Khairat A, Elhassanat H, Mosleh A, Hamad B, Elzomer J, Elkaabi A. Postnatal management of antenatally diagnosed ureteropelvic junction obstruction. J Ped Urol 2006; 2:163–168
2. Peters CA. Urinary tract obstruction in children. J Urol 1995; 154:1874
3. Rodriguez LV, Lock J, Kennedy WA, Shortliffe, LD. Evaluation of sonographic renal parenchymal area in the management of hydronephrosis. J Urol 2001; 165:548

Q 143

Antonio Savanelli, Emanuela Giordano, and Barbara Greco

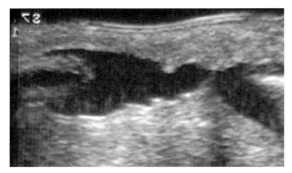

Fig. 1

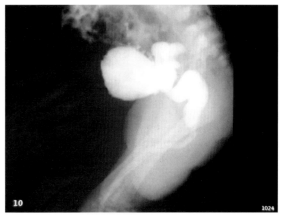

Fig. 2

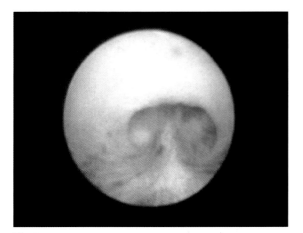

Fig. 3

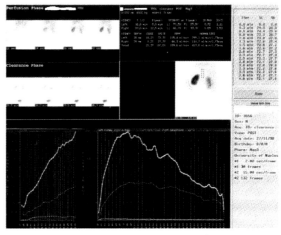

Fig. 4

A 6-day-old baby was prenatally diagnosed with hydronephrosis and bilateral megaureter. The postnatal ultrasound investigation showed the presence of a bilateral pyelocalyceal dilatation, megaureters with tortuous course, and distended bladder with thickened bladder wall (Fig. 1). Blood test results showed acute kidney failure.

- Based on Fig. 1, what could the pathological condition be?
- What is the second instrumental investigation to be performed?

- What does Fig. 2 show?
- What is the therapeutic approach?
- What does Fig. 3 show?
- What will the therapeutic approach be in the case of persistent acute kidney failure or eventual complications?
- What is the follow-up for this condition?
- What does Fig. 4 show?

A 143

Hydronephrosis and bilateral megaureter suggest the presence of several pathologies: vesicoureteral reflux (VUR), bilateral obstructive megaureter, and posterior urethral valves (PUVs). The finding of a distended bladder with thickened bladder wall on the ultrasound scan suggests the presence of cervical–ureteral obstructive pathology as well as PUVs (Fig. 1). PUV is a congenital condition that occurs only in boys and consists in a situation where the urethral valves, which are small leaflets of tissue, have a narrow, slit-like opening that partially impedes urine outflow. In fact, this pathological condition represents the most common cause of severe congenital obstruction of the lower urinary tract. When there are PUVs the ultrasound scan, occasionally, shows a dilated posterior urethra or bright kidneys with loss of corticomedullary differentiation.

The second instrumental investigation is the *micturating cystourethrogram (MCUG)*. This diagnostic test may be performed via urethral or suprapubic catheter and requires the introduction of iodate intravenous urography agents into the bladder. Radiographs are taken when the bladder is full and while the patient passes urine. The position and integrity of the bladder and the urethra are clearly shown during this examination. MCUG is very important in analyzing the evacuation of the bladder and the filling of the urethra and in searching for a possible VUR, bladder outline, or a dilated obstructed posterior urethra.

Figure 2 shows the patient's MCUG with PUVs: the bladder dilatation and anomalies, such as bladder diverticula, and a very large ectasia of the posterior urethra are seen. There is no presence of VUR.

When planning the therapy, first of all, it is important to pay attention to the young patient's fluid and the electrolyte and acid-base balance. It is also important to achieve an adequate provisional urinary drainage by inserting a fine urethral catheter and, subsequently, to ablate the valve through a diagnostic and therapeutic cystoscopy.

Figure 3 shows the results of the *cystoscopic investigation*. A small cystoscope is introduced in the urethral external meatus up to the urethra and, when possible, in the bladder. In the present case, there is the presence of a perforated urethral membrane below the verumonta-

num in the posterior urethra (type III valves according to Young's classification; believed to originate from incomplete canalization between the anterior and posterior urethra) (Fig. 3).

In the case of complications or no improvement, it will be necessary to perform *vesicostomy*.

The patient is monitored with:

(a) Laboratory tests to check the renal function.
(b) Ultrasound of the loins and urinary tracts after 6 months to check the dilatation of the upper urinary tracts.
(c) MCUG after 6 months to check the urethral gauge or the persistence of PUVs after ablation.
(d) Renal scintigraphy (diuresis renography), which is a valuable tool in the evaluation of renal function and washout, once the patient is 1 month older.
(e) Urodynamic testing, which is a functional test of the bladder and bladder outlet function. It is very important to perform this test in order to check for the eventual presence of urinary incontinence, which occurs in patients treated by valve ablation with an incidence of 13%–38%.

Figure 4 shows the *renal scintigraphy* after the treatment of the PUVs.

Diuresis renography should be performed only when the patient is at least 1 month old. ^{99m}Tc MAG-3 is the recommended radiopharmaceutical, at a dose of 1.85 MBq/kg (50 µCi/kg) and a minimum dosage of 37 MBq (1 mCi). ^{99m}Tc MAG-3 yields higher extraction from the kidneys than ^{99m}Tc DTPA, which is another less preferred agent used in diuresis renography. Renal uptake by ^{99m}Tc MAG-3 is 55% compared with 20% uptake by ^{99m}Tc DTPA. This higher extraction results in better images for qualitative and quantitative analysis, and this is of particular benefit in the pediatric period, when renal function is immature. In this case the MAG-3 scan shows normal renal function of the left kidney and a decrease in the function of the right side (Fig. 4).

In *urodynamic testing* the bladder has a good capacity with a good compliance: max. vol. 186 ml; leak point pressure (LPP) 30 cm H_2O; max. pressure of emptying 50 cm H_2O.

Suggested Reading

1. Gatti JM, Kirsch AJ. Posterior urethral valve. Pre and postnatal management. Current Urology Reports 2001; 2:138
2. Glassberg KI. The valve bladder syndrome: 20 years later. J Urol 2001; 166:1406
3. Lopez Pereira P, Martinez Urrutia Mj, Espinosa L et al. Bladder dysfunction as a prognostic factor in patients with posterior urethral valves. BJU International 2002; 90:308

Q 144

Bruno Cigliano

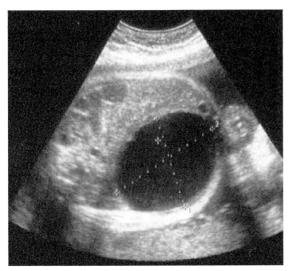

Fig. 1

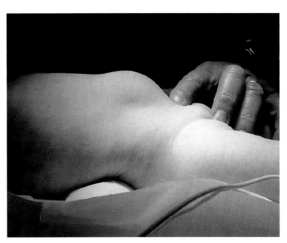

Fig. 2

A full-term female newborn had a large intra-abdominal cystic lesion, which was detected on ultrasound performed during the third trimester of pregnancy (Fig. 1). At birth, her abdomen was distended (Fig. 2) and a large soft mass was palpable. Ultrasound was performed showing a large cystic mass containing a smaller cystic lesion, with no relationship with the kidneys, liver, or spleen (Fig. 3). An intestinal duplication was suspected and a pediatric surgeon was called to evaluate her condition.

- What does Fig. 3 show?
- What is the possible diagnosis in this baby?
- What other diagnostic examinations do you recommend to establish a correct diagnosis?
- What is the most appropriate management in this case?

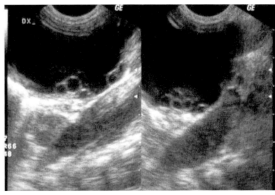

Fig. 3

A 144

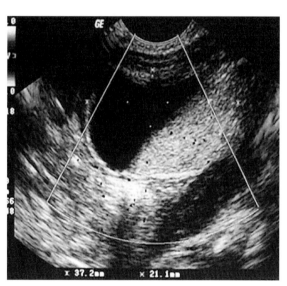

Fig. 4

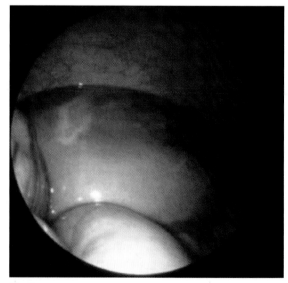

Fig. 5

Fig. 6

Figure 3 shows a large cystic lesion in the abdomen that has no relationship with the kidneys, liver, or spleen. There are various diagnostic possibilities (mesenteric cyst, urachal cyst, intestinal duplication, ovarian cyst etc.), but the presence of the "daughter sign" is strongly suggestive of an ovarian cyst.

Ovarian cysts are the most common intraperitoneal masses found in female newborns.

The management of these lesions depends on their dimension, evolution, and ultrasonographic appearance.

Ultrasonography is generally sufficient for diagnosis; it is also accurate in predicting complicated cases and is recommended for monitoring spontaneous resolution. Usually, cysts that are 4–5 cm in diameter or larger, not decreasing in size, or complicated (Fig. 4) are treated. Treatment may consist of US-guided needle aspiration, surgery (Fig. 5), or laparoscopy (Fig. 6). Laparoscopic treatment is a safe and quick technique in neonates and in our opinion is the best treatment.

Q 145

Craig T. Albanese

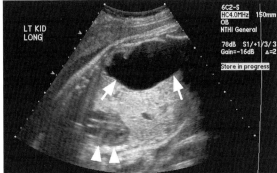

Fig. 1

Fig. 2

A routine prenatal ultrasound at 18 weeks' gestation was performed. The left kidney (*arrows*) is pictured (Fig. 1) as is the fetal heart (*arrowheads*).

- What are the findings?

Figure 2 is another view of the kidney (*between arrows*). MR imaging was performed (Fig. 3), showing the fetal kidney (*arrow*) and lung (*asterisk*).

- What is the diagnosis?

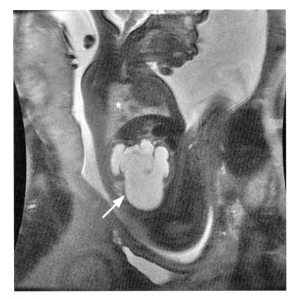

Fig. 3

A 145

This child has a unilateral ureteropelvic junction (UPJ) obstruction. There is marked hydronephrosis. Since it was unilateral, there was no impact on amniotic fluid production (i.e., there was no oligohydramnios).

The child underwent a dismembered pyeloplasty at 4 months of life.

Suggested Reading

1. Boubaker A, Prior JO, Meyrat B, Bischof Delaloye A, McAleer IM, Frey P. Unilateral ureteropelvic junction obstruction in children: long-term follow-up after unilateral pyeloplasty. J Urol 2003 Aug; 170(2 Pt 1):575–9

2. Perez-Brayfield MR, Kirsch AJ, Jones RA, Grattan-Smith JD. A prospective study comparing ultrasound, nuclear scintigraphy and dynamic contrast enhanced magnetic resonance imaging in the evaluation of hydronephrosis. J Urol 2003 Oct; 170(4 Pt 1):1330–4

3. Rodriguez LV, Spielman D, Herfkens RJ, Shortliffe LD. Magnetic resonance imaging for the evaluation of hydronephrosis, reflux and renal scarring in children. J Urol 2001 Sep; 166(3):1023–7

Q 146

François Becmeur

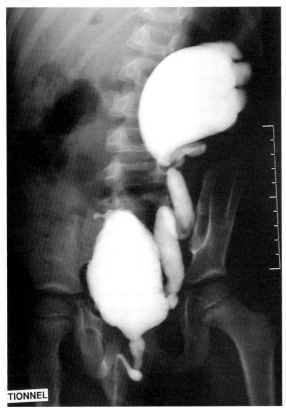
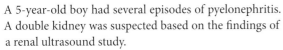

Fig. 1

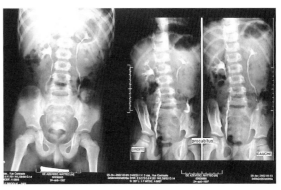

Fig. 2

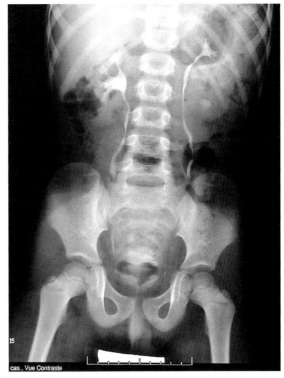

Fig. 3

A 5-year-old boy had several episodes of pyelonephritis. A double kidney was suspected based on the findings of a renal ultrasound study.

Cystography (Fig. 1) was performed. The pediatrician asked for intravenous urography (Figs. 2–5) in order to complete the data acquired from the renal ultrasound (Fig. 6). Finally, a DMSA renal scan was necessary to specify the functional characteristics of each kidney (Fig. 7).

- Describe the figures.
- Which therapeutic approach do you propose?

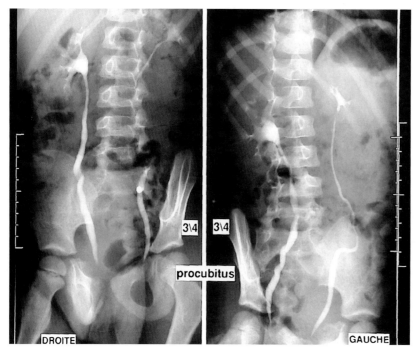

Fig. 4

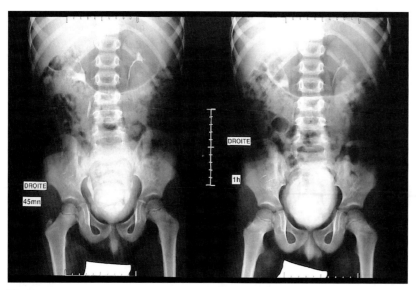

Fig. 5

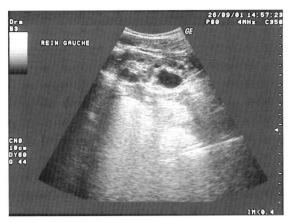

Fig. 6

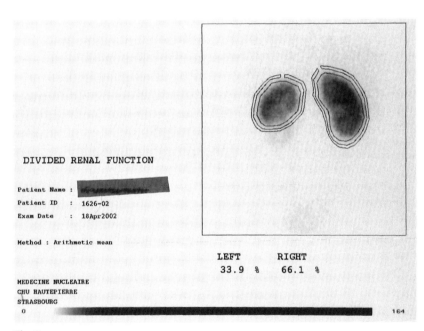

Fig. 7

A 146

The micturating cystography shows the existence of a major vesicoureteral reflux on the left side of the lower pole.

It was important to know whether the lower left renal pole was functional. The answer would determine the choice of treatment. Indeed, if the lower pole were functional, a preserving treatment should be proposed: medical, endoscopic, or surgical. To specify the functional anatomy of the kidneys, the pediatrician decided to perform intravenous urography and renal scanning with DMSA.

Intravenous urography makes it possible to assess, during the first minutes of the examination, a functional right kidney and a functional upper left pole. The late opacification (45 min and 1 h) of the lower pole was due to retrograde flow because of vesicorenal reflux. The renal DMSA scan confirms the absence of functionality of the left lower pole.

Left lower polar nephrectomy is the only treatment indicated for this child. Partial nephrectomy can be carried out by retroperitoneoscopy.

Suggested Reading

1. Blumenthal I. Vesicoureteric reflux and urinary tract infection in children. Postgrad Med J 2006 Jan; 82(963):31–5
2. Darge K, Riedmiller H. Current status of vesicoureteral reflux diagnosis.World J Urol 2004 Jun; 22(2):88–95
3. Garin EH, Olavarria F, Garcia Nieto V, Valenciano B, Campos A, Young L. Clinical significance of primary vesicoureteral reflux and urinary antibiotic prophylaxis after acute pyelonephritis: a multicenter, randomized, controlled study. Pediatrics 2006 Mar; 117(3):626–32
4. Heidenreich A, Ozgur E, Becker T, Haupt G. Surgical management of vesicoureteral reflux in pediatric patients. World J Urol 2004 Jun; 22(2):96–106
5. Riccabona M, Fotter R. Modern imaging technology for childhood urinary tract infection Radiologe 2005 Dec; 45(12):1078–8

Q 147

François Becmeur

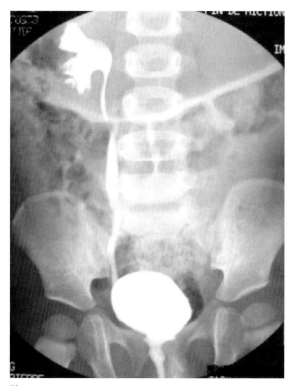

Fig. 1

Fig. 2

A 7-year-old girl had a fever of 39.5°C, right lumbar pains, and burning micturition.

- Which examinations do you suggest in emergency?
- Which treatment do you propose?

During the last 3 years, the child had several episodes of fever.

- What is the probable cause?
- What do you see on the retrograde cystogram (Fig. 1)?
- How can you evaluate the repercussions of this pathological condition on renal function (Fig. 2)?
- Which treatment do you propose for this condition?
- What is its effect on renal function?

A 147

This girl probably has acute pyelonephritis.

In emergency, urine analysis and renal ultrasound must be performed. The diagnosis of pyelonephritis will be confirmed by urine culture and the bacteria will be identified; ultrasonography will eliminate renal abscess, lithiasis, or hydronephrosis.

For antibiotic treatment, intravenous antibiotic therapy is indicated consisting in beta-lactamine+aminosides for 48 h, followed by oral administration according to the antibiogram for 10 days.

Vesicoureteral reflux must be investigated with retrograde cystography.

The cystography shows a grade-3 vesicoureteral reflux in the inferior pole with a complete ureteric duplication on the right.

Renal function can be evaluated by a renal DMSA scan, which in this case shows a relative function of 36% on the right kidney and of 64% on the left one. We observed the late effects of pyelonephritis of the inferior third of the right kidney.

Surgical treatment of the reflux either by endoscopic or by a ureterovesical reimplantation is indicated. For this treatment, we recommend certain hygienic and dietetic measures with abundant drink and regular micturition in the course of the day.

The function of the right kidney will not recover, but should remain stable if the patient does not have any episodes of UTI.

Suggested Reading

1. Capdevila Cogul E, Martin Ibanez I, Mainou Cid C, Toral Rodriguez E, Cols Roig Mf, Agut Quijano T, Caritg Bosch J, Camarasa Pique F. First urinary tract infection in healthy infants: epidemiology, diagnosis and treatment An Esp Pediatr 2001 Oct; 55(4):310–4

2. Halevy R, Smolkin V, Bykov S, Chervinsky L, Sakran W, Koren A. Power Doppler ultrasonography in the diagnosis of acute childhood pyelonephritis. Pediatr Nephrol 2004 Sep; 19(9):987–91

3. Kirsch AJ, Grattan-Smith JD, Molitierno JA Jr. The role of magnetic resonance imaging in pediatric urology. Curr Opin Urol 2006 Jul; 16(4):283–90

4. de La Vaissiere B, Castello B, Quinet B, Cohen R, Grimprel E. Management of acute pyelonephritis in patients older than 3 months: survey conducted in 39 paediatric emergency departments of the Ile de France Region in 2004 Arch Pediatr 2006 Mar; 13(3):245–50

5. Lin KY, Chiu NT, Chen MJ, Lai CH, Huang JJ, Wang YT, Chiou YY. Acute pyelonephritis and sequelae of renal scar in pediatric first febrile urinary tract infection. Pediatr Nephrol 2003 Apr; 18(4):362–5

Q 148

Antonio Savanelli, Francesca Alicchio, and Pier Francesco Rambaldi

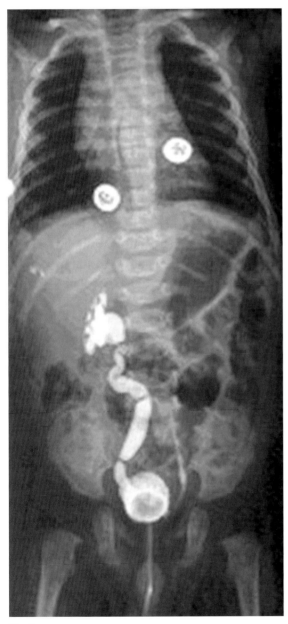

Fig. 1

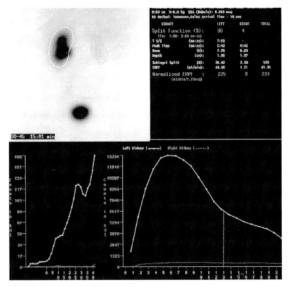

Fig. 2

A 15-day-old baby presented with loss of weight and urinary tract infection (UTI). On the ultrasound scan, only a reduction in the volume of the right kidney was evident without dilatation of the urinary tract.

- Which diagnosis is suspected?
- Which instrumental examination could be performed?
- What does Fig. 1 show?
- What is the treatment for vesicoureteral reflux (VUR) in the newborn and what does Fig. 2 show?
- What do you think the next step in follow-up should be?

The patient, at 16 months of age, continued to have insufficient weight gain and recurrent UTI.

- Which treatment should be indicated?

A 148

The patient could be affected by a congenital bilateral VUR.

This condition represents the most frequent uropathy in the pediatric age. It can be either primitive due to a congenital malformation or a delay of development of the vesicoureteral junction or secondary due to anatomical or functional vesical or ureteral factors.

In 26% of cases, the antenatal ultrasound does not show dilatation of the upper urinary tract.

The examination in Fig. 1 is a cystourethrogram (CUGM) that shows bilateral VUR of a severe degree on the right and moderated degree on the left.

The treatment of VUR in a baby comprises antibiotic prophylaxis of UTI. The examination in Fig. 2 shows a renal scintigram with MAG-3 that demonstrates a remarkable reduction in right renal function.

The next diagnostic step in the follow-up is nuclear cystography, which in this case demonstrates the same situation, and renal scintigraphy with MAG-3 confirms the finding of a nonfunctioning right kidney (Fig. 3).

Surgical treatment is indicated. We performed right retroperitoneoscopic nephrectomy (Fig. 4) and endoscopic treatment of the VUR by Deflux (Fig. 5).

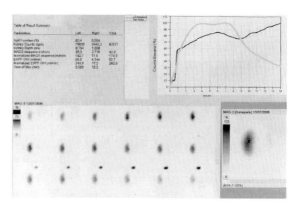

Fig. 3

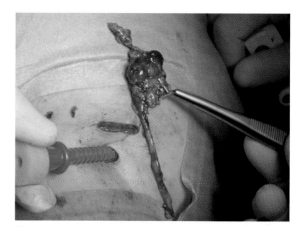

Fig. 4

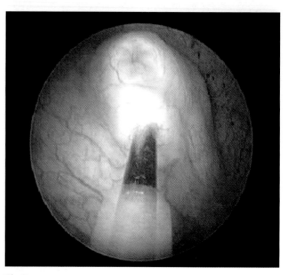

Fig.5

Suggested Reading

1. Badwan KH, Diamond DA. Vesicoureteral reflux: diagnosis and management. J Med Liban 2005 Apr–Jun; 53(2):61–5
2. Bhide A, Sairam S, Farrugia MK, Boddy SA, Thilaganathan B. The sensitivity of antenatal ultrasound for predicting renal tract surgery in early childhood. Ultrasound Obstet Gynecol 2005 May; 25(5):489–92
3. Cohen AL, Rivara FP, Davis R, Christakis DA. Compliance with guidelines for the medical care of first urinary tract infections in infants: a population-based study. Pediatrics 2005 Jun; 115(6):1474–8
4. Dillon MJ, Goonasekera CD. Reflux nephropathy J Am Soc Nephrol 1998 Dec; 9(12):2377–83
5. Smellie JM, Barratt TM, Chantler C, Gordon I, Prescod NP, Ransley PG, Woolf AS. Medical versus surgical treatment in children with severe bilateral vesicoureteric reflux and bilateral nephropathy: a randomised rial. Lancet 2001 Apr 28; 357(9265):1329–33

Q 149

Antonio Savanelli, Barbara Greco, and Concetta De Luca

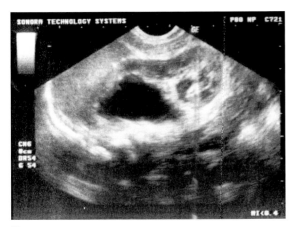

Fig. 1

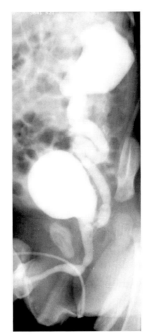

Fig. 2

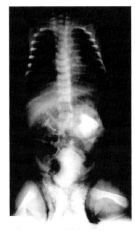

Fig. 3

A newborn was antenatally diagnosed with a renal cyst of the upper renal pole. The perinatal ultrasound showed a left ureteral duplication with dilatation of the ureteral and upper segment system.

- What does the ultrasound (Fig. 1) show?
- What is the possible diagnosis?

- What other examinations are necessary?
- What does Fig. 2 show?
- What does Fig. 3 show?
- What is the final diagnosis?
- What is the treatment?
- What is the follow-up?

A 149

The ultrasound (Fig. 1) shows a duplex kidney with dilatation of the upper left segment. Dilatation of the upper tract in ureteral duplication and a normal lower urinary tract are compatible with the diagnosis of ectopic ureter and ureterocele. The absence of a ureterocele in the bladder on the ultrasound scan confirms the diagnostic suspicion of ectopic ureter. Today, ultrasound may be able to trace the ureter into the pelvis and into an abnormally low position beyond the bladder.

In this case, we needed to perform voiding cystourethrography, excretory urography with renography, and cystoscopy.

The cystography shows reflux in the left ectopic ureter. The cystoscopy demonstrates the ectopic ureter.

Figure 3 shows a urogram. A normal right kidney and left duplex kidney can be seen. The ureter and the upper pelvis are dilated.

The diagnosis is refluxing ectopic ureter in the left duplex kidney.

Management of the upper segment of the ectopic renoureteral unit most often involves surgical treatment. The procedure is dependent on the function of the ectopic segment. In this case, a pyeloureterostomy (upper segment ureter to lower segment pelvis) was preferred over partial nephrectomy, and partial left ureterectomy was performed. The distal ureteral stump should be left as short as possible.

Follow-up includes ultrasound, cystography, and a MAG-3 renogram at 6 months.

At follow-up the patient showed an improved dilatation of the upper pelvis and persistent refluxing ureteral stump, which had determined a UTI. The reflux into the refluxing ectopic ureteral stump (Fig. 4) was treated successfully by endoscopic injection of macroplastic material.

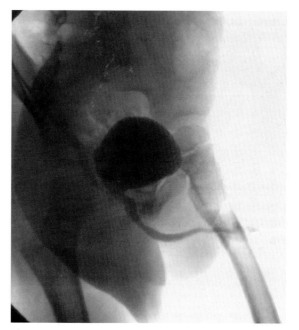

Fig. 4

Suggested Reading

1. Bieri M, Smith CK, Smith AY, Borden TA. Ipsilateral uretero-ureterostomy for vesicoureteral reflux in duplicated ureters. J Urol 1998; 159:3,1016

2. De Caluwe D, Chertin B, Puri P. Long-term outcome of the retained ureteral stump after lower pole heminephrectomy in duplex kidneys. Eur Urol 2002; 42(1):63

3. el Ghoneimi A, Miranda J, Truong T, Monfort G. Ectopic ureter with complete ureteric duplication: conservative surgical treatment. J Pediatr Surg 1996, 31:467

Q 150

Brice Antao and Azad Najmaldin

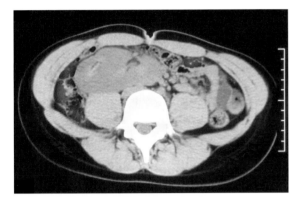

Fig. 1

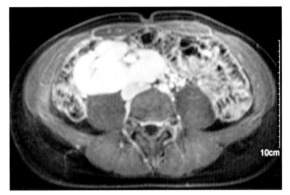

Fig. 2

A 15-year-old girl presented to the Accident and Emergency department with sudden onset of right-sided abdominal pain. She was known to have an antenatal diagnosis of solitary right kidney. On examination she was pyrexial at 38°C and had a tender palpable mass on the right side of her abdomen.

- What is the differential diagnosis?
- What initial investigations would you request?
- What are the findings in Fig. 1 that support the diagnosis?
- What is the investigation shown in Figs. 2 and 3, and why was it performed?
- What is the diagnosis and how do you manage this condition?
- What are the potential complications of this condition and how can these be managed?

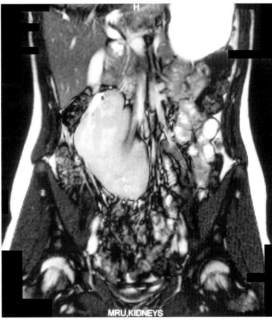

Fig. 3

A 150

The differential diagnoses include appendix mass, mass associated with Crohn's disease, intestinal duplication cyst, hepatobiliary mass, torted ovarian cyst, pyelonephritis, hydronephrosis, obstructing urinary calculi, infected lymphatic cysts, and tumors.

A baseline blood and urine analysis may prove helpful. The patient had a high white blood cell count and C-reactive protein and her urine analysis confirmed a coliform infection. Ultrasonography is easily available, noninvasive, and often informative. Figure 4 confirmed an absent left kidney and an abnormally long and enlarged right renal mass and an unusual but nondilated collecting system. No other abnormality was identified in the abdomen and pelvis.

A CT scan of the abdomen (Fig. 1) clearly demonstrated features of a cross-fused renal ectopia in the right side of abdomen and no other abnormalities.

Figures 2 and 3 are MR urography images. This investigation provides anatomical and functional evaluation of the urinary tract in a single examination without the use of ionizing radiations. T2 sequences in coronal and axial section with contrast enhancement demonstrated a cross-fused ectopia. The right moiety lies superior–laterally, while the left moiety which lies inferior–medially has a bifid collecting system. There is no evidence of hydroureter or hydronephrosis.

The diagnosis is an infected right crossed renal ectopia. The management is conservative and includes: intravenous antibiotics, possible intravenous fluids, analgesia, and close monitoring (pulse, respiration, urine output, degree of pain, tenderness and size of the mass). Repeat ultrasonography is also used to monitor progress. The patient responded well to the above regimen and was allowed home after 4 days. She was reviewed in the clinic with repeat ultrasonography after a few days, weeks, and months.

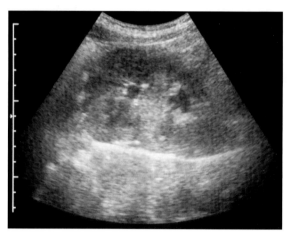

Fig. 4

The potential complications include recurrent infection and scaring. Malignancy has also been reported, albeit sporadically. Regular ultrasonography to monitor the size of the collecting system and ureter may prove helpful in the long term. A DMSA scan may be necessary to assess scaring and function. An isotope micturating cystourethrogram or a formal contrast cystogram with or without cystoscopy will add more information and exclude vesicoureteric reflux as an associated problem. An acutely infected kidney associated with significant hydronephrosis may require percutaneous drainage. Subsequent surgery will depend on whether or not the patient remains symptomatic or has associated problems such as obstruction, reflux, or a nonfunctioning symptomatic moiety.

Suggested Reading

1. Grattan-Smith JD, Perez-Bayfield MR, Jones RA, et al. MR imaging of kidneys: functional evaluation using F-15 perfusion imaging. Pediatr Radiol 2003; 33:293–304

2. Stimac G, Dimanovski J, Ruzic B, Spajic B, Kraus O. Tumors in kidney fusion anomalies-report of five cases and review of the literature. Scand J Urol Nephrol 2004; 38(6):485–9

3. Taweel W, Sripathi V, Ahmed S. Crossed fused renal ectopia with hydronephrosis. Aust NZ J Surg 1998; 68(11):808–9

Q 151

Gianluca Terrin, Annalisa Passariello, and Hana Dolezalova

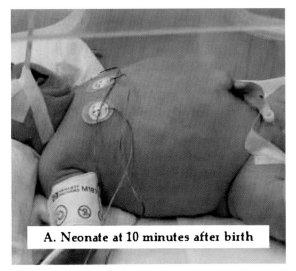

A. Neonate at 10 minutes after birth

Fig. 1a

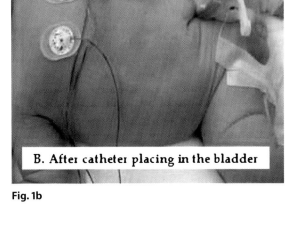

B. After catheter placing in the bladder

Fig. 1b

A routine prenatal ultrasound scan performed at 20 weeks' gestational age on a consanguineous 31-year-old woman (gravida 1) revealed marked bladder distension, hydroureteronephrosis, polyhydramnios, and ascites. A dilated posterior urethra was not identified on subsequent ultrasound studies. Two in-utero bladder evacuative punctures were performed during pregnancy. A normal 46 XX karyotype was detected at amniocentesis. The maternal Coombs test was negative.

- In this case, is it possible to distinguish obstructive from nonobstructive in-utero bladder distension?
- What is megacystis microcolon intestinal hypoperistalsis syndrome (MMIHS)?

The neonate was born at 35 weeks (birth weight 4,350 g). Physical examination showed laxity of the abdominal musculature and a renal bladder ultrasound revealed megacystis with bilateral hydroureteronephrosis. Shortly after delivery the child required intubation and mechanical ventilation (Fig. 1). After placing a catheter in the bladder, more than 800 ml of urine was drained and re-inspection of the abdominal wall revealed a prune aspect (Fig. 2). The cyst rapidly refilled after aspiration. Acute renal failure was observed. Oral feeding was started on day 1 of life and suspended on day 7 for feeding intolerance. A urinary and gastrointestinal tract radiological examination was performed.

- What do Figs. 2–4 show?

This clinical condition suggests a diagnosis of MMIH syndrome such as prune belly syndrome (PBS).

- Describes the main features used to distinguish between these two entities.

Bladder distension persisted, associated with recurrent urinary tract infections. Enteral feeding intolerance persisted and total parenteral nutrition was adopted. On day 28 the presence of intestinal malrotation was diagnosed by a laparoscopic procedure. Subsequently, vesicostomy and correction of an intestinal malrotation were performed. Histological examination showed a normal number of ganglia in the autonomic intestinal plexus and normal acetylcholinesterase staining. Inadequate bladder specimens were obtained.

- Is it possible to differentiate MMIHS from PBS on the basis of the intestinal histological examination?
- Describe the prognosis of MMIHS.

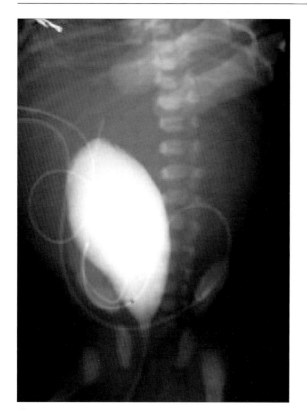

Fig. 2

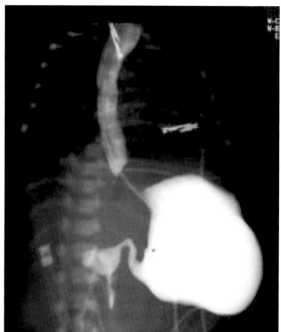

Fig. 3

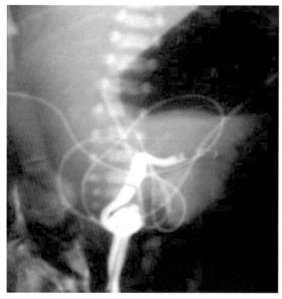

Fig. 4

A 151

Congenital anomalies of the genitourinary system are detected in about 1:500 fetuses during routine prenatal ultrasound screening. The bladder forms one of the most readily identified structures in the fetus and is seen at 12 weeks of gestation. Prenatal differentiation between obstructive and nonobstructive megacystis is mainly based on the amount of amniotic fluid, renal echogenicity, and bladder wall thickness. The presence of oligohydramnios, progressive bladder wall thickening, and dilated posterior urethra is suggestive of obstructive uropathy (e.g., urethra valves). A normal amount of amniotic fluid suggests a nonobstructive bladder distention. Nonobstructive forms of megacystis are seen in isolated congenital megacystis, in nonrefluxing–nonobstructive megaureter–megacystis, and in MMIHS. The former, in this clinical setting, is the most probable diagnostic hypothesis, because the presence of polyhydramnios suggests an intestinal implication.

MMIHS is an inherited disorder transmitted in an autosomal recessive fashion, causing a functional obstruction of both the gastrointestinal and genitourinary tracts. Polyhydramnios is the major prenatal feature indicating gut involvement. Recent evidence suggests that MMIHS is a result of the functional deficiency of the α-3 or β2/β4 subunits of the nicotinic-acetylcholine receptor (nAChR) in peripheral autonomic and enteric ganglia. A defective cholinergic signal determines the fate of a functional bladder and intestinal hypoperistalsis and, additionally, the α-3 subunits seem to be involved in direct cell-to-cell communication during fetal maturation and differentiation of the involved organs.

Figure 2 shows an enlarged bladder without reflux, while Fig. 3 demonstrates a dilated stomach associated with delayed gastric emptying time. Figure 4 shows a dilated stomach and narrow microcolon.

Findings in PBS and MMIHS may overlap. PBS, which usually presents in male infants, is characterized by the triad of laxity of the abdominal wall musculature, hydroureteronephrosis, and cryptorchidism. In females, as in males in whom not all of the triad is present, the condition is referred to as pseudo-PBS. In PBS the bladder is capacious and urethral abnormalities with an obstructive enlarged bladder may coexist. Intestinal malrotation and Hirschsprung's disease have been described in association with PBS. The current hypothesis regarding the etiopathogenesis of PBS proposes a mesodermal arrest between the 6th and 10th weeks of gestation or an in utero urethral obstruction. Consequently, fetal megacystis development determines the increase of intra-abdominal pressure that induces laxity of the abdominal musculature and a defect of intestinal fixation and rotation.

Pathological findings in MMIHS vary considerably and include changes of the neural tissue and muscle of the bowel wall. This variability may be due to the focal nature of some of the pathological findings reported or may reflect pathological heterogeneity within MMIHS. More recently, a marked reduction of contractile and cytoskeleton proteins in smooth muscle cells combined with reduced expression of intramuscular interstitial cells of Cajal, pacemaker cells coordinating intestinal motility, in the gut were reported. Excessive smooth muscle glycogen storage and vacuolar degeneration on histological bladder examination of patients affected by MMIHS were also described. Interestingly, in both syndromes abundant fibrocytes and collagen are present in the gastrointestinal tract; moreover, in PBS excessive fibrous tissue associated with both increased musculature and defective or dysplastic muscles of the urinary tract have been identified. Immunohistochemical and ultrastructural studies on urinary tract smooth muscle cells in patients with PBS have not been reported.

The prognosis in MMIHS is generally poor. To date, up to about 10% of children have survived and the majority required total parenteral nutrition. Postoperative complications, sepsis, and liver failure are the most common causes of death. Intestinal transplantation was adopted in a limited number of cases of MMIHS. The prenatal diagnosis of this condition remains a challenge, and the contribution of prenatal ultrasound is limited. Recently, digestive enzyme measurement of the amniotic fluid has been proposed to differentiate MMIHS from other forms of megacystis during the prenatal period. Molecular genetics may contribute significantly to the prenatal diagnosis and to familial counseling. High-frequency polymorphisms in neuronal nicotinic acetylcholine receptor genes have been reported. Although no loss-of-function mutations have been identified, these genes remain strong candidates for involvement in MMIHS.

Suggested Reading

1. Lev-Lehman E, Bercovich D, Xu W, Stokton DW, Beaudet A. Characterization of the human β-4 nAChR gene and polymorphisms in CHRNA3 and CHRNB4. J Hum Genet 2001; 46:362–66

2. Levin TL, Soghier L, Blitman NM, Vega-Rich C, Nafday S. Megacystis-microcolon intestinal hypoperistalsis and prune belly: overlapping syndromes. Pediatr Radiol 2004; 34:995–98

3. McHugo J, Whittle M. Enlarged fetal bladders: aetiology, management and outcome Prenatal Diagn 2001; 21:958–63

4. Richardson CE, Morgan JM, Jasani B, Green JT, Rhodes J, Williams GT, Lindstrom J, Wonnacott S, Thomas GAO, Smith V. Megacystis-microcolon intestinal hypoperistalsis syndrome and the absence of the α3 nicotinic acetylcholine receptor subunit. Gastroenterology 2001; 121:350–57

5. White SM, Chamberlain P, Hitchcock R, Sullivan PB, Boyd PA. Megacystis-microcolon intestinal hypoperistalsis syndrome: the difficulties with antenatal diagnosis. Case report and review of the literature. Prenatal Diagn 2000; 20:697–700

5

Cardiovascular Disorders

Introduction

A congenital heart defect (CHD) is an abnormality that is present at birth. Congenital heart surgery was practiced before the heart–lung machine was developed as surgeons started to work on abnormalities of the arteries of the heart. Dr. John Streider at the Massachusetts General Hospital in Boston tied off a patent ductus arteriosus in a child on 6 March 1937.

The human heart begins to develop at the end of the first month of fetal life and takes about another 8 weeks before it resembles an adult heart. During this period, about 8 out of every 1,000 newborns develop some form of congenital heart defect ranging from very mild to quite severe. The incidence of CHD ranges between 2.5% and 12%, being one of the most common congenital anomalies in human beings. Of these, ventricular septal defects and atrial septal defects are the most frequently diagnosed, with about 15.6/10,000 birth survivors in the former, and around 4/10,000 in the latter. However, the real incidence of CHD seems to be higher, according to data that 10%–25% of fetal deaths are due to CHD.

The exact cause of CHD is unknown, but recent information suggests there may be genetic influences involved. In some cases, they are associated with other medical conditions, such as the mother contracting German measles (rubella) while pregnant. It has been estimated that 25% of CHD cases are encountered within complex congenital syndromes, and the cause of CHD can be attributed to the pathogenetic factor responsible for the syndrome; almost 6% of CHDs are due to environmental teratogenic factors; finally, metabolic diseases and collagenopathies of the mother are frequently encountered in CHD. However, the vast majority of CHD cases still do not have a clarified complex etiopathogenesis, in which genetic, environmental, and maternal factors are implicated.

CHDs are traditionally classified into five general groups:

1. CHDs with excessive pulmonary blood flow: these diseases are characterized by a left-to-right shunt of a variable quantity of circulating blood, due to an anomalous intra- and/or extracardiac connection between the systemic and pulmonary circulation. This results in an augmented pulmonary flow with right and then left chamber overload, depending on the site of the anomalous connection, the age of the diagnosis, and the presence of hypertensive pulmonary disease (e.g., atrial septal defects, anomalous pulmonary venous return, ventricular septal defect, patent ductus arteriosus, atrioventricular septal defects, aortopulmonary window, truncus arteriosus).

2. CHDs with reduced pulmonary blood flow: these are characterized by a reduced pulmonary flow, secondary to a right ventricular obstruction, with arterial hypo-oxygenation directly related to the degree of pulmonary flow reduction (e.g., tetralogy of Fallot, Ebstein disease).

3. CHD with parallel circulations: in these pathological conditions, unoxygenated systemic venous return directly enters into the systemic arterial circulation, whereas oxygenated pulmonary return re-enters into the pulmonary bed. A typical example is the transposition of the great arteries, in which the aorta arises from the right ventricle, and the pulmonary trunk from the left ventricle. In these cases, survival is warranted by the presence of an anomalous communication between the two circulations, aimed at ensuring an adequate mixing between oxygenated and unoxygenated blood. The greater the communication, the higher the mixing and the capability to prolong survival. These CHD cases are commonly associated with other types of CHD, which involve the sites of the mixing, such as a patent ductus arteriosus, an atrial septal defect, and sometimes a ventricular septal defect.

4. Ductus-dependent CHDs: all CHDs with severe obstructions to the right or left ventricular flow, therefore requiring a patent ductus to assure an adequate pulmonary or systemic flow (e.g., critical aortic valve stenosis, critical pulmonary valve stenosis, severe aortic coarctation, pulmonary atresia, aortic arch interruption).

5. CHDs with ventricular outflow obstructions: all the CHDs in which the symptoms depend on the presence of an obstruction, at different levels, to the right or left ventricular flow. However, in these cases the degree of obstruction is not so dependent on a patent ductus to have a sufficient pulmonary or systemic flow. These obstructions cause a pressure overload to the involved ventricle. (e.g., noncritical pulmonary and aortic valve stenosis, supravalvular and subvalvular aortic stenoses, aortic coarctation).

Some CHDs are diagnosed shortly after birth or even while the fetus is in the uterus by using ultrasound or echocardiography. They may be diagnosed later when the child is of school age, or in rare circumstances, the congenital cardiac defect remains hidden until adulthood. If one omits all patients born before 1990 and those not diagnosed in the first year of life, assuming stable mortality in early adulthood, nearly 760,000 adults will have CHD by 2020.

When signs or symptoms of CHD are considered, one indicator of some types of CHD in a newborn is a faint bluish color of the skin. Some children with heart defects may not thrive, and many suffer from congested lungs, which may be related to heart failure. However, the two main signs raising suspicion for CHD are cyanosis and congestive heart failure. Congestive heart failure is responsible for delayed growth, fatigue, effort breathlessness, dyspnea, cough, re-entrant intercostal spaces, recurrent respiratory infections, palpitations from paroxysmal atrial tachycardia, and atrial fibrillation. Right heart failure furthermore causes fluid retention, hepatomegaly, sometimes distal edemas, and finally severe cardiac cachexia. Physical examination shows the delay of somatic and often mental growth, heart murmurs, splitting of the second heart sound, hyposphygmic femoral pulses, hepatomegaly, etc.

If a defect in a newborn is suspected, the pediatrician will recommend an electrocardiogram and probably an echocardiogram.

1. Electrocardiography may suggest CHD or, on the contrary, be almost normal. Generally, signs of CHD are left or right ventricular hypertrophy, left or right deviation of the QRS axis, intraventricular delay, or bundle branch blocks (often right bundle block). Atrial enlargement may be responsible for supraventricular tachycardias, atrial flutter, or fibrillation.

2. Chest radiography is still important when there is a significant suspicion of CHD. First of all, the localization of the left ventricular apex together with the gastric bulla is important so as to define the "situs": a right-sided apex and bulla are defined as a "situs inversus," often associated with CHD. Cardiomegaly (cardio/thoracic ratio >0.50) is suggestive of ventricular overload and/or congestive heart failure. CHD with excessive pulmonary blood flow shows typical enlargement of the pulmonary trunk shadow on the left margin of the cardiac silhouette, as well as enlargement of the right and left pulmonary arteries to the periphery of the lung field. In general, pulmonary vascular markings are increased or plethoric. Often the shadow of the aortic arch is abnormally small, due to the left-to-right shunt. On the other hand, CHD with reduced pulmonary blood flow demonstrates an atypical reduction or absence of the pulmonary trunk shadow, hypoperfusion of the pulmonary fields, or sometimes, due to the development with age of high-flow systemic-to-pulmonary collaterals, an altered pulmonary blood flow pattern in one or both lungs (i.e., plethora of one lung or part of it and oligemia of the other). Typical radiological signs such as calcified patent ductus arteriosus or boot-shaped heart shadow in tetralogy of Fallot are diagnostic.

3. Echocardiography is certainly the most important examination with which to correctly define the CHD affecting the patient. Two-dimensional Doppler echocardiography has the advantage of being reproducible, easy, safe, and with its transthoracic, or in more complex cases, transesophageal approach it not only helps define the diagnosis, but also indicates the therapeutic approach (medical, interventional, surgical, palliation/correction, etc.). Its use in pediatric cardiology requires a strict methodology: first, the cardiologist must define the position of the heart within the chest. Then, the sequential definition of the "situs" (solitus/inversus), of the veno-atrial concordance, of the atrio-ventricular concordance, of the spatial relation of the two ventricles, of the ventricular-arterial concordance, and of the spatial relationship of the great arteries represents the next step of the echocardiographic evaluation. The addition of Doppler color-flow imaging allows a reasonable estimate of the Qp/Qs ratio to be made (pulmonary to systemic output ratio, useful to discriminate between CHD with excessive and CHD with reduced pulmonary blood flow). The recent introduction of three-dimensional echocardiography has the potential of providing a three-dimensional reconstruction of the cardiac chambers and of the CHD, which is of great interest for the surgical approach.

4. Cardiac catheterization, besides echocardiography, is a gold standard diagnostic tool for all CHDs. In particular, it plays a key role in determining the stage of the CHD, by measuring intra-atrial, intraventricular, intrapulmonary, and intra-aortic pressures. Moreover, contrast-enhanced imaging strictly defines the morphology of the CHD. Moreover, it allows the calculation of pulmonary and systemic flow (Qp/Qs) and of pulmonary resistances, and it identifies the sites of shunts by blood gaseous analysis at different levels of sampling. Moreover, direct administration of vasodilators into the pulmonary bed also defines the reversibility of a pre-existing pulmonary hypertension. Finally, this technique is also crucial in the therapeutic management, since it is possible to carry out:

   a. Septostomy, to improve arteriovenous blood mixing in the transposition of the great arteries

b. Balloon valvuloplasty in pulmonary or aortic valve stenosis

c. Balloon angioplasty with stent release in vascular stenoses (first of all in the coarctation of the aorta)

d. Atrial and ventricular septal defect closure with umbrella-shaped devices

e. Coil embolization to occlude patent ductus arteriosus, arteriovenous fistula, and systemic-to-pulmonary collaterals

f. Myocardial biopsies to diagnose cardiomyopathy or to evaluate acute/subacute/chronic rejection in heart transplant recipients

Other tests increasingly used to diagnose CHDs today include CT and MR imaging. CT scan is generally employed in left ventricular obstruction, mainly in supra-aortic valve stenosis and, more frequently, in coarctation of the aorta. It precisely defines the anatomy and the degree of aortic narrowing. Vascular rings are another possible field of application.

Finally, the use of MR imaging is growing in daily practice because of its precise anatomic and functional cardiovascular definition, its noninvasiveness, its high sensitivity, and its objectiveness. It can be stated that there is no type of CHD which cannot be diagnosed with MR imaging, and in which MR imaging is not useful in the functional, preoperative, postoperative, and prognostic evaluation.

Q 152

Juan A. Tovar

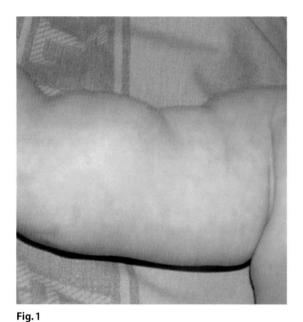

Fig. 1

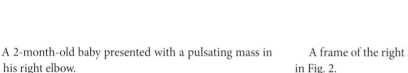

Fig. 2

A 2-month-old baby presented with a pulsating mass in his right elbow.

He was born after an uneventful delivery weighing 1,500 g. He had respiratory distress requiring ventilatory assistance for 1 week. During this period and in the ensuing days he had several venous punctures in both arms for blood sampling.

His respiratory condition improved and he was discharged without major problems. Two weeks after discharge, the parents noticed the mass in his right arm.

A frame of the right humeral angiography is depicted in Fig. 2.

He was treated via a transarterial route. The pulsating mass disappeared and the radial pulse was preserved.

- Describe what you see in Fig. 1.
- What is the difference between aneurysm and pseudoaneurysm?
- What sort of procedures may be indicated in these cases?
- Are there any sequelae to be expected?

A 152

This baby had a humeral artery pseudoaneurysm.

Arterial injuries in children, and particularly in young babies, are most often iatrogenic. The progressively more aggressive approach to the treatment of various neonatal conditions requiring frequent venous sampling, arterial monitoring, or central lines has increased the risk of arterial, venous, or arteriovenous lesions.

A false aneurysm or pseudoaneurysm is the result of extravasation of blood through a partially ruptured arterial wall. The space created by the spillage heals forming a false vascular wall that is devoid of the normal arterial wall layers and that becomes more or less dilated and pulsatile.

Arteriography or angio-MR imaging depicts the anatomy of the lesion and orient the treatment.

In this case the pseudoaneurysm has a neck and the main artery is patent.

Treatment consisted in percutaneous transarterial embolization.

Several substances are indicated for this purpose, including thrombin. Open surgery with anatomical repair is also a valid option.

Most patients can be cured without permanent sequelae.

Suggested Reading

1. Gow KW, Mykytenko J, Patrick EL, Dodson TF. Brachial artery pseudoaneurysm in a 6-week-old infant. Am Surg 2004; 70:518–21
2. Pezzullo JA, Wallach MT. Successful percutaneous thrombin injection of a brachial artery pseudoaneurysm in a neonate. AJR Am J Roentgenol 2002; 178:244–5
3. Rey C, Marache P, Watel A, Francart C. Iatrogenic false aneurysm of the brachial artery in an infant. Eur J Pediatr 1987; 146:438–9

Q 153

Francesco Onorati, Giacomo Sica, and Attilio Renzulli

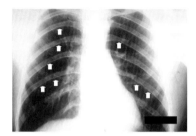

Fig. 1

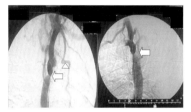

Fig. 3

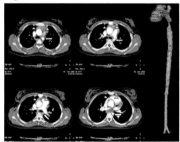

Fig. 4

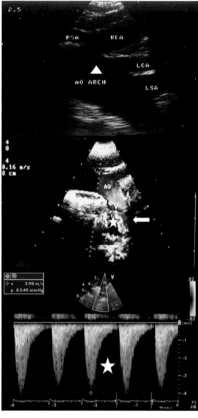

Fig. 2

A 17-year-old boy complaining of headache and dyspnea during submaximal efforts was referred to our department. He had no medical problems until the age of 15 years, after which he progressively developed recurrent headache, fatigue, and ongoing shortness of breath for maximal efforts. He also reported a few episodes of nose bleeding.

Physical examination showed systemic hypertension in the upper body (180/110 mmHg in the arms), with femoral hypotension (90/55 mmHg in the limbs).

- Which congenital heart disease could be suspected according to the blood pressure pattern?

The patient underwent chest radiography (PA projection), as shown in Fig. 1.

- What are the typical rib findings (*arrows*) of this disease?

A mono-2D Doppler echocardiography image is shown in Fig. 2.

- What is the anomaly of the aortic image?
- What are the main findings on echocardiography?
- Which other investigations should be performed in this case?

Angiography was also performed as shown in Fig. 3.

- Why was preoperative angiography carried out and what is indicated by the *arrow* and the *triangle*?

A CT scan is shown in Fig. 4.

- Which anatomic structures are pathological?
- What are the therapeutic options?

A 153

The patient was affected by coarctation of the aorta (AoCo), a congenital narrowing of the aortic isthmus (Fig. 5, *arrow*). Depending on the grade of the aortic narrowing and the patency of the ductus arteriosus, signs and symptoms develop at different ages: severe narrowing characterizes neonatal and infant AoCo, the less severe forms present in childhood or adulthood.

AoCo causes high blood pressure in the ascending aorta and aortic arch branches, leading to systemic hypertension with headache and nasal bleeding. Hypertension also causes progressive dilation of the ascending aorta and left ventricular hypertrophy, leading to cardiomegaly and congestive heart failure. Similarly, the isthmic narrowing explains why physical examination demonstrated hypertension of the upper body and hypotension with poor femoral pulses in the lower body.

Chest radiography shows the typical "rib notching," caused by the hypertrophy of the intercostal arteries, due to a collateral circulation through the intercostal and mammary arteries between the upper and lower thoracic aorta. Ectatic ascending aorta and aortic arch can be noted in long-lasting AoCo.

2D echocardiography can depict AoCo, particularly in neonates and small infants. Associated intracardiac defects or other congenital anomalies can be easily detected. The severity of AoCo can often be assessed through color Doppler signaling (*star*, Fig. 2). Figure 2 shows a parasternal view of the AoCo (*arrow*) and a moderate aortic arch dilation (*triangle*), with the origins of the innominate and left carotid arteries.

With the advent of CT or MR imaging, cardiac catheterization and aortography are nowadays rarely performed. However, cardiac catheterization with aortography still remains a good diagnostic tool with which to better define the anatomy of the lesion and collateral circulation as well as any associated congenital cardiac lesions; it also provides hemodynamic data. Moreover, in selected cases AoCo can be treated with interventional cardiology, stenting the narrowed area.

The CT scan demonstrated progressive narrowing of the descending thoracic aorta (*arrow*). Other findings suggestive of AoCo are dilated intercostal and mammary circulation (*triangle*). Collaterals are better appreciated on 3D-rendered images.

Besides interventional techniques, the gold standard is still surgical therapy. The aim of surgery is to restore a normal aortic flow, resecting the narrowed aorta and all the surrounding apoptotic tissue. Therefore, depending on the extension of the narrowing and the age of the patient, surgery varies from resection of the AoCo and direct reconstruction (end-to-end anastomosis) with wide mobilization of the aortic arch and ascending aorta in newborns, infants, and young children, to an enlargement or replacement of the descending aorta with a diamond-shaped or tubular Dacron graft. Figure 5 shows an intraoperative view of the CoA (*arrow*) and the completion of the operation. Several operations have been reported for bypassing the lesion with a Dacron tube: subclavian-to-descending aorta (Clagett operation) or aortic–aortic bypass. In complex cases of multiple obstructions to the left ventricular outflow, an ascending-to-supradiaphragmatic aorta bypass and apico-aortic conduit can be performed.

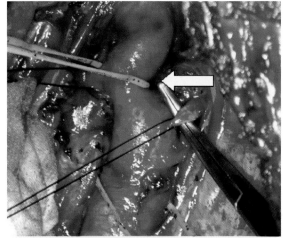

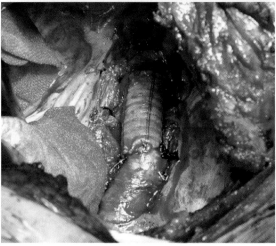

Fig. 5

Q 154

Francesco Onorati, Giacomo Sica, and Attilio Renzulli

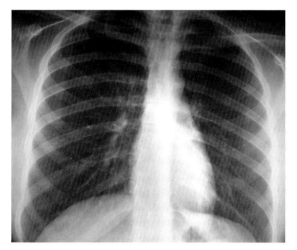

Fig. 1

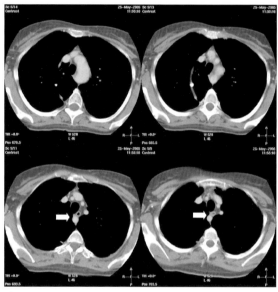

Fig. 2

A 17-year-old girl was admitted to our institution complaining of a persistent barking cough, with a few episodes of apnea causing cyanosis and one episode of unconsciousness. The patient reported progressive dysphagia in the last 5 years. She recently fed poorly and therefore felt quite sick; in particular, the patient reported great difficulties in swallowing liquids and solids, with episodes of choking and regurgitation.

Physical examination did not show any relevant signs, apart from expiratory wheezing.

- Does the chest radiograph (PA projection, Fig. 1) show any abnormality?

Immediately thereafter, the patient underwent CT scanning as demonstrated in Fig. 2.

- What is the main finding of the CT imaging depicted by the *arrow*?

Cardiac catheterization and aortography were performed (Fig. 3).

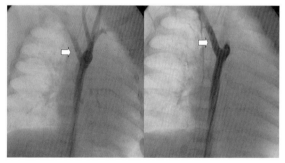

Fig. 3

- Why did the patient undergo aortography?
- Which vascular structure has an abnormal course?
- What pathological condition is affecting the patient?
- What is the treatment of choice?

A 154

The patient had so-called right lusoria subclavian artery—a congenital malformation belonging to a particular group of vascular anomalies defined as "vascular rings." Vascular rings are congenital anomalies in which the aortic arch and its branches completely or incompletely compress either the trachea, or the esophagus, or both by encircling them. Vascular rings are caused by inappropriate persistence or resorption of the six pairs of aortic arches connecting the ventral and dorsal aortae during embryological development. These arches variously recede, fuse, and remodel to form the typical left-sided aortic arch and its major branches.

In this case the right subclavian artery arises from the posterior wall of the aortic arch, next to the origin of a normal-positioned left subclavian artery. The aberrant artery compresses the esophagus and partially the trachea to reach the right arm. Furthermore, esophageal compression causes tracheobronchial hyper-reactivity. Because of this, the patient reported some signs and symptoms of respiratory impairment (cough, apnea, cyanosis, unconsciousness, and expiratory wheezing). Moreover, the right-sided course of the artery posterior to the esophagus causes its compression that has been traditionally blamed for the digestive symptoms (dysphagia, choke, and regurgitation).

The plain chest radiograph in the frontal view appeared normal. No relevant signs of cardiac or vascular pathologies could be detected. This is a common finding in right lusoria subclavian artery disease. On the contrary, other vascular rings, such as double aortic arch or right-sided aortic arch, can be easily suspected on chest radiographs (upper mediastinal shadow enlargement).

The clinical suspicion of right lusoria subclavian artery disease was confirmed. The CT scan clearly defined the anatomy of the origin and course of the supra-aortic branches. An isolated right common carotid course from the arch to the neck is shown, as well as a normal position of the left common carotid and of the left subclavian artery; in particular, the aberrant right subclavian artery arises as the last branch of the aortic arch from the posterior wall, running behind and thus compressing the esophagus. The retroesophageal artery in dysphagia lusoria is frequently visible on unenhanced scans even if intravenous contrast medium administration clearly detects the anomaly.

Alternatively, high-field (1.5 T) MR angiography should be preferred in children and adolescents, since it has a comparable clear definition of the anatomy, but avoids patient exposure to ionizing radiation and the use of nephrotoxic contrast medium.

In order to exclude associated cardiac and/or vascular malformations, the patient underwent cardiac catheterization and aortography (Fig. 3), which excluded congenital cardiac diseases, confirming the posterior origin of the right subclavian artery from the aortic arch.

Surgery is the only therapy for symptomatic cases. Surgical exploration did not show a constraining ligamentum arteriosus, but demonstrated the vascular nature of the esophageal compression: surgery therefore consisted of the repositioning of the aberrant right subclavian artery to the aortic arch through a prosthetic graft interposition. Postoperatively, the patient experienced immediate resolution of her dysphagia.

Suggested Reading

1. Cameron D (2004). Congenital anomalies of the aortic arch. In: Gardner TJ, Spray TL (eds) Operative Cardiac Surgery 5th Edition. Oxford University Press, Oxford, 851–861
2. Kamiya H et al. Surgical treatment of aberrant right subclavian artery (arteria lusoria) aneurysm using three different methods. Ann Thorac Surg 2006; 82:187–190
3. Woods RK et al. Vascular anomalies and tracheoesophageal compression: a single institution's 25-year experience. Ann Thorac Surg 2001; 72:434–439

Q 155

Francesco Onorati, Giacomo Sica, and Attilio Renzulli

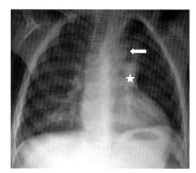

Fig. 1

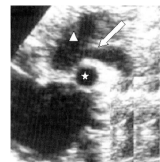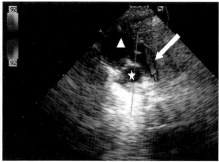

Fig. 2

A 6-year-old boy was admitted to hospital complaining of recurrent pneumonia, progressive dyspnea for mild to moderate efforts, and fatigue. Case-history findings revealed the patient was small for gestational age and his weight at birth was below the 5th percentile. Physical examination demonstrated a loud continuous murmur, which was maximal over the pulmonary artery and radiated upward beneath the mid-third of the clavicle. An electrocardiogram (ECG) demonstrated left ventricular hypertrophy.

A chest radiograph is shown in Fig. 1.
- What relevant findings on the left edge of the mediastinal shadow can be appreciated?
- How do the pulmonary fields appear?

Thereafter, the patient was scheduled for echocardiography, as shown in Fig. 2.
- What is the main finding of the study?
- Which vessel is indicated by the *arrow*?
- Which anatomic structures are indicated by the *triangle* and the *star*?

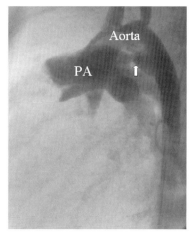

Fig. 3

The patient then underwent angiography, as shown in Fig. 3.
- What was the main indication for aortography?
- What pathological condition is affecting this child?
- Which technique is employed to treat this disease?

A 155

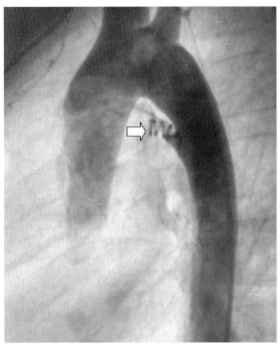

Fig. 4

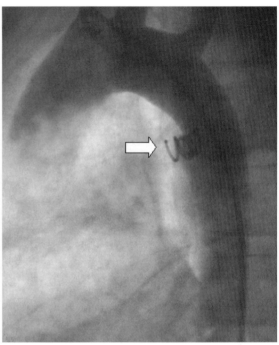

Fig. 5

The patient had a patent ductus arteriosus (PDA). PDA is an abnormal persistence of a patent lumen in the fetal ductus arteriosus, which usually connects the upper descending aorta with the proximal portion of the left pulmonary artery.

Symptoms and signs of PDA are due to left-to-right shunting, with increased pulmonary flow eventually leading to pulmonary hypertension. This hemodynamic abnormality is responsible for the recurrent pneumonia and progressive dyspnea reported by the patient. Chronic pulmonary hypertension leads to biventricular hypertrophy and finally to congestive heart failure.

A chest radiograph in PA view (Fig. 1) shows moderate cardiomegaly, with enlargement of the first (aortic, *arrow*) and second (pulmonary artery, *star*) left arches, and increased pulmonary vascularization.

In adults, a calcified PDA can sometimes be appreciated.

Echocardiography was performed to confirm the suspicion of a PDA, as well as to rule out associated cardiac abnormalities. The patient did not have any associated lesion, but a large PDA was clearly demonstrated on the sagittal view of the high parasternal window; in particular, a large PDA continuing into the upper de-

scending thoracic aorta is seen (*arrow*), together with the enlarged left pulmonary artery (*star*). An ascending aorta is also detected (*triangle*). Doppler signaling can be helpful in demonstrating the PDA and the direction of the shunt (*arrow*). Pulmonary pressure can be assessed with a noninvasive method through Doppler echocardiography.

In newborns, attempts should be made to close the PDA with medical treatment (indometacine).

Cardiac catheterization and aortography are no longer indicated in the diagnosis of PDA. However, the possibility to treat patients with an interventional cardiology technique through coil-embolization of the PDA makes angiography a useful technique for diagnosing and treating a PDA in the same session. Aortography (Fig. 3) showed the large PDA, contrasting both the descending thoracic aorta and, in a retrograde fashion, the common (*PA*) and the two main pulmonary arteries; furthermore, following percutaneous coil embolization (Figs. 4, 5) the PDA was successfully treated, with no residual shunting from the aorta to the pulmonary artery. Surgery can be performed with very low operative risks on patients not responding to less invasive techniques or on patients with associated cardiac abnormalities.

Q 156

Francesco Onorati, Giacomo Sica, and Attilio Renzulli

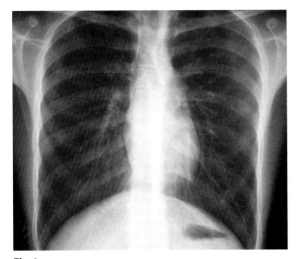

Fig. 1

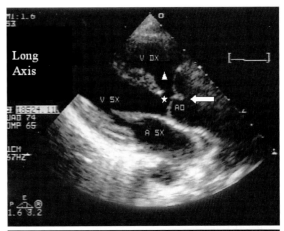

Fig. 2

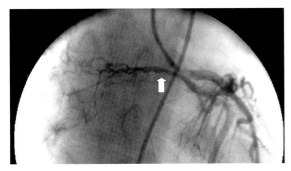

Fig. 3

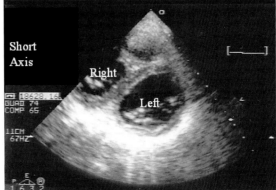

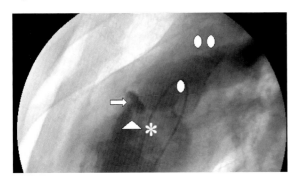

Fig. 4

A 13-year-old boy weighing 34 kg and complaining of cyanosis, shortness of breath, and hypoxic spells was referred to our institution. The child frequently resorted to the "squatting" position (knee–chest position).

On physical examination, he showed intense cyano-sis and clubbing of the fingers and toes. A systolic murmur in the second intercostal space was found.

An electrocardiogram (ECG) showed moderate right ventricular hypertrophy.

Blood analysis demonstrated polycythemia, with a hemoglobin (Hb) value above 20 g/dl, and hyperbilirubinemia (3.2 mg/dl).

A chest radiograph is shown in Fig. 1.

- Are the pulmonary fields hypoperfused?

Following chest radiography, the patient underwent transthoracic echocardiography, as shown in Fig. 2.

- What does Fig. 2 shows?

Cardiac catheterization and angiography (Figs. 3, 4) were then performed.

- Why is cardiac catheterization mandatory before surgical therapy?
- What kind of congenital heart disease is affecting this patient?
- What is the best way to manage this condition?

A 156

The patient had tetralogy of Fallot (TOF). TOF is a malformation characterized by displacement of the infundibular septum and its malalignment, leading to right ventricle outflow tract stenosis or atresia, and a large ventricular septal defect (VSD). Malalignment generates a subaortic VSD with an overriding aorta onto the right ventricle. The pulmonary valve is congenitally stenosed. Distal stenoses in the pulmonary arteries can be found.

Severe obstruction of the right outflow tract leads to right ventricular hypertrophy. Cyanosis depends on the severity of the pulmonary stenosis and is caused not only by the VSD but mainly by the overriding aorta. Cyanosis, furthermore, leads to polycythemia and clubbing of fingers and toes.

The chest radiograph showed hypoperfused pulmonary fields with a normal heart size due to the lack of pulmonary blood flow, congestive heart failure, and a decreased pulmonary vascularization.

Transthoracic echocardiography clearly showed the VSD (*star*) and aortic overriding (*arrow*) and narrowing of the right ventricle infundibulum (*triangle*) secondary to infundibular hypertrophy in parasternal long axis; the parasternal short axis depicted a comparable right and left ventricular hypertrophy, due to equalized intraventricular pressures secondary to the large VSD.

Although surgery can be performed on the basis of the echocardiographic findings alone, cardiac catheter-ization and angiography are useful for planning the surgical strategy and ruling out stenoses of the pulmonary branches and coronary anomalies (anterior descending artery running transversely on the right ventricular infundibulum), often associated with TOF. Finally, the "stop-flow" technique shows any systemic-to-pulmonary collaterals.

In this case, coronary angiography also demonstrated a circumflex-to-left bronchial artery coronary fistula (Fig. 3, *arrow*). The main pulmonary artery (Fig. 4, *circle*), overriding aorta (*double circle*), infundibular (*triangle*) and pulmonary valve (*arrow*) stenosis, as well as the misaligned septum (*asterisk*) are shown.

Surgery still remains the only treatment for TOF. The main steps of surgical treatment are: closure of VSD and resection of the parietal band through a right atrial approach; relief of the pulmonary valve stenosis; and assessment of the pulmonary annulus, main pulmonary artery, and infundibulum by Hegar dilators. In the case of hypoplastic pulmonary valve annulus, a transannular patch should be implanted.

In very sick infants with other associated abnormalities and pulmonary valve atresia, an initial palliative approach through a modified Blalock–Taussig shunt can be performed.

Suggested Reading

1. Bernardes RJ et al. A comparison of magnetic resonance angiography with conventional angiography in the diagnosis of tetralogy of Fallot. Cardiol Young 2006; 16:281–288
2. Dorfman AL and Geva T. Magnetic resonance imaging evaluation of congenital heart disease: conotruncal anomalies. J Cardiovasc Magn Reson 2006; 8:645–659
3. Karl TR and Brizard CPR (2004). Tetralogy of Fallot. In: Gardner TJ, Spray TL (eds) Operative Cardiac Surgery 5th Edition. Oxford University Press, Oxford, 689–705

Q 157

Francesco Onorati, Giacomo Sica, and Attilio Renzulli

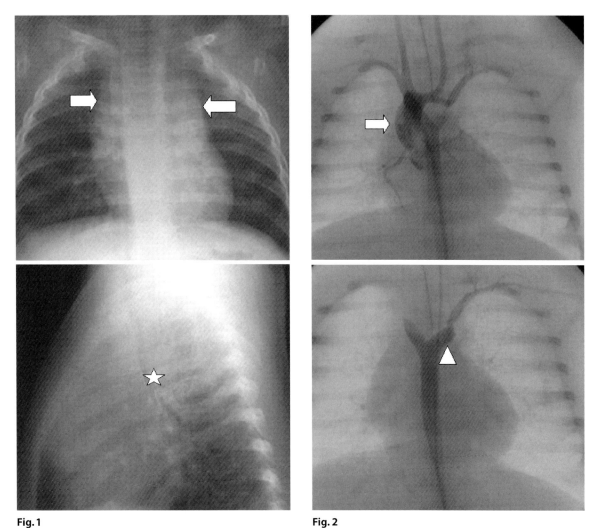

Fig. 1

Fig. 2

A 3-year-old boy was admitted to hospital because of recurrent episodes of cyanosis leading to unconsciousness. The patient had a history of asthma treated with bronchodilators. His parents reported that he had developed stridor during the last year, exacerbated when the child lay on his back, and noisy breathing during the night. They also reported recurrent respiratory infections. Physical examination demonstrated tachypnea and expiratory wheeze.

Chest radiography (AP, LL projections) was performed. Thereafter, according to the radiology findings,

cardiac catheterization and angiography were carried out.
- What abnormality of the mediastinal shadow can be detected on the chest radiograph?

Cardiac catheterization and aortic angiography (Fig. 2) led to the final diagnosis.
- What is the anatomy of the aortic arch on aortography?
- What pathological condition is affecting this child?
- Are CT scanning and MR imaging useful to correctly diagnose this congenital anomaly?

A 157

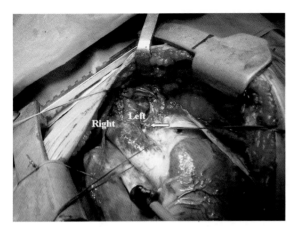

Fig. 3

The patient had a double aortic arch, a rare congenital malformation consisting of a normal ascending aorta, with a normal aortic valve, which divides into two arches as it leaves the pericardial sac; a left and right aortic arch can be identified, joining together again posteriorly, forming a normal descending aorta. This malformation belongs to the so-called vascular rings, where an arterial ring surrounds the esophagus, aorta, or both. In this case, an intraoperative (Fig. 3) examination showed a left aortic arch passing anteriorly and to the left of the trachea and being joined by the ductus arteriosus (ligated, *white arrow*), where it becomes the descending aorta, and a right arch, which passes posteriorly and to the right of the esophagus to reach the left-sided descending aorta, thus forming a complete vascular ring.

Signs and symptoms are related to the tracheoesophageal compression. Our patient demonstrated mainly respiratory symptoms, due to a predominant tracheal compression, secondary to a well-developed left arch, but no esophageal symptoms, due to a less-developed right arch.

Enlargement of the upper mediastinal shadow on a chest radiograph of a child with respiratory difficulties or dysphagia should alert one to the likelihood of a vascular ring. Figure 1 shows an enlarged upper mediastinal shadow (*arrow*), suggesting the presence of a right-sided aortic arch; the lateral view of this chest radiograph demonstrates a narrow tracheal air column (*star*), suggesting extrinsic compression of the trachea.

Cardiac catheterization is no longer mandatory because CT techniques (Fig. 4) have shown good sensi-

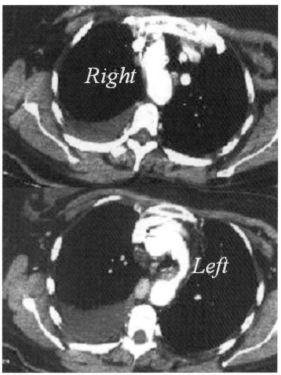

Fig. 4

tivity and specificity. However, the variety of the lesion and the complexity of the anatomy generally lead to a full angiographic examination in order to better define the anatomy and to rule out any other associated cardiac pathology. The study in Fig. 2 clearly defined the anatomy of the malformation with a right (*arrow*) and left (*triangle*) arch, and it confirmed the normal aortic valve function.

Suggested Reading

1. Cameron D (2004). Congenital anomalies of the aortic arch. In: Gardner TJ, Spray TL (eds) Operative Cardiac Surgery 5th Edition. Oxford University Press, Oxford, 851–861
2. Sivanandam S et al. Prenatal diagnosis of conotruncal malformations: diagnostic accuracy, outcome, chromosomal abnormalities, and extracardiac anomalies. Am J Perinatol 2006; 23:241–245
3. Weinberg PM. Aortic arch anomalies. J Cardiovasc Magn Reson 2006; 8:633–643

Q 158

Masayuki Fujioka, Carl Muroi, Nadia Khan and Yasuhiro Yonekawa

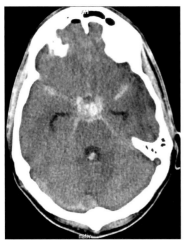

Fig. 1

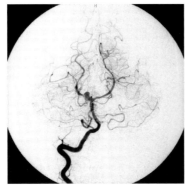

Fig. 2

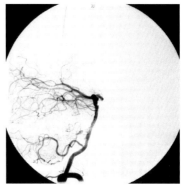

Fig. 3

A 15-year-old boy had a bitemporal headache of sudden onset with subsequent vomiting and consciousness disturbance when he was watching TV at home.

He was transferred to the emergency room of the hospital.

On his arrival at the hospital he was unconscious (Glasgow Coma Scale 6) with weak spontaneous respiration and with his right pupil dilated.

- What cranial nerve disturbance should be suspected and what mechanism should be considered as a possible cause at first?

CT scanning of the head was performed (Fig. 1).

- What does the CT scan show?

Cerebral angiography was performed immediately after the CT scanning.

- What do Figs. 2 and 3 show?
- What is the best way to manage this condition?

A 158

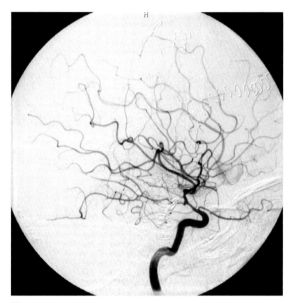

Fig. 4

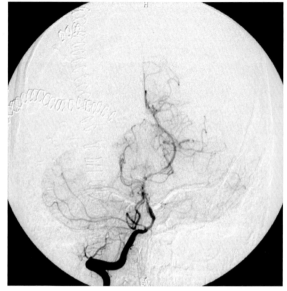

Fig. 5

The right pupil dilatation on arrival at the hospital represents right oculomotor nerve palsy. If the cause of the anisocoria is brainstem (midbrain) compression, emergency surgery would be required for decompression. The presence of brain herniation, therefore, should be investigated first.

The CT scan (Fig. 1) shows a subarachnoid hemorrhage (SAH) resulting from the rupture of the brain vascular structure. The distribution of the SAH seems symmetrical with a localization in the basal cistern and in the fourth ventricle. The CT scan shows no intracerebral hemorrhage leading to brain herniation. Several conditions (vascular anomaly including cerebral aneurysm, arteriovenous malformation, and venous angioma) should be investigated as the possible cause of the SAH.

Cerebral angiography (Figs. 2, 3) shows the cerebral aneurysms at the top of the basilar artery and at the proximal portion of the right posterior cerebral artery (P1 segment). The ruptured aneurysm(s) seemingly damages the peripheral portion of the oculomotor nerve that runs between the posterior cerebral artery and the superior cerebellar artery.

Aneurysmal clipping surgery (pterional craniotomy) with ventricular drainage was performed to prevent aneurysmal re-rupture. Barbiturate therapy and hypother-

mia therapy for brain protection were initiated in the intensive care unit after the surgery.

The CT scans obtained 7 days after the clipping showed large low-dense areas in the right cerebellar hemisphere and the right cerebral occipital lobe. The delayed brain infarcts after SAH suggested the presence of cerebral vasospasm.

The postoperative cerebral angiography (Figs. 4, 5) showed severe vasospasm of the right internal carotid artery, the right vertebral artery, the basilar artery, and the bilateral posterior cerebral arteries. Intra-arterial infusion of papaverine was performed at the same time.

After a 6-month follow-up, this boy is independent in his daily life, although the mild ataxia in the right extremities and the left homonymous hemianopsia remain. The pediatric case of cerebral aneurysm is considered rare compared to adult cases. In general, multiple aneurysms are present in around 20%–30% of adult cases of SAH. In the pediatric cases, around 10% of patients have multiple aneurysms. Hypertension is one of the most important factors associated with the multiplicity. In our case, the radiological studies (chest radiograph, CT angiography, MR angiography, and aortic angiography) suggested and showed the coarctation of the aorta that is known to be associated with cerebral aneurysm.

Q 159

Masayuki Fujioka, Carl Muroi, Nadia Khan and Yasuhiro Yonekawa

A 9-year-old boy presented with a severe throbbing headache of sudden onset with nausea and projectile vomiting. This was followed by deterioration in consciousness, reaching a score of 7 on the Glasgow Coma Scale (GCS), and by seizures. On arrival to our emergency room, he had a GCS score of 4. A CT scan of his brain showed an intracerebral hemorrhage in the left frontal lobe with its breakthrough into the ventricular system. Ventricle drainage was performed immediately.

Four-vessel cerebral angiography was performed as shown in Fig. 1.

- What is the cause of hemorrhage?
- What is the therapeutic possibility for this 9-year-old child?

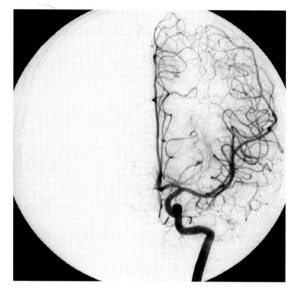

Fig. 1

A 159

The left internal carotid artery angiography (Fig. 1) shows an aneurysm of 3-mm diameter arising from the artery of Huebner that originates from the distal segment of the left A1 portion. This cerebral aneurysm caused the intracranial hemorrhage.

The cerebral aneurysm was treated with a polyvinyl alcohol embolization by selective catheterization of the origin of the Huebner artery (Fig. 2).

Figure 3 shows the follow-up angiography after the intravascular treatment of the aneurysm.

Suggested Reading

1. Huang J, McGirt MJ, Gailloud P, Tamargo RJ. Intracranial aneurysms in the pediatric population: case series and literature review. Surg Neurol 2005; 63:424–323
2. Jain P and Mehta V. Anteriorcommunicating artery aneurysm in a 3-year-old girl. Child's Nervous System 2002; 18:71–73

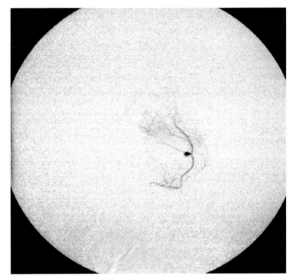

Fig. 2

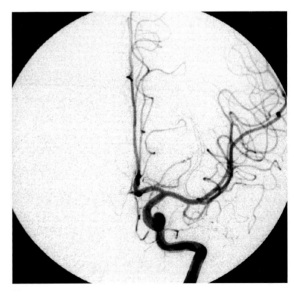

Fig. 3

Q 160

Masayuki Fujioka, Carl Muroi, Nadia Khan and Yasuhiro Yonekawa

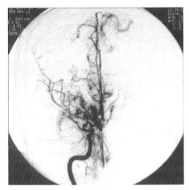

Fig. 1

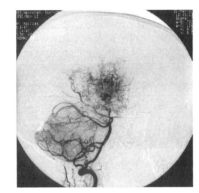

Fig. 2

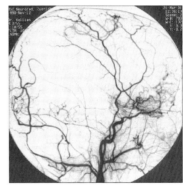

Fig. 3

A 5-year-old boy presented with a cortical infarct in the right middle cerebral artery territory. Cerebral angiography showed stenotic changes of the bilateral internal carotid arteries (ICA) and the right middle cerebral artery (MCA) (Fig. 1). A vertebral angiogram showed stenosis of the posterior cerebral artery (PCA; Fig. 2).

- What are these typical collateral formations called that appear in the regions of the lenticulostriate arteries (Fig. 1) and of the thalamoperforators (Fig. 2)?

After demonstration of the external carotid circulation on lateral view, a typical ethmoidal collateral circulation and a transdural anastomosis are observed in Fig. 3.

- What is the angiographic diagnosis of this patient?

The child had no other systemic disease and his general examination was normal.

- What is the clinical diagnosis?
- What is the common clinical presentation of this disease in children?
- What other single examination is required to plan a cerebral revascularization procedure?

A 160

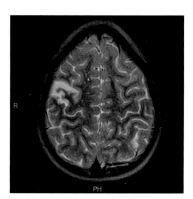

Fig. 4

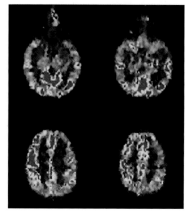

Fig. 5

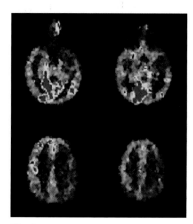

Fig. 6

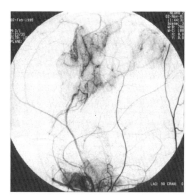

Fig. 7

This 5-year-old boy presents the typical collateral vessel formations usually observed in moyamoya angiopathy. These collateral vascular networks usually develop (a) at the site of stenosis or occlusion of the ICA (Fig. 1) with formation of the lenticulostriatal moyamoya or "puff of smoke" vessels or (b) at the site of PCA stenosis (Fig. 2) with moyamoya collateral formation in the thalamoperforators. Transdural anastomoses are also characteristically seen when the disease is well advanced (Fig. 3).

The angiographic diagnosis is moyamoya angiopathy.

The clinical diagnosis is moyamoya disease but not moyamoya syndrome.

Signs and symptoms of repeated cerebral ischemia or infarcts as seen in Fig. 4 are the most common presentation of this disease in children.

A cerebral perfusion scan using $H_2^{15}O$ PET to demonstrate the cerebral perfusion reserves (Fig. 5 baseline and Fig. 6 after a Diamox challenge) is mandatory to tailor the number, the side (right vs. left), and the location (MCA, ACA, or PCA arterial distribution) of the cerebral revascularization procedure (Fig. 7).

This boy underwent left STA–MCA bypass surgery (superficial temporal artery–middle cerebral artery) because the PET scan showed cerebral hypoperfusion in the left cerebral hemisphere. He is doing fine at 6 months after the surgery.

Q 161

Masayuki Fujioka, Carl Muroi, Nadia Khan and Yasuhiro Yonekawa

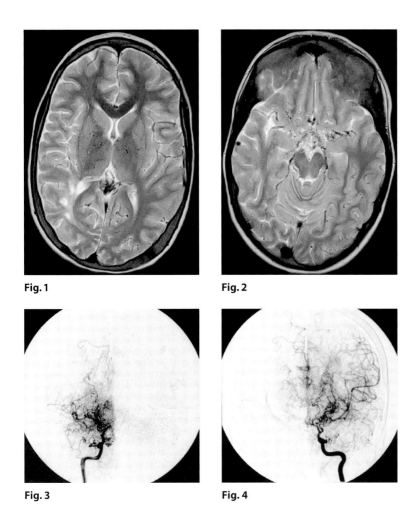

Fig. 1

Fig. 2

Fig. 3

Fig. 4

A 10-year-old girl presented with deteriorating neurological symptoms of increasing frequency of bifrontal headaches along with periodic temporary weakness of both upper extremities, especially the left side. She had her first headache attack at the age of 5 years. She was diagnosed as having hemolytic anemia at the age of 4 months due to a rare unstable hemoglobinopathy with abnormal oxygen affinity called "Hb Alesha." MR imaging of her brain at the age of 5 years was normal.

- What is the possible diagnosis?
- What do the repeat T2-weighted MR images (at 10 years of age) show (Figs. 1, 2)?
- What is the angiopathy demonstrated on the right and left internal carotid angiograms (AP views, Figs. 3, 4)?
- What is the clinical diagnosis of this case?

A 161

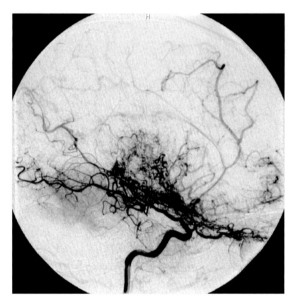

Fig. 5

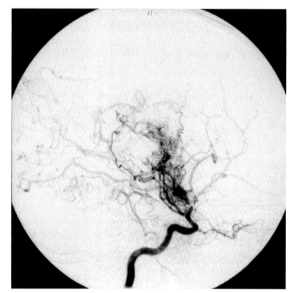

Fig. 6

This 10-year-old girl was considered to have repeated transient ischemic attacks in the form of headaches and transient weakness of the bilateral sides.

The MR images show collateral vessel formations at the level of the basal ganglia bilaterally (Figs. 1, 2).

The internal carotid angiography (Figs. 3, 4) confirms the diagnosis of "moyamoya angiopathy" characterized by the typical internal carotid artery (ICA) stenosis in the supraclinoid segment and by the typical "moyamoya collaterals" at the level of the basal ganglia ("puff of smoke").

Figures 5 and 6 also demonstrate the moyamoya collaterals on the ICA angiograms (lateral views).

This case is an example of "moyamoya syndrome." Moyamoya syndrome represents a typical moyamoya angiopathy accompanying systemic diseases.

The patient is doing fine and returned to school 6 months after the bilateral STA–MCA anastomosis surgery.

Suggested Reading

1. Khan N, Schuknecht B, Boltshauser E, Capone A, Buck A, Imhof HG, Yonekawa Y. Moyamoya disease and Moyamoya syndrome: experience in Europe; choice of revascularisation procedures. Acta Neurochir (Wien) 2003; 145(12):1061–71
2. Yonekawa Y, Taub E. Moyamoya disease: Status 1998. The Neurologist 1999; 5:13–23
3. Yonekawa Y, Goto Y, Ogata (1992). Moyamoya disease: Diagnosis, Treatment, Recent Achievement: In: Barnett HJM et al. (eds): Storke Pathophysiology, Diagnosis and Management Churchill Livingstone, New York, 721–47

Q 162

Frédéric Gauthier, Sophie Branchereau, and Chiara Grimaldi

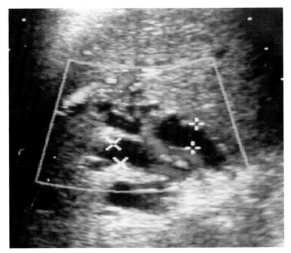

Fig. 1

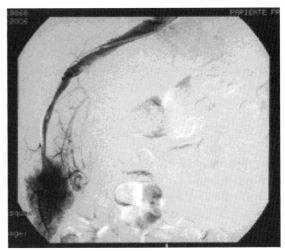

Fig. 2

A 1.5-year-old girl had a clinical history of prematurity (28 gestational weeks) and neonatal bacterial meningitis that needed an umbilical venous catheter. She was referred to our department for the first time at 8 months of age for hematemesis and melena.

• How do you manage this patient?

We performed an abdominal color Doppler US that is shown in Fig. 1. The child required a surgical intervention.

• What do you need to know in order to plan the operation?
• Figure 2 shows the suprahepatic phlebography: how do you interpret it?
• Which is your surgical management?

A 162

In managing this patient, you have to assess the degree of anemia and the presence of esophageal varices with gastroesophageal endoscopy. In this case, we found grade-4 esophageal varices and portal hypertension gastropathy.

In Fig. 1, we can see a portal anechogenic biliary tree dilation contrasting with the colored blood vessels of the cavernoma.

When planning surgery, you need to know whether the intrahepatic portal system and the mesenteric system are patent.

Figure 2 shows the right intrahepatic portal system without communication with the left intrahepatic portal system.

According to the phlebography findings, it is not possible to perform a mesorex shunt. Since there was a patent superior mesenteric vein, we decided to perform a mesocaval shunt with jugular graft interposition.

Suggested Reading

1. Gauthier-Villars M, Franchi S, Gauthier F, Fabre M, Pariente D, Bernard O. Cholestasis in children with portal vein obstruction. J Pediatr 2005; 146(4):568–73
2. Valayer J, Hay JM, Gauthier F, Broto J. Shunt surgery for treatment of portal hypertension in children. World J Surg 1985; 9(2):258–68

Q 163

Christophe Chardot and Sylviane Hanquinet

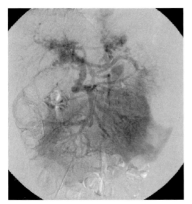

Fig. 1

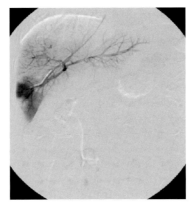

Fig. 2

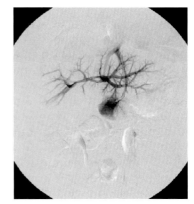

Fig. 3

An 18-month-old boy, who was born after a normal pregnancy and normal delivery, presented with a 2-month history of repeated episodes of melena. Clinical examination showed a baby in good general condition, with pale lips but without jaundice. Significant splenomegaly (5 cm below the costal margin) was found, without hepatomegaly. Blood count showed microcytic anemia, with a hemoglobin level of 83 g/l. Routine liver test results (ASAT, ALAT, GGT, bilirubin, INR) were normal.

- What is the most likely diagnosis?
- What is abdominal US likely to show?
- Which investigation is most likely to identify the origin of the gastrointestinal (GI) bleeding?
- What findings are expected, according to the clinical presentation?
- Which additional questions should be asked to the parents regarding familial history and the neonatal period, in order to find a cause of the current problem?

- The platelet count is 80,000/mm³. How do you interpret this finding? In addition to blood group and standard coagulation tests, which other hematological investigation is needed before considering surgery?
- Apart from the risk of GI bleeding, what main complications may arise in this condition?
- How can these potential complications be detected?
- What is the ideal treatment in such a case? Why?
- What are the anatomical prerequisites and which investigations are needed to assess them?
- Figure 1 represents the venous sequence of a superior mesenteric arteriography. How do you interpret it?
- Figure 2 represents a retrograde transparenchymal portography through the right hepatic vein. How do you interpret it?
- Where is the recessus of Rex located on this retrograde portography (Fig. 3)?
- How do you interpret the postoperative US Doppler study of the shunt (Fig. 4)?

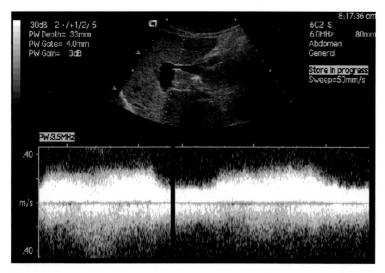

Fig. 4

A 163

The association of upper GI bleeding, normal liver, and significant splenomegaly suggests prehepatic portal hypertension whose main cause is portal vein obstruction with subsequent portal cavernoma.

An abdominal US is likely to show:
— A normal liver (Fig. 5)
— Varices of the liver hilum and nonvisualization of the portal vein (Figs. 5, 6)
— Increased thickness of the hepatogastric omentum (more than the aortic diameter) due to varices (Fig. 7)
— Splenomegaly
— Retroperitoneal varices and possibly spontaneous splenorenal shunts

Upper GI endoscopy is required after upper GI bleeding in order to identify the origin of the bleeding. Endoscopy is likely to show signs of portal hypertension: esophageal (Fig. 8) and/or gastric varices (Fig. 9), and/or hypertensive gastropathy.

Portal vein obstruction in infancy is due to portal vein thrombosis, whose main causes are: infection or thrombosis of an umbilical catheter; umphalitis; and inherited prothrombotic coagulopathy.

Therefore, the neonatal history of the child should be precisely known, and familial cases of thrombotic diseases should be sought.

Thrombocytopenia is due to hypersplenism. In order to exclude prothrombotic coagulation disorders, a detailed investigation of coagulation is advisable, including protein C, protein S, antithrombin 3 levels, and the search for mutations of factors II or V.

The main risk of portal vein obstruction is GI bleeding. Other complications may arise:

— Bile duct compression by varices in the liver hilum, causing cholestasis, intrahepatic bile duct dilatation, and liver fibrosis. This complication can be detected by liver tests and abdominal US.
— Liver nodules (adenomas or nodular regenerative hyperplasia) due to the modifications of intrahepatic portal flow. This can be detected by abdominal US.
— Pulmonary arteriovenous shunts. This complication is supposedly due to excessive opening of the pulmonary capillaries secondary to the action of intestinal vasoactive substances that are no longer eliminated by the liver and directly arrive to the lungs via portosystemic shunts. Pulmonary shunts can be detected by oxymetry (hypoxia) and be confirmed by pulmonary perfusion scintigraphy. Figure 10 shows a normal scintigram on the left and severe pulmonary shunts on the right.
— Pulmonary hypertension: Intestinal vasoactive substances may cause spasm of the small pulmonary arteries. This complication can be detected by echocardiography (signs of pulmonary hypertension) and confirmed by heart catheterism.

The ideal treatment of portal vein obstruction with portal cavernoma is to restore a physiological portal flow towards the liver. This relieves portal hypertension and avoids the long-term complications of portosystemic shunts. Restoration of a physiologic portal flow may be achieved by shunting the obstructed portal vein, usually between the superior mesenteric vein and the intrahepatic left portal vein (Rex recessus) with an internal jugular vein of the patient. The anatomical prerequisites are:
— Normal liver parenchyma without severe fibrosis or cirrhosis (liver biopsy).

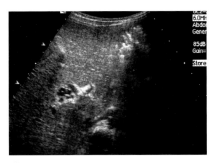

Fig. 5

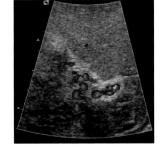

Fig. 6

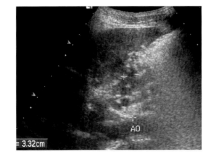

Fig. 7

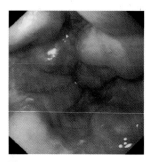 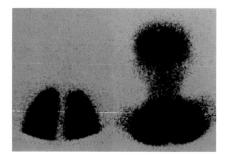 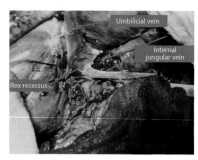

Fig. 8   **Fig. 9**   **Fig. 10**

– Patent intrahepatic portal system: this may be seen on US. In cases where US does not show the intrahepatic portal system, its patency has to be assessed by either hepatic retrograde portography (retrograde opacification of the portal system via hepatic veins and liver parenchyma), percutaneous transhepatic portography, or intraoperative portography.
– Patent intra-abdominal portal system, ideally with patent splenic vein, superior mesenteric vein, and splenomesenteric confluence. This can be seen on abdominal US Doppler, and if needed on angio-CT scan, MR imaging, or arteriography.
– Patent internal jugular veins, allowing retrieval of one of them (US).

Figure 1 shows a patent mesenteric vein (on the right side of the aortic catheter), as well as a splenic vein and splenomesenteric confluence. The portal vein is obstructed. Numerous varices are seen in the liver hilum and in front of the stomach.

Figure 2 shows the catheter in the right hepatic vein (introduced from the right jugular vein), the area of pa-

renchymography in the right liver, and the retrograde opacification of a complete intrahepatic portal system (right and left branches opacified). The portal system is slightly hypoplastic, but will re-expand after restoration of a physiologic portal flow.

The recessus of Rex is the area where the left portal vein divides into portal branches to segments 2, 3, and 4, and to the umbilical vein. In Fig. 3, the catheter comes from the left hepatic vein, with the area of parenchymography in the left lobe, and opacification of a large recessus of Rex connected to the portal branches of segments 2, 3, and 4 as well as to the left portal vein. The umbilical vein is not opacified. Figure 10 shows an intraoperative view of the anastomosis between the autologous jugular vein and the recessus of Rex.

The US Doppler (Fig. 4) shows a patent shunt, with a satisfactory blood flow: blood velocity is between 15 and 30 cm/s with variations according to respiratory movements. The liver is normal. Note that after a Rex shunt, the flow in the left portal vein is reversed.

Suggested Reading

1. de Ville de Goyet J, Alberti D, Clapuyt P, Falchetti D, Rigamonti V, Bax NM et al. Direct bypassing of extrahepatic portal venous obstruction in children: a new technique for combined hepatic portal revascularization and treatment of extrahepatic portal hypertension. J Pediatr Surg 1998; 33(4):597–601

2. de Ville de Goyet J, Alberti D, Falchetti D, Rigamonti W, Matricardi L, Clapuyt P et al. Treatment of extrahepatic portal hypertension in children by mesenteric-to-left portal vein bypass: a new physiological procedure. Eur J Surg 1999; 165(8):777–81

Q 164

Giovanni Esposito, Ciro Esposito, and Giuseppe Amici

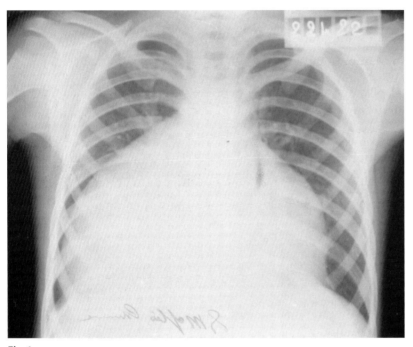

Fig. 1

A 10-year-old child, without any previous medical problems, pricked the anterior side of his left thorax with a nail while playing. After a few hours he began experiencing respiratory difficulties with dyspnea and later retrosternal pain appeared. Chest radiography was performed, after which the child was admitted to our hospital. On physical examination, he presented dyspnea, a fast pulse rate, augmentation of the heart flatness, distant heart sounds, and subcyanosis of the lips and fingers. Laboratory tests showed a slight anemia (RC 3,800,000 and Hb 11.3).

After some more examinations, the diagnosis was made and treatment was planned.
- What does the chest radiograph demonstrate (Fig. 1)?
- What was the suspected diagnosis?
- Which other examinations were performed and what were their results?
- What was the evolution of the disease?
- What was the treatment?
- What was the follow-up?

A 164

The chest radiograph shows an augmentation of cardiac volume with a classic "fiasco" image.

The suspected diagnosis was pericardial effusion.

An ECG and a pericardiocentesis were carried out. The ECG showed the presence of a low-voltage complex like a pericardial effusion. The pericardiocentesis, performed under local anesthesia via the subxiphoid route, led to drainage of 150 ml of blood.

Based on these results and clinical outcome, the diagnosis of traumatic hemopericardium was made. The condition improved after the first drainage, but there was a recurrence of symptoms which required new blood drainage (200 ml). Therefore, surgery was proposed.

The treatment consisted in a left thoracotomy at the fifth intercostal space through which the pericardium was opened and 700 ml of blood came out. On heart examination, no wounds were found and the etiological hypothesis was of a laceration of the pericardial vessels. A pericardial flap was resected and a partial suture was performed leaving a small hole inferiorly.

The postoperative course was regular and the ECG normalized. Following a radiographic checkup (Fig. 2), the patient was discharged 7 days after surgery.

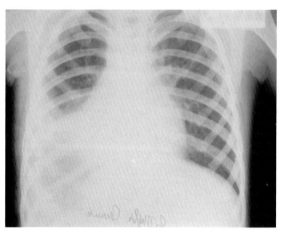

Fig. 2

Suggested Reading

1. Bowers P, Harris P, Truesdell S, Stewart S. Delayed hemopericardium and cardiac tamponade after unrecognized chest trauma. Pediatr Emerg Care 1994 Aug; 10(4):222–4
2. Cil E, Senkaya I, Tarim O. Delayed hemopericardium due to trivial chest trauma. Cardiol Young 1998 Jul; 8(3):390–2
3. Tulzer G, Lechner E, Gitter R. Emergencies in pediatric cardiology. Ther Umsch 2001 Feb; 58(2):76–9
4. Mok GC, Menahem S. Large pericardial effusions of inflammatory origin in childhood. Cardiol Young 2003 Apr;13(2):131-6
5. Atar S, Chiu J, Forrester JS, Siegel RJ. Bloody pericardial effusion in patients with cardiac tamponade: is the cause cancerous, tuberculous, or iatrogenic in the 1990s? Chest 1999 Dec;116(6):1564-9
6. Tsang TS, Barnes ME, Hayes SN, Freeman WK, Dearani JA, Butler SL, Seward JB. Clinical and echocardiographic characteristics of significant pericardial effusions following cardiothoracic surgery and outcomes of echo-guided pericardiocentesis for management: Mayo Clinic experience, 1979-1998. Chest 1999 Aug;116(2):322-31
7. Palatianos GM, Thurer RJ, Pompeo MQ, Kaiser GA. Clinical experience with subxiphoid drainage of pericardial effusions. Ann Thorac Surg 1989 Sep;48(3):381-5

Q 165

Giovanni Esposito, Ciro Esposito and Alessandro Settimi

A full-term 3-month-old infant, born after a normal pregnancy, presented with splenomegaly. On physical examination the spleen was palpable in the left iliac fossa exceeding the xiphoumbilical line. The child had a pained look, his skin was pale, and the subcutaneous tissue was scanty. Laboratory tests yielded the following results: RBC 2,740,000; Hb 7.5;WBC 8,500; PLT 70,000; glutamyl oxaloacetic transaminase (GOT) 195 U/l; glutamyl pyruvic transaminase (GPT) 99 U/l; immunoglobulin G (IgG) 1,130; IgM 196; IgA 142. TORCH (Toxoplasma, Rubella, Cytomegalovirus, Herpes), venereal disease, and hepatitis markers were negative. Splenoportography was performed (Fig. 1), after which the patient underwent surgical treatment.

- What does the splenoportography show?
- What was the diagnosis and the possible cause?
- Which operation was performed?
- Which examinations were carried out during the follow-up?

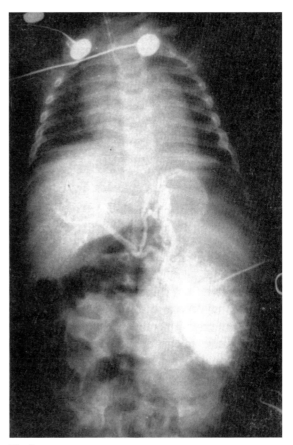

Fig. 1

A 165

The splenoportography shows the obstruction of the splenic vein, the patency of the portal vein, and the presence of a collateral circle that drains the splenic blood in the portal vein through the gastric veins and the coronary vein of the stomach. Splenomanometry revealed an endosplenic pressure of 25 cm H_2O.

Based on these findings, the suspected diagnosis was of a thrombosis of the splenic vein probably due to sepsis developed during intrauterine or perinatal life causing splenic vein thrombosis and impairment of hepatic function (as demonstrated by the anemia, platelet count decrease, and increase of IgM and GOT).

Splenectomy was performed followed by the implantation of splenic tissue on the right rectum muscle in order to avoid postsplenectomy sepsis.

The postoperative course was uneventful. The follow-up, which included a clinical examination and laboratory tests, demonstrated normal growth of the child. After 1 year, a splenic scintiscan with 99mTc-marked red blood cells (Fig. 2) was carried out and revealed a good function of the splenic tissue graft.

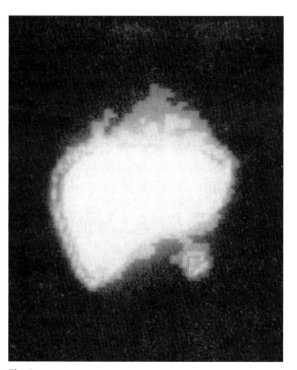

Fig. 2

Suggested Reading

1. Berk DR, Ahmed A. Portal, splenic, and superior mesenteric vein thrombosis in a patient with latent essential thrombocythemia and hyperhomocysteinemia. J Clin Gastroenterol 2006 Mar; 40(3):227–8

2. Gupta N, Sahni V, Singh P, Das A, Kar P. Spontaneous bacterial peritonitis in isolated splenic vein thrombosis with portal hypertension. Indian J Gastroenterol 2006 Sep–Oct; 25(5):263–4

3. Hiraiwa K, Morozumi K, Miyazaki H, Sotome K, Furukawa A, Nakamaru M, Tanaka Y, Iri H. Isolated splenic vein thrombosis secondary to splenic metastasis: a case report. World J Gastroenterol 2006 Oct 28; 12(40):6561–3

4. Ikeda M, Sekimoto M, Takiguchi S, Yasui M, Danno K, Fujie Y, Kitani K, Seki Y, Hata T, Shingai T, Takemasa I, Ikenaga M, Yamamoto H, Ohue M, Monden M. Total splenic vein thrombosis after laparoscopic splenectomy: a possible candidate for treatment. Am J Surg 2007 Jan; 193(1):21–5

5. Reddy B, Gonzalez-Angulo AM, Kemmerly SA. Splenic vein thrombosis presenting as Fusobacterium nucleatum bacteremia. J La State Med Soc 2006 Jul–Aug; 158(4):183–5

Q 166

Vincenzo Farina, Claudia Tiano, Selvaggia Lenta, and Luigi Scippa

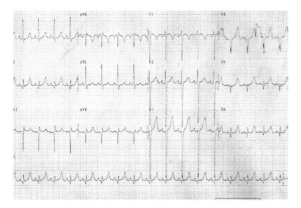

Fig. 1

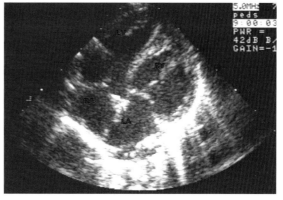

Fig. 2

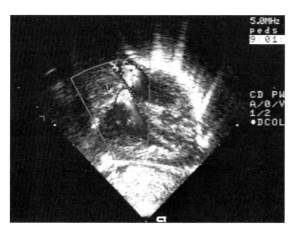

Fig. 3

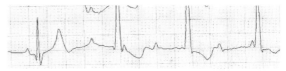

Fig. 4

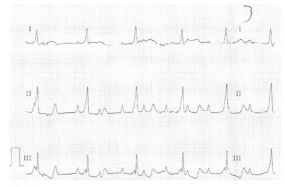

Fig. 5

A systolic murmur of grade-2 (of 6) intensity was found in a newborn girl, without any symptoms.

The cardiologist performed the examinations shown in Figs. 1–3.

- What do Figs. 1–3 show?
- What pathological condition is affecting this child?
- Why did the cardiologist repeat the examinations approximately every 6 months?
- What does Fig. 4 show?
- Did the condition change during the follow-up?

When the girl was 7 years old the mother reported an episode of severe dyspnea during physical exercise.

- Which examination did the doctors decide to perform?
- What did they find (Fig. 5)?
- What is the best way to manage this condition?

A 166

During the first cardiac examination, this child underwent an ECG and an echocardiography.

As you can see in Fig. 1, the ECG shows a left axial deviation and prominent Q waves in the inferior and right precordial leads, with absent left precordial Q waves. The echocardiography shows corrected transposition of the great arteries (c-TGA): double discordance between the atria and ventricles (Fig. 2) and between the ventricles and great arteries with aortic left positioning (Fig. 3); a moderate ventricular septal defect; stenosis of the pulmonary valves; right ventricle dilatation without contractility abnormalities; moderate homologous A-V valve insufficiency.

c-TGA is a rare congenital cardiac pathology with an incidence of less than 1%. In 95% of cases, an association with other cardiac abnormalities such as ventricular septal defects, pulmonary valves stenoses, A-V valve insufficiency and, with longer follow-up, dysrhythmias is reported in the literature. All patients should be seen periodically in order to evaluate their clinical, imaging, and hemodynamic conditions and to decide the right treatment.

Six months after the diagnosis, the child underwent another cardiac evaluation and, as shown in Fig. 3, the ECG revealed a Mobitz I A-V block with Luciani-Wenckebach periodism alternated with AVB 2:1; the echocardiographic findings did not change. When she was 1 year old, we witnessed a complete regression of the pulmonary valve stenosis and the spontaneous clo-

sure of the ventricular septal defect. The child continued with the follow-up, undergoing periodically ECG, Holter-ECG, and echocardiography. At 6 years of age it was decided to start therapy with an ACE inhibitor because of dilatation and thickening of the right ventricle and because of the increase in episodes of Mobitz II A-V block.

At 7 years of age, on the basis of the mother's report of an episode of dyspnea occurring during physical exercise, the cardiologist decided to repeat the routine examinations (ECG, Holter-ECG, and echocardiography) and to also perform an ergometric test. This test, as shown in Fig. 5, revealed a complete A-V block as early as the third minute.

Consequently, the doctors decided to evaluate the child with an electrophysiologic study and to consider her for a pacemaker implantation.

Many patients with c-TGA have survived to adulthood even without surgical correction; however, the dysrhythmias frequently occur with age and are associated with deterioration of RV function. Surgical treatment should be considered at the earliest sign of RV dysfunction. All patients should be seen periodically to evaluate their condition and decide on the right therapeutic approach. Patients diagnosed as having c-TGA with or without cardiac defects should be followed up carefully during their clinical course to identify and treat different type of dysrhythmias that can appear anytime and that can represent a high risk of death.

Suggested Reading

1. Harska V, Duncan BW, Maver JE Jr, Freed M, del Nido PJ, Jonas RA. Long term outcome of surgical treated patients with corrected transposition of the great arteries. Circulation 2005; 10:1987–91
2. Lange R, Horer J, Kostolny M, Cleuziou J, Vogt M, Busch R, Holper K, Meisner H, Hess J, Schreiber C. Presence of a ventricular septal defect and the Mustard operation are risk factors for late mortality after the atrial switch operation: thirty years of follow-up in 417 patients at a single center. Circulation 2006 Oct 31; 114(18):1905–13
3. Warnes CA. Transposition of the great arteries. Circulation 2006 Dec 12; 114(24):2699–709

Q 167

Vincenzo Farina, Claudia Tiano, Selvaggia Lenta, and Luigi Scippa

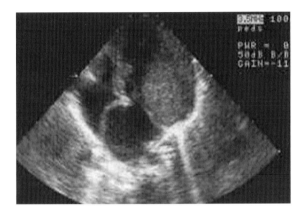

Fig. 1

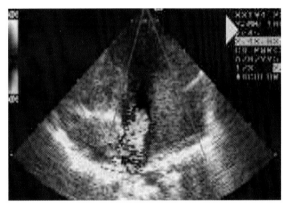

Fig. 2

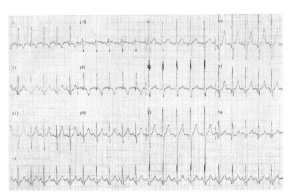

Fig. 3

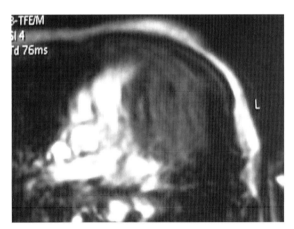

Fig. 4

A 3-month-old girl was admitted to our department because of the presence of a holosystolic murmur, of grade-3 intensity (of 6), at the apex. Physical examination results and her growth were normal.

The cardiologist performed the examinations shown in Figs. 1–3.

- What do Figs. 1 and 2 show?
- What does Fig. 3, during follow-up, show?
- Which therapy was started?
- Which other diagnostic examinations need to be performed in this case (Figs. 4, 5)?
- What pathological condition is affecting this child?
- What is the best way to manage this condition?

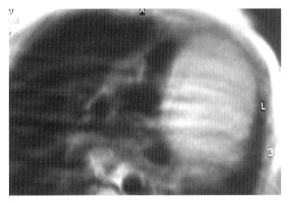

Fig. 5

A 167

This child is affected by cardiac rhabdomyoma.

Figures 1 and 2 show a highly echogenic well-circumscribed mass (4×2.5 cm) with a posterior intraventricular location that leads to distortion of the posterior leaflet of the mitral valve (secondary moderate mitral insufficiency) with a moderate increase of the blood flow across the valve, but not interfering with cardiac output.

During follow-up, the ECG (Fig. 3) shows signs of left ventricular hypertrophy and the echocardiographic study shows atrial enlargement (20 mm) with mild tricuspid insufficiency.

Despite the absence of clinical signs related to the pathology of origin, in order to increase the flow across the mitral valve, the patient started therapy with an ACE inhibitor.

Because of the close association between cardiac rhabdomyomas and tuberous sclerosis (TS) syndrome reported in 86% of cases, the patient underwent screening for TS including ophthalmologic and neurological tests, abdominal ultrasonography, laboratory tests, and brain CT, which all yielded normal results.

In accordance with the oncologist, to better define the mass characteristics, the patient underwent cardiac MR imaging (Figs. 4, 5), showing an increase in the size of the cardiac mass (5.5×4.1 cm) with involvement of the cardiac apex and disruption of the right cardiac chamber.

The patient was affected by isolated cardiac rhabdomyoma, which, without life-threatening hemodynamic instability or arrhythmias, is not an absolute indication for surgery.

There are reports in the literature that large rhabdomyomas may significantly regress in size or disappear completely. In our patient, the mass increased during follow-up and the only possible therapy was excision of the mass or cardiac transplantation. At the time of writing the girl is 2 years old and surgical intervention is not indicated; however, the child is being monitored for early detection of arrhythmias or flow hemodynamic abnormalities.

Suggested Reading

1. De Wilde H, Benatar A. Cardiac rhabdomyoma with long-term conduction abnormality: Progression from pre-excitation to bundle branch block and finally complete heart block. Med Sci Monit 2007 Jan 18; 13(2):CS21–23

2. Durairaj M, Mangotra K, Makhale CN, Shinde R, Mehta AC, Sathe AS. Cardiac rhabdomyoma in a neonate: application of serial echocardiography. Echocardiography 2006 Jul; 23(6):510–2

3. Uzun O, Wilson DG, Vujanic GM, Parsons JM, De Giovanni JV. Cardiac tumours in children. Orphanet J Rare Dis 2007 Mar 1; 2(1):11 [Epub ahead of print]

6

Musculoskeletal Disorder

Introduction

During the last 30 years the focus of pediatric orthopedics has changed considerably as a result of many important studies. From a situation where diagnosis was founded on clinical expertise, now there is an increased use of sophisticated imaging and surgical techniques that require a precise knowledge of the anatomy of skeletally immature bone. Important issues faced in this field include an understanding of the behavior of growth cartilage together with how it interacts with the developing blood supply and the factors that can lead to necrosis.

One of the most important steps forward in the treatment of pediatric orthopedic diseases was the development of noninvasive diagnosis and prophylaxis of one of the most frequent congenital diseases of the musculoskeletal apparatus: developmental displacement of the hip. As the result of a worldwide ultrasound screening program, the incidence of serious dislocation and the need for invasive surgical intervention have been reduced considerably.

Another key development in this field has been the application of more advanced imaging techniques. Thus, in addition to the use of ultrasonography, MR imaging has considerably improved the evaluation of soft tissue diseases by enhancing the visibility of cartilage. This tissue is clearly of great musculoskeletal interest, but previously was not detectable by any other noninvasive investigative techniques. MR imaging and CT have revolutionized bone and soft tissue investigation in a way similar to the use of radiographs as a standard radiological tool following Roentgen's discovery of x-rays.

Arthroscopy has become a high-performance technique that improves the diagnosis and the treatment of articular pathologic problems such as meniscus or ligament tears and cartilage damage that is idiopathic or secondary to trauma and to changes in blood supply. In these applications, the performance of arthroscopy continues to improve with time, according to the increasing skill of the operator and the technological improvements of the instruments and surgical tools.

In the field of tumoral and tumor-like lesions of bone and soft tissue, important progress has been made in the establishment of the limb-sparing technique for malignant bone tumors to avoid amputation and the associated damaging psychological problems. Also, the minimally invasive radiological embolization technique has been a vital step forward in the treatment of, for example, large, benign, but apparently aggressive aneurysmal bone cysts.

Last but not least, it is important to stress that a combination of progress made in anesthesia and the widespread application of minimally invasive surgical techniques has lad to a huge improvement of this pediatric surgical specialization. It has opened up the real possibility to cure any disease of the musculoskeletal system, be it congenital, acquired, genetic, malformative, infectious, or posttraumatic, as well as benign and even malignant tumors of uncertain prognosis.

Q 168

Francesco Sadile and Fabrizio Cigala

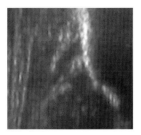 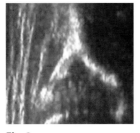 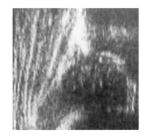 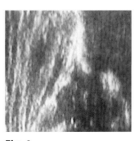

Fig. 1   Fig. 2   Fig. 3   Fig. 4

A 1-month-old girl was born at term with no clinical at-risk features of orthopedic disease; the Ortolani-Barlow test result was normal at birth and 2 weeks later.

Her mother was referred to an orthopedic specialist because of a retrieved familial history of developmental displacement of the hip (DDH) not previously reported.

An ultrasound examination of both hips was performed at 45 days of life.

- What do Figs. 1 (right hip) and 2 (left hip) show at 45 days of age?
- Which pathological condition is affecting this child?
- Why did the specialist perform the second ultrasound examination?
- What do Figs. 3 (right hip) and 4 (left hip) show at 3 months of age?
- What is the best way to manage this condition?
- What are the results at mid-term follow-up?

A 168

This child is affected by developmental dysplasia of the right hip (DDH).

Frequently at birth, clinical tests such as the Ortolani-Barlow click sign and limitation of hip abduction yield normal results, whereas 1 month later clinical examination is more effective.

In particular, the clinical evaluation made at birth should be repeated every 2 weeks to check and to avoid false-negative or false-positive ultrasonographic findings.

Furthermore, together with a clinical examination, an anamnestic history of DDH is particularly important in cross-linked cases difficult to detect in a postpartum interview: it is recommended that a form is filled in every time.

According to Graf's ultrasound hip examination method, Fig. 1 shows a type-IIC hip and Fig. 2 a type-IIB hip.

Even if the natural history of these cases is benign, i.e., complete maturation within 3 or 4 months of age, a different evolution may be seen both clinically and sonographically.

In particular, type IIC is classified as at-risk hip with no abduction device.

Figures 3 and 4 at 3 months of age show an apparently good restoration of the alpha and beta angles according to Graf's method, but the right hip was clinically unstable and Ortolani's maneuver was positive.

In instances of clinical and ultrasonographic dissociation, it is mandatory to perform a standard or frog-leg radiography of the pelvis.

Normally, a frog-leg position after birth is advisable for all newborns so as to facilitate a complete and stable acetabular maturation; in cases of immature or worse hips, as in this example, an abduction device is indicated such as the Milgram type in Fig. 5, which shows, on the right, a worsening of the right acetabulum, hypoplasia of the ossification center, but a full hip centering at 5 months after detection of right hip instability.

The mid-term results of hips treated with abduction devices are similar to what is shown in Fig. 6, a progressive restoration and maturation of hip parameters, confirmed by long-term results shown in Fig. 7.

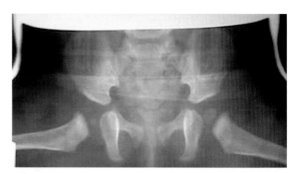

Fig. 5

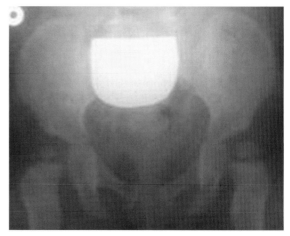

Fig. 6

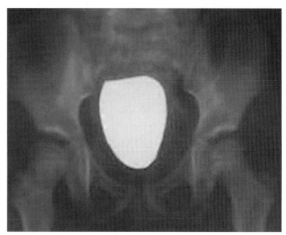

Fig. 7

Q 169

Francesco Sadile and Fabrizio Cigala

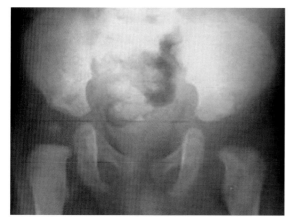

Fig. 1

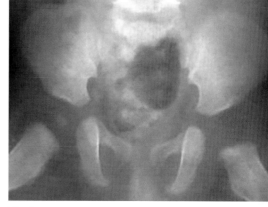

Fig. 2

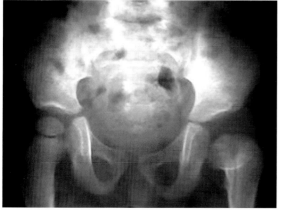

Fig. 3

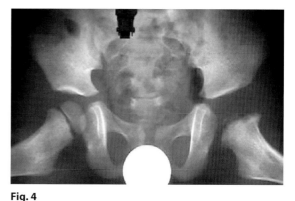

Fig. 4

A boy was born at full term, weighing 3,050 kg and measuring 48 cm, with no at-risk signs of orthopedic disease.

At 50 days of life, culture of synovial fluid led to the diagnosis of septic arthritis of the right knee caused by *Candida albicans*. Parenteral therapy with Ambisone was started for a period of 30 days.

Just before starting this therapy, the pediatric orthopedic consultant noticed a painful stiff contralateral hip, but hip radiographs did not show anything of importance.

At the 5-month follow-up, the right knee was clinically normal, whereas the left hip showed a limitation of abduction and internal rotation.

- What do Figs. 1 and 2 show at 5 months?
- Is a harness indicated in this case to prevent hip subluxation?
- What do Figs. 3 and 4 show at 3 years?
- What are the results at long-term follow-up?

A 169

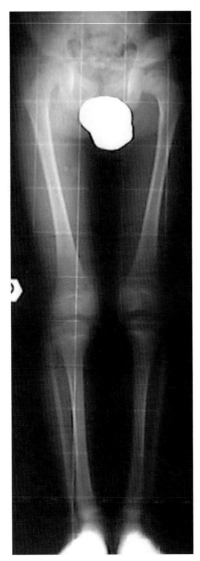

Fig. 5

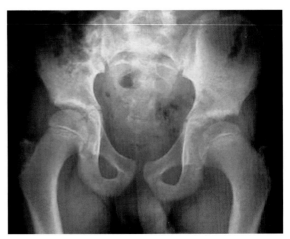

Fig. 6

mal femoral metaphysis, and partial extrusion from the cavity with no sign of acetabular dysplasia.

The Milgram abduction harness prevents any other degree of subluxation within 4 months.

Figures 3 and 4 show an initial ossification of the proximal femoral head, an enlargement of the proximal femoral metaphysis, and no sign of acetabular dysplasia.

Figures 5 (at 6 years of age) and 6 (at 11 years of age) show the positive evolution of skeletal growth of the lower limbs; in particular, Fig. 5 shows axial normality of the right knee and Fig. 6 demonstrates the very good remodeling of the left hip, particularly when compared with Fig .3.

This child is affected by mycotic septic arthritis of the left hip and right knee.

Frequently at birth, the knee is flexed and somewhat stiff, whereas the hip should be stable with a range of motion that tends to improve with skeletal growth.

In particular, passive articular motion should not cause any pain or crying in a newborn with apyretic subcutaneous swelling.

Figures 1 and 2 show a hypoplasia of the proximal femoral center of ossification, an osteolysis of the proxi-

Suggested Reading

1. Cigala F, Lotito FM, Sadile F. La terapia ortopedica negli esiti di artrite settica. In: Nuove frontiere in pediatria medica e chirurgica CIC Eds 1986; 149–153
2. Hechard P, Carlioz H. Méthode pratique de prévision des inégalités de longueur des membres inférieurs. Rev Chir Orthop 1979; 7:373–375
3. Nade S. Acute arthritis in infancy and childhood J Bone Joint Surg 1983; 65B:234–241
4. Paterson D. Septic arthritis of hip joint. Orthop Clin North Am 1978; 9:135–142
5. Zamzam MM. The role of ultrasound in differentiating septic arthritis from transient synovitis of the hip in children. J Pediatr Orthop 2006; 15B:418–422

Q 170

Francesco Sadile and Fabrizio Cigala

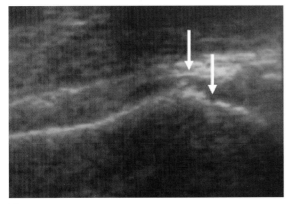

Fig. 1

A 13-year-old girl was referred to an orthopedic institution suffering from left hip pain 1 year after undergoing a right hip operation not clearly reported to the specialist at the time of the visit.

At the time of the first episode of right hip pain, the contralateral side was clinically painless with a complete range of motion (ROM) and was radiographically normal on both views.

- Generally, what is the clinical presentation at the onset of any hip disease?
- Which diagnostic examinations are necessary in these cases?
- What does Fig. 1 show?
- Which radiological examinations should be performed?
- Which pathological condition is affecting this child on the left side?
- What are the results at long-term follow-up?

A 170

This child was affected by slipped capital femoral epiphysis (SCFE) bilaterally with sequential onset of the disease from right to left.

At the onset of any developmental juvenile hip disease the clinical signs are (1) stiff hip in flexion (positive Thomas's maneuver), (2) limitation of internal rotation, and (3) limitation of abduction.

Frequently, at the onset of a SCFE, these clinical signs are not found at the contralateral side and there are no objective radiographic predictive signs, which in the literature is known as "so-called contralateral sound hip."

In particular, a clinical evaluation should be made more frequently and any variations from normal are to be considered at-risk signs of subsequent bilateral occurrence of SCFE.

At a very early phase of femoral head slipping, as shown in Fig. 1, an anterior ultrasonographic hip view can show an initial sign of the posterior slipping of the femoral proximal epiphysis (note how the *arrow*—femoral head—slips from up to down).

The first orthopedic surgeon in agreement with part of the scientific surgical community, preferred to cure only the hip affected by slipping because there was no true diagnosis of this condition on the other side yet.

Figures 2 and 3 are radiographs showing the right hip fixation and the slipping of the contralateral left hip.

Figures 4 and 5 show the contralateral left Knowles pinning.

Long-term results depend on the severity of the slipping; in mild and moderate cases (<50°), especially in young patients with a great potential of bone remodeling, good results occur in the majority; in severe cases (>50°) the results depend on the type of corrective osteotomy, such as cervical osteotomy according to Dunn and intertrochanteric according to Southwick's procedure, and on the complications, such as avascular head necrosis and chondrolysis, respectively.

Suggested Reading

1. Bidwell TA, Susan Stott N. Sequential slipped capital femoral epiphysis: who is at risk for a second slip? ANZ J Surg 2006; 76:973–976
2. Cigala F, Sadile F. Southwick's osteotomy in the treatment of chronic slipped upper femoral epiphysis. Fixation with AO blade plate. Italian J Orthop and Traum 1984; 10:461–468
3. Cigala F, Sadile F, Lotito FM, Coppola C. Southwick's osteotomy in the treatment of chronic slipped capital femoral epiphysis fixed by AO blade-plate at 130°. Long-term results. Mapfre Medicina 10 Suppl 1999; 1:138–145

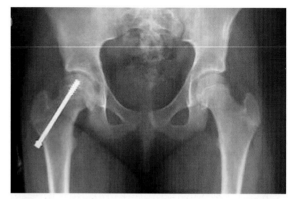

Fig. 2

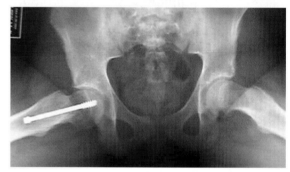

Fig. 3

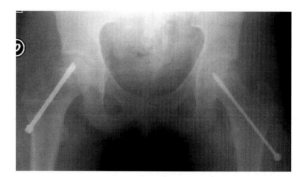

Fig. 4

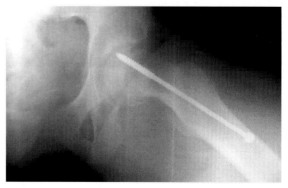

Fig. 5

Q 171

Francesco Sadile and Fabrizio Cigala

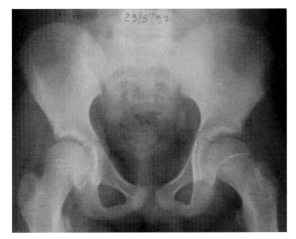

Fig. 1

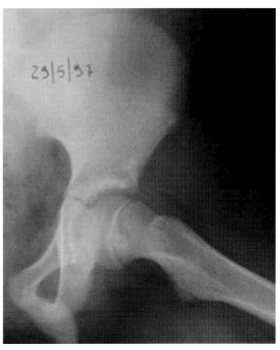

Fig. 2

An 11-year-old fast-growing boy suffered from occasional left knee pain for 4 months.

In the last month, he complained of limping especially after a walk or sports activity. A radiograph of the left knee was normal.

On hospital admission, a pelvic radiograph was acquired in the AP and "frog leg" view.

- What do Figs. 1 and 2 show?
- What pathological condition is affecting this child?
- Why did the child complain of knee pain initially?
- What is the best way to manage this condition?
- What is the natural history of this condition if untreated?

A 171

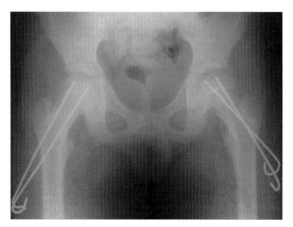

Fig. 3

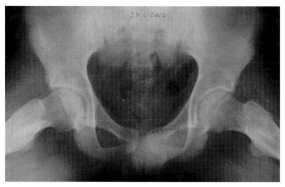

Fig. 4

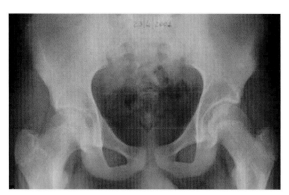

Fig. 5

Fig. 6

This child is affected by chronic slipped capital femoral epiphysis of the left hip (SCFE).

SCFE can occur in acute or chronic form.

Chronic SCFE is classified into slight, mild, and severe types according to the gravity of the slipping: <30°, from 30° to 50°, and >50°, respectively, according to Southwick's radiological method.

Figures 1 and 2 show an asymmetry of the Klein line on the left side in relation to the right one as seen in the AP and frog leg views.

Knee pain as an expression of early hip pain is explained on an anatomical basis as a short circuit mediated by a full canal by-pass from the obturator sensory branch of the ischiatic nerve and the medial saphenous sensory branch of the femoral nerve.

In the slight and mild types, the choice of therapy is cartilage pinning with Knowles rods or similar devices such as Kirchner wires, depending on the patient's age (see Figs. 3, 4).

If untreated the head tends to fall step by step medially and posteriorly causing severe deformity of the hip and consequently early osteoarthritis. Thus, it is mandatory to treat these patients early so as to achieve the best results, like those shown in Figs. 5 and 6 at the end of treatment.

Q 172

Francesco Sadile and Fabrizio Cigala

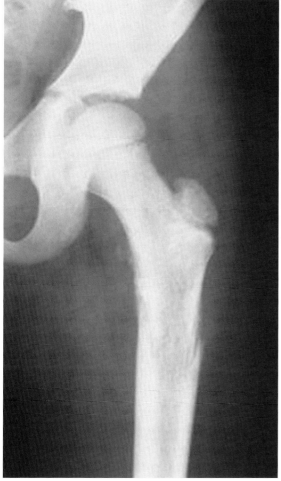

Fig. 1

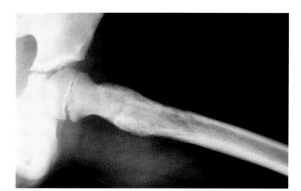

Fig. 2

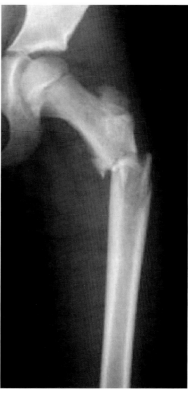

Fig. 3

A 10-year-old boy suffered from left hip pain for 4 months. He underwent radiography of the left femur in AP and lateral views.

• What do Figs. 1 and 2 show?

On the same day, the boy fell and was taken to hospital.

• What does Fig. 3 show?
• What should the correct diagnosis have been?
• Which diagnostic procedures should have been initiated?

A 172

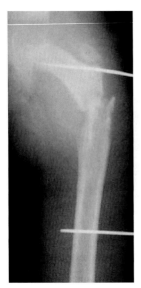

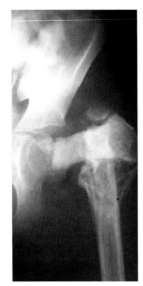

Fig. 4   **Fig. 5**

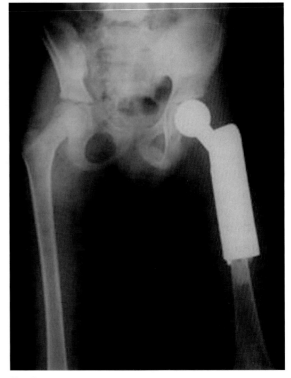

Fig. 6

Figures 1 and 2 show osteoporosis and cortical erosion of the proximal femoral metaphysis.

The correct diagnosis, by examining the radiograph in Fig. 3, should have been "pathological fracture at the femoral neck."

As shown in Fig. 4, in the emergency room the fracture was treated percutaneously with Kirchner wires and immobilized in a plaster of Paris cast.

Once a risk fracture was established at this level, the procedures that should have been initiated include plaster cast immobilization and fine-needle aspiration or open biopsy. The diagnosis of Ewing sarcoma would

have been made 2.5 months earlier. Total-body scintigraphy, thoracic CT, and MR imaging of the hip would have been required.

The child was treated preoperatively according to an adjuvant chemotherapeutic protocol.

Subsequently, as shown in Figs. 5 and 6, a proximal femoral resection (Fig. 5) was carried out with a custom-made prosthesis (Fig. 6).

At the 5-year follow-up the child was free of disease. The prosthesis was working well and showed no lines of radiolucency. The limb was about 6 cm short.

Suggested Reading

1. Campanacci M. Tumori dell'osso e della parti molli. A.Gaggi Ed. Bologna 1990
2. Huvos AG. Bone tumors. Diagnosis treatment and prognosis. W Saunders Ed. Philadelphia 1990
3. Iaccarino V, Sadile F, Vetrani A, Fulciniti F, Troncone G, Riccio R, Misasi N. Percutaneous intralesional brushing of cystic lesions of bone: a technical improvement of diagnostic cytology. Skeletal Radiology 1990; 19:187–190
4. Mirra JM. Bone tumors. Diagnosis and treatment. JP Lippincott Philadelphia 1991

Q 173

Giovanni Esposito and Ciro Esposito

A 7-year-old girl fell down and sustained an injury to the right arm. She had pain in the upper third of the right arm and functional impotence. After radiography (Fig. 1) was performed, she underwent surgery.

- What does the radiograph show?
- What was the diagnosis?
- What was the treatment?
- What did the disease consist in?
- What was the follow-up?

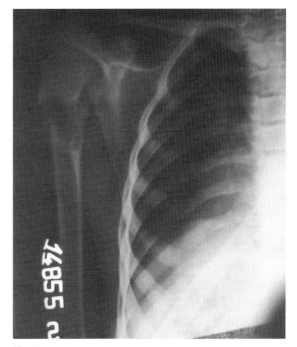

Fig. 1

A 173

The radiograph shows a fracture of the upper third of the humerus over a bone cyst with some displacement of the fragments. The cyst resembles an osteolysis with cleanly incised margins and a thinning or ballooning cortex, traversed by bone septum.

The diagnosis was bone cyst complicated by a traumatic fracture.

The treatment comprised surgical curettage of the cyst, reduction of the fracture, and a homologous bone graft. After surgery the arm was immobilized for 4 weeks.

After removing the plaster, the radiographic checkup revealed that bone union had taken place. After 2 years, there were no signs of recurrence.

Unicameral bone cysts are due to atrophic and degenerative phenomena that may present asymptomatically or with a local pain. They occur more frequently in the metaphysis of the humerus as in the case illustrated here or in the metaphysis of the femur, tibia, and rarely in the ribs, ileum, calcaneum, and talus. They may be complicated by a fracture, both spontaneous or traumatic. When a fracture complicates a symptomatic cyst the pain becomes continuous and it is accompanied by the symptoms of the fracture.

When the cyst is intact, treatment includes curettage of the cavity followed by an intracystic injection of cortisone and by a bone graft or radical subperiosteal excision of the cyst followed by an autologous or homologous bone graft. When a fracture is present, the treatment is like the one illustrated in our case.

Suggested Reading

1. Bhatnagar R, Nzegwu NI, Miller NH. Diagnosis and treatment of common fractures in children: femoral shaft fractures and supracondylar humeral fractures. J Surg Orthop Adv 2006 Spring; 15(1):1–15
2. Carmichael KD, Joyner K. Quality of reduction versus timing of surgical intervention for pediatric supracondylar humerus fractures. Orthopedics 2006 Jul; 29(7):628–32
3. Hart ES, Grottkau BE, Rebello GN, Albright MB. Broken bones: common pediatric upper extremity fractures–part II. Orthop Nurs 2006 Sep–Oct; 25(5):311–23
4. Scaglietti O, Marchetti PG, Bartolozzi P. The effect of methylprednisone acetate in the treatment of bone cysts. Results of three years follow-up. J Bone Joint Surg 1979; 61:200-3
5. Schroeden B. The results of treatment of simple cysts with curettage and cryotherapy. J Pediatr Orthop 1996; 47: 27-30

Q 174

Giovanni Esposito, Ciro Esposito, and Alessandro Settimi

A young girl, without any previous medical problems, suffered from pain in the lower third of the left thigh with functional impotence of the left leg. In the same site, a painless, hard, consistent swelling had appeared 2 months earlier. After radiography of the femur (Fig. 1) and other examinations, she underwent surgery.

- What does the radiograph of the femur demonstrate?
- Which other examination were necessary?
- What was the diagnosis?
- What was the treatment?
- What was the follow-up?

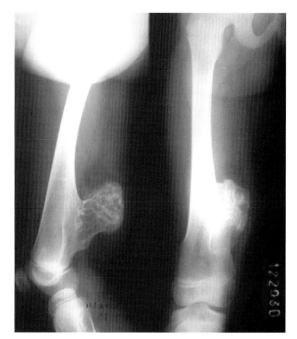

Fig. 1

A 174

The radiograph shows an osteocartilaginous mass with a large base and fungus shape in the supracondyle region of the femur.

The diagnosis was very simple: a huge exostosis of the femur. Exostosis is a hyperplasia of cartilaginous tissue projecting from the surface of a bone, generally long ones. It is usually a benign and asymptomatic disease that can appear with pain accompanied by a mass in the same region.

When there is an exostosis the entire skeleton should be examined for other localizations. In our case, there were two exostoses of the femur (a bigger one in the medial side, the other in the lateral side of the upper third of femur), and in addition two other exostoses were located in the right humerus (Fig. 2). The definitive diagnosis was multiple exostoses disease. This entity is characterized by a dominant inheritance and it is more frequent in males. In general, exostosis is accompanied by segmentary deformities and growth decrease in the length of the affected bone.

The treatment consists in removing the exostosis, because of its potential malignant transformation into osteochondroma. In our case, we resected only the large exostosis located in the femur. The small exostosis of the femur and the exostosis of the humerus were excised 6 months later at another institution.

The postoperative course was uneventful and the girl was discharged following a radiographic evaluation 10 days after surgery (Fig. 3).

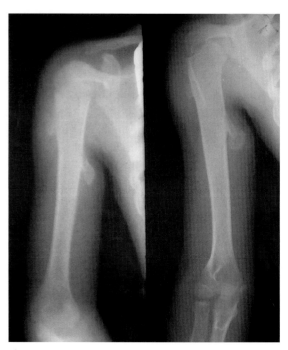

Fig. 2

Suggested Reading

1. Alvarez C, Tredwell S, De Vera M, Hayden M. The genotype-phenotype correlation of hereditary multiple exostoses. Clin Genet 2006 Aug; 70(2):122–30
2. Darilek S, Wicklund C, Novy D, Scott A, Gambello M, Johnston D, Hecht J. Hereditary multiple exostosis and pain. J Pediatr Orthop 2005 May–Jun; 25(3):369–76
3. Porter DE, Lonie L, Fraser M, Dobson-Stone C, Porter JR, Monaco AP, Simpson AH. Severity of disease and risk of malignant change in hereditary multiple exostoses. A genotype-phenotype study. J Bone Joint Surg Br 2004 Sep; 86(7):1041–6

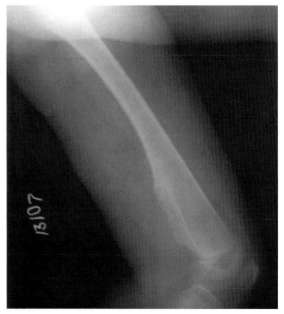

Fig. 3

Q 175

Craig T. Albanese

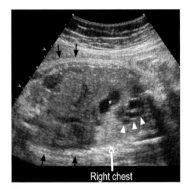

Fig. 1

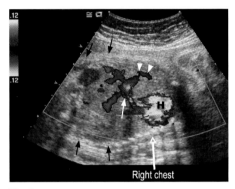

Fig. 2

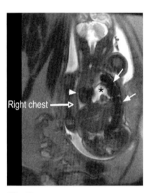

Fig. 3

A routine prenatal coronal ultrasound through the fetal chest and abdomen at 21 weeks' gestation is presented in Fig. 1 (abdomen, *black arrows*; stomach, *asterisk*; heart, *arrowheads*). Color flow Doppler (Fig. 2) demonstrates a branch of the left hepatic vein (*arrowhead*) above the level of the diaphragm (abdomen, *black arrows*; infra-diaphragmatic inferior vena cava, *arrow*; heart, *H*).

The abnormality was imaged with MR imaging (Figs. 3, 4).

- What is the diagnosis?

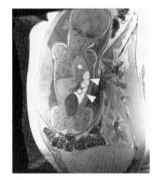

Fig. 4

A 175

The ultrasound demonstrates a left congenital diaphragmatic hernia. The left lobe of the liver and the stomach are herniated into the left hemithorax. Subsequent fetal MR imaging (Fig. 3) with a fluid-sensitive sequence demonstrates the stomach (*asterisk*) and colon (*arrows*) herniated into the left hemithorax. The heart (*arrowhead*) is displaced into the right chest. Fetal MR imaging (Fig. 4) with an iron-sensitive sequence demonstrates the left lobe of the liver (*asterisk*) herniated into the left hemithorax. The herniated colon is also depicted (*arrowheads*).

A postnatal chest radiograph (Fig. 5) shows a large left-side diaphragmatic hernia involving the stomach (*asterisk*), liver, and intestines, with secondary mediastinal shift to the right. At birth, this child had severe respiratory failure, required extracorporeal membrane oxygenation support, and succumbed from pulmonary hypoplasia and pulmonary hypertension at 16 days of life.

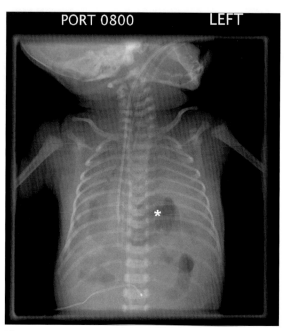

Fig. 5

Suggested Reading

1. Deprest J, Jani J, Van Schoubroeck D, Cannie M, Gallot D, Dymarkowski S, Fryns JP, Naulaers G, Gratacos E, Nicolaides K. Current consequences of prenatal diagnosis of congenital diaphragmatic hernia. J Pediatr Surg 2006 Feb; 41(2):423–30

2. Dillon E, Renwick M, Wright C. Congenital diaphragmatic herniation: antenatal detection and outcome. Br J Radiol 2000 Apr; 73(868):360–5

3. Jani J, Keller RL, Benachi A, Nicolaides KH, Favre R, Gratacos E, Laudy J, Eisenberg V, Eggink A, Vaast P, Deprest J. Antenatal-CDH-Registry Group. Prenatal prediction of survival in isolated left-sided diaphragmatic hernia. Ultrasound Obstet Gynecol 2006 Jan; 27(1):18–22

Q 176

Giovanni Esposito and Ciro Esposito

An 8-year-old child, without a significant medical history, fell from a tree. At the emergency unit, a lacerated wound of the left parieto-occipital region, contusion of the left shoulder, and concussion were found.

After radiography of the head (Fig. 1), the boy was transferred to a neurosurgical unit. A few minutes later the child had several epileptic Jacksonian crises. Consequently, he underwent urgent surgical treatment.

- What did the radiograph show?
- What was the diagnosis?
- What was the treatment?
- What was the follow-up?

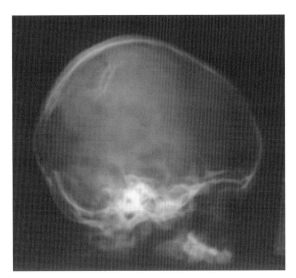

Fig. 1

A 176

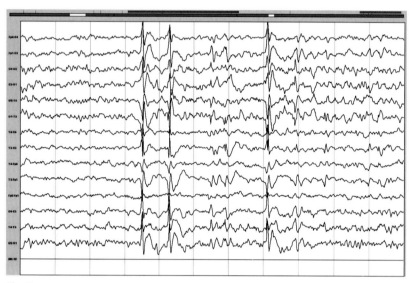

Fig. 2

This patient had a skull fracture. The radiography showed a diastatic fracture of the left parietal bone.

The diagnosis was cranial fracture complicated by a compression of the brain due to splinters. Other diagnostic procedures that can be performed in this case are a MRJ and an EEG.

The treatment consisted in craniotomy with removal of the splinters.

The postoperative course was uneventful with a gradual disappearance of the epileptic crisis and a good recovery (as shows the EEG in Fig. 2); the child was discharged 10 days later.

Suggested Reading

1. Adamsbaum C, Rolland Y, Husson B. Pediatric neuroimaging emergencies. J Neuroradiol 2004 Sep; 31(4):272–80
2. Da Dalt L, Marchi AG, Laudizi L, Crichiutti G, Messi G, Pavanello L, Valent F, Barbone F. Predictors of intracranial injuries in children after blunt head trauma. Eur J Pediatr 2006 Mar; 165(3):142–8
3. Fischer B, Wit J. Emergency ward management of traumatic head injury in children. Unfallchirurg 2006 Nov 23
4. Jankowitz BT, Adelson PD. Pediatric traumatic brain injury: past, present and future.
5. Dev Neurosci 2006; 28(4–5):264–75
6. Kim KA, Wang MY, Griffith PM, Summers S, Levy ML. Analysis of pediatric head injury from falls. Neurosurg Focus 2000 Jan 15

Q 177

Juan A. Tovar

A boy was born to a 31-year-old primiparous woman after a long, cephalic delivery. He weighed 4.3 kg and did not require resuscitation.

Immediately after birth, a bulge in his left clavicle was seen. This area was obviously painful and the baby cried upon mobilization. He was otherwise normal and started feeding a few hours after birth.

A plain radiograph of the left clavicle is depicted in Fig. 1.

- Can you describe the lesion shown in Fig. 1?
- Can you suggest the best form of treatment in these cases?
- What is the best moment for operation?
- Describe the sequelae that can be expected.

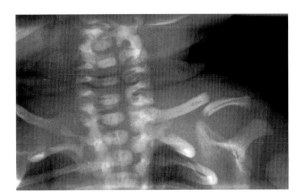

Fig. 1

A 177

This baby has a fracture of the clavicle.

This is a rather common lesion after delivery of large babies, when shoulder dystocia occurs, or in premature deliveries. However, most cases are seen after normal deliveries of normal-weight babies.

Figure 1 shows a mid-clavicular fracture with displacement of the fragments and conservation of the clavicular axis.

These lesions do not require specific treatment. Several forms of bracing and contentions are advised but, in fact, none is necessary since this mesenchymal bone heals rapidly and without sequelae.

In no case is surgery justified.

Suggested Reading

1. Chez RA, Carlan S, Greenberg SL, Spellacy WN. Fractured clavicle is an unavoidable event. Am J Obstet Gynecol 1994; 171:797–8

2. Gonen R, Spiegel D, Abend M. Is macrosomia predictable, and are shoulder dystocia and birth trauma preventable? Obstet Gynecol 1996; 88:526–9

3. Kaplan B, Rabinerson D, Avrech OM, Carmi N, Steinberg DM, Merlob P. Fracture of the clavicle in the newborn following normal labor and delivery. Int J Gynaecol Obstet 1998; 63:15–20

Q 178

Francesco Sadile and Fabrizio Cigala

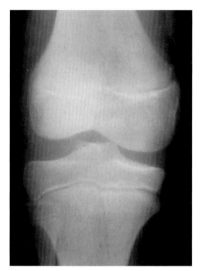 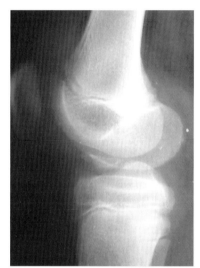

Fig. 1   **Fig. 2**

A 9-year-old girl was born at term with no clinical at-risk signs of orthopedic disease.

Her parents were referred to our orthopedic institution because she suffered indirect trauma in the right knee during a handball game.

Figures 1 and 2 show two radiographic planes of the knee examination performed on admission to the emergency unit.

- What do Figs. 1 (anteroposterior view) and 2 (lateral view) show?
- How would you classify this secondary pathological condition affecting the patient?
- What is the best way to manage this condition?
- What are the results at long-term follow-up?

A 178

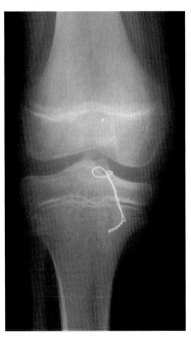

Fig. 3

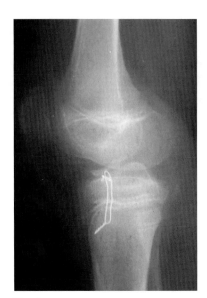

Fig. 4

This girl is affected by posttraumatic fracture of the anterior tibial prominence (tibial spine avulsion).

Figures 1 and 2 show a detachment of the anterior portion of the intercondylar prominence with a complete loss of bone continuity of the fracture fragment from the tibial floor.

This particular fracture is categorized as fracture–dislocation of the anterior ligament that requires fracture and ligament fixation. The latter produces knee laxity characterized clinically by a positive Lachman test (anterior tibial translation at almost 15°–20° of passive flexion) and by anterior subluxation of the lateral condyle at jerk or pivot shift testing.

According to Meyer's and McKeever's classification, type I fractures are defined as incomplete or minimally displaced spine avulsion, type II is a complete fracture

rotated with the posterior aspect still in place, whereas type III represents a completely displaced fracture clearly visible on radiographs.

In our case, the trauma is classified as type III, i.e., requiring surgical reduction and fixation to restore the normal biomechanics of the knee.

Normally, in types I and II the gold standard treatment is a conservative plaster cast of the lower limb with the knee in slight flexion (20°–30°) for 3 or 4 weeks.

Figures 3 and 4 at 3-month follow-up show an apparently good surgical reduction by an arthroscopically assisted wire-fixation method.

The mid- and long-term results are very satisfactory from an anatomic as well as a functional point of view. The anterior laxity disappears very quickly, as demonstrated by knee testing at follow-up.

Q 179

Francesco Sadile and Fabrizio Cigala

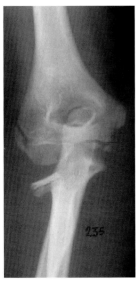

Fig. 1

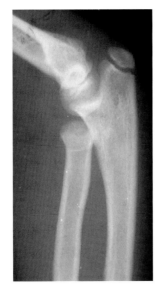

Fig. 2

An 8-year-old boy was referred to our orthopedic institution because of an indirect trauma on his right wrist following a bad tumble during a running game with his friends.

Figures 1 and 2 show two radiographic planes of the elbow examination performed on admission to the emergency unit.

- What do Figs. 1 (anteroposterior view) and 2 (lateral view) show?
- How would you classify this secondary pathological condition affecting the child?
- What is the best way to manage this condition?
- What are the results at long-term follow-up?

A 179

This boy is affected by fracture of the neck of the right radius.

Figures 1 and 2 show a complete fracture–dislocation of the head of the radius.

This particular fracture is categorized as fracture–dislocation at the elbow requiring surgical open reduction and fixation.

According to Judet's classification, type I and II fractures are defined as incomplete or minimally displaced fracture of the neck of the radius up to 30°, type III is defined as having more than 30°–60° tilt with a variable degree of displacement, whereas type IV represents a completely displaced fracture clearly visible on radiographs.

In our case, the trauma is classified as type IV, i.e., requiring surgical reduction and fixation to restore the normal elbow anatomy and function.

Normally, in type I a plaster cast is sufficient for complete healing of the trauma; for types II to III the gold standard method is closed reduction—under general anesthesia—and a conservative plaster cast of the elbow for 3–4 weeks with rehabilitation.

Figures 3 and 4 show the postoperative follow-up with complete good surgical reduction using Kirchner's wire fixation method.

The mid- and long-term results are very satisfactory but generally depend on the amount of growth cartilage damage (type IV) and blood supply interruption (type IV), which are not easy to assess just after trauma; in fact, no method can predict the prognosis of this type of fracture. Accurate analysis of the radiographs and appropriate classification along with the best choice of treatment (closed or open) contribute to achieving good results with no necrosis and no limitation of the articular function of the elbow.

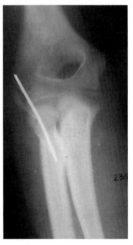 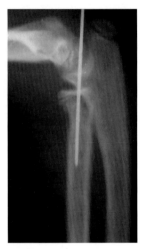

Fig. 3   **Fig. 4**

Suggested Reading

1. Weber GB, Brunner Ch, Freuler F. Treatment of fractures in children and adolescents. Springer-Verlag Berlin Heidelberg New York 1980

7

Emergency
and Trauma

Q 180

Juan A. Tovar

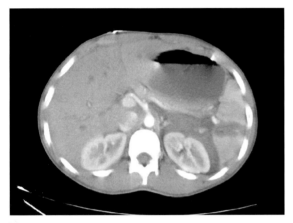

Fig. 1

A 7-year-old boy fell from his bicycle on the curb and hit his lower thorax and upper abdomen.

He was admitted to hospital with good vital signs, moderate tachycardia, and bruises in the lower thoracic wall.

His blood hemoglobin level was 10 g/dl and blood gases and electrolytes were normal. Serum amylase and glutamic-oxaloacetic-transaminase (GOT) and glutamic-pyruvic-transaminase (GPT) levels were slightly increased.

He was admitted to the ICU, where a central line and nasogastric and urinary catheters were inserted.

A section of the CT scan with contrast, performed 2 h after the trauma, is depicted in Fig. 1.

Over the ensuing hours the abdomen became distended and painful, hemoglobin levels fell to 7g/dl, urine output decreased, and tachycardia developed.

Blood was given at 25 ml/kg until vital signs stabilized and urine output was normalized.

- What does Fig. 1 show?
- Are the kidneys normal?
- What additional tests would you order?
- What would your therapeutic approach be at this stage?

A 180

This child had splenic rupture, a rather common lesion, that caused retroperitoneal hemorrhage and moderate hemoperitoneum.

It is not unusual to have some increase of serum liver and pancreatic enzymes because these organs are also traumatized, although mildly.

In Fig. 1, the splenic hilum is disrupted and a complete separation of both splenic halves is seen.

However, parenchymal vascularization remains good and the splenic artery is well depicted.

The pancreas is displaced forward and the kidneys look normal.

Additional tests are probably not necessary, except for repeated hemoglobin measurements. The splenic lesion can be monitored by ultrasonography.

The symptoms of hemodynamic instability and the decrease in hemoglobin show that bleeding continued until stabilization.

The therapeutic approach should be close observation and replacement of blood loss. These hemorrhages are generally low-pressure ones and subside when intraperitoneal pressure increases with hemoperitoneum.

The spleen heals nicely in the vast majority of these cases with full preservation of function.

Surgery is only indicated when significant blood loss continues (requiring more than 40 ml/kg of blood). In such cases, repair of the organ is not always possible and splenectomy may be unavoidable.

Splenectomy is potentially dangerous particularly in early childhood because the patient becomes more prone to suffering OPSI (overwhelming postsplenectomy infection).

Suggested Reading

1. Brown RL, Irish MS, McCabe AJ, Glick PL, Caty MG. Observation of splenic trauma: when is a little too much? J Pediatr Surg 1999; 34:1124–6

2. Ein SH, Shandling B, Simpson JS, Stephens CA. Nonoperative management of traumatized spleen in children: how and why. J Pediatr Surg 1978; 13:117–9

3. Schwartz MZ, Kangah R. Splenic injury in children after blunt trauma: blood transfusion requirements and length of hospitalization for laparotomy versus observation. J Pediatr Surg 1994; 29:596–8

4. Sjovall A, Hirsch K. Blunt abdominal trauma in children: risks of nonoperative treatment. J Pediatr Surg 1997; 32:1169–74

5. Wesson DE, Filler RM, Ein SH, Shandling B, Simpson JS, Stephens CA. Ruptured spleen—when to operate? J Pediatr Surg 1981; 16:324–6

Q 181

Juan A. Tovar

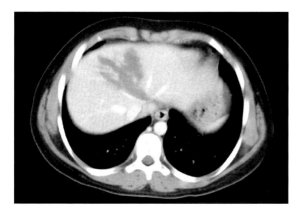

Fig. 1

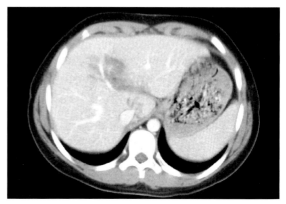

Fig. 2

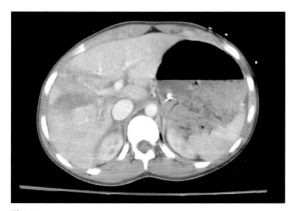
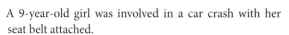

Fig. 3

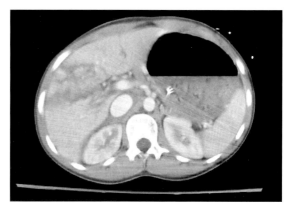

Fig. 4

A 9-year-old girl was involved in a car crash with her seat belt attached.

She was admitted to hospital with tachycardia and several bruises in various parts of her body.

Urine output was reduced, blood pressure was stable, and she had severe abdominal pain. No neurological signs or limb fractures were detected.

Hematocrit was 30%, serum glutamic-oxalacetic transaminase (SGOT) and serum glutamate-pyruvate transaminase (SGPT) levels were increased, and total bilirubin was slightly increased. Amylases were normal.

Several IV contrast-enhanced CT scan sections are shown in Figs. 1–4.

Over the following 2 days, the abdomen remained distended and tender, hemoglobin levels fell to 7 g/dl, urine output was maintained, and tachycardia disappeared.

Blood transfusion was not required.

- What do Figs. 1–4 show?
- What would your therapeutic approach be at this stage?

A 181

This child had liver rupture that caused retroperitoneal hemorrhage and moderate hemoperitoneum.

It is usual to have increased serum liver enzymes because of the crushed parenchyma and cell damage.

Figures 1–4 show that there was no intrapleural blood, that the upper part of the liver was obliquely severed to the left of the inferior vena cava, which was intact, that the wound crossed to the right side along the axis of the right portal vein, which was also undamaged, and that there was blood between the right kidney and the liver. Both kidneys seem intact.

Close monitoring is necessary, and ultrasonography is very useful for this purpose.

Most of these patients stabilize and do not require any operative treatment. Hemorrhages are generally low-pressure ones and the bleeders as well as the bile ducts are sealed. If this does not happen, bile collections may be seen in the ensuing days. In this case, percutaneous drainage may suffice.

Surgery in only indicated when significant blood continues, when there are associated hollow viscus lesions, and when massive bile leaks occur.

Secondary surgery or percutaneous procedures may be indicated in a few cases for treating persistent bile or pus collections or hemobilia, but most heal without major operative procedures.

Suggested Reading

1. Ameh EA, Chirdan LB, Nmadu PT. Blunt abdominal trauma in children: epidemiology, management, and management problems in a developing country. Pediatr Surg Int 2000; 16:505–9

2. Avanoglu A, Ulman I, Ergun O, et al. Blood transfusion requirements in children with blunt spleen and liver injuries. Eur J Pediatr Surg 1998; 8:322–5

3. Hendren WH, Warshaw AL, Fleischli DJ, Bartlett MK. Traumatic hemobilia: non-operative management with healing documented by serial angiography. Ann Surg 1971; 174:991–3

4. Kumar R, Holland AJ, Shi E, Cass DT. Isolated and multi-system hepatic trauma in children: the true role of non-operative management. Pediatr Surg Int 2002; 18:98–103

5. Landau A, van As AB, Numanoglu A, Millar AJ, Rode H. Liver injuries in children: the role of selective non-operative management. Injury 2006; 37:66–71

6. Ozturk H, Dokucu AI, Onen A, Otcu S, Gedik S, Azal OF. Non-operative management of isolated solid organ injuries due to blunt abdominal trauma in children: a fifteen-year experience. Eur J Pediatr Surg 2004; 14:29–34

Q 182

Juan A. Tovar

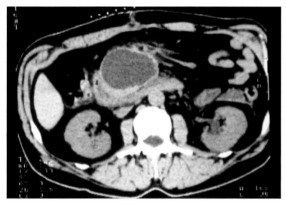

Fig. 1

A 9-year-old boy fell while riding a bicycle. Upon physical examination, the abdomen was tender and a round bruise was visible above the umbilicus.

His hematocrit was normal but he had leukocytosis and high serum amylase and lipase levels.

Abdominal ultrasonography revealed a thickened body of the pancreas.

He was kept NPO and improved over the next few days. Amylase levels decreased but they increased again on day 8.

A CT scan was performed and one of the sections is shown in Fig. 1.
- Describe Fig. 1.
- Describe the different therapeutic options in cases like this one.
- What would your therapeutic approach be at this stage?
- In which circumstances would you indicate an operation?

A 182

This child had a blunt abdominal trauma. The handlebar bruise demonstrates that there was severe pressure on the organs located between the anterior abdominal wall and the spine.

Under these circumstances the pancreas is crushed and the parenchyma and ducts may be disrupted.

Enzymes are released and the pancreas is inflamed. If ductal lesions are relatively large, exocrine secretion accumulates leading to a pseudocyst.

The CT scan section in Fig. 1 depicts one of these pseudocysts located in front of the pancreas. The parenchyma does not look fractured. Endoscopic retrograde cholangiopancreatography (ERCP) or magnetic RCP may be of interest in theses cases.

Nonoperative treatment is generally successful. Under pancreatic rest, the pseudocyst usually regresses and the lesions heal.

Other therapeutic options are puncture and external drainage as well as cystogastrostomy via a transgastric, laparoscopic, or endoscopic approach.

However, when major disruption of the Wirsung duct occurs, the cyst may be very large and without tendency to heal. In these cases the parenchyma may be severed between the head and the body. More extensive operative treatment may be required in these rare cases. Distal pancreatectomy with preservation of the spleen when possible is an option. Pancreaticojejunal anastomosis may help to preserve the entire pancreas in cases of complete body disruption.

Suggested Reading

1. Bosboom D, Braam AW, Blickman JG, Wijnen RM. The role of imaging studies in pancreatic injury due to blunt abdominal trauma in children. Eur J Radiol 2006; 59:3–7
2. Canty TG Sr, Weinman D. Management of major pancreatic duct injuries in children. J Trauma 2001; 50:1001–7
3. Canty TG Sr, Weinman D. Treatment of pancreatic duct disruption in children by an endoscopically placed stent. J Pediatr Surg 2001; 36:345–8
4. Patty I, Kalaoui M, Al-Shamali M, Al-Hassan F, Al-Naqeeb B. Endoscopic drainage for pancreatic pseudocyst in children. J Pediatr Surg 2001; 36:503–5
5. Saad DF, Gow KW, Cabbabe S, Heiss KF, Wulkan ML. Laparoscopic cystogastrostomy for the treatment of pancreatic pseudocysts in children. J Pediatr Surg 2005; 40:e13–7
6. Stringer MD. Pancreatic trauma in children. Br J Surg 2005; 92:467–70

Q 183

Jean Stephane Valla

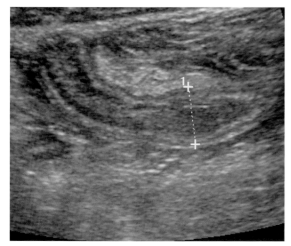

Fig. 1

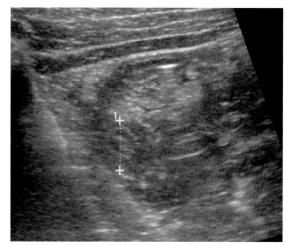

Fig. 2

A 9-year-old boy suffered from sudden pain in the peri-umbilical area, with subsequent localization of the pain to the right lower quadrant. The pain was constant and was made worse by movement. After some hours he was vomiting and had a low-grade fever. The boy was referred to us in emergency 24 h after the onset of symptoms.

- What is the suspected pathological condition affecting this child?
- What is the most important component of the diagnostic work-up?

The surgeon performed the examinations shown in Figs. 1–3.

- What do Figs. 1–3 show?
- Which other diagnostic examinations are necessary in this case?
- What is the best way to manage this condition?

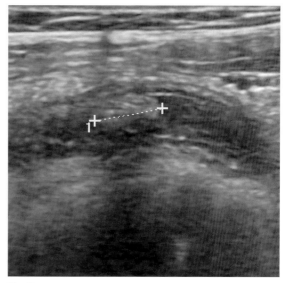

Fig. 3

A 183

This child is suspected of suffering from acute appendicitis because symptoms are typical of this condition. However, the presentation may be variable, depending on the patient's age and other factors. The diagnosis is often difficult in the following patients: toddlers, adolescent girls, obese patients, immunosuppressed children etc.

Physical examination is the most important component of the diagnostic work-up: localized tenderness in a child is due to appendicitis unless proved otherwise. Despite many advances in imaging and diagnostic modalities, appendicitis remains largely a clinical diagnosis.

Ultrasonographic findings in acute appendicitis include:
- Appendiceal distension with a diameter greater than 6 mm (Fig. 1)
- "Target sign" (Fig. 2)
- Appendicolith (stercolith in appendiceal lumen) (Fig. 3)
- High periappendiceal echogenicity and peritoneal fluid in the pericecal area or pouch of Douglas

In this case no other diagnostic examinations are necessary; in doubtful cases, the following examinations could be useful:
- Blood samples: white blood cells count, neutrophil count, and C reactive protein are poor sensitive diagnostic tests in children with symptoms that have been present for less than 24 h. Transaminase and amylase levels should be measured to rule out hepatitis or pancreatitis.

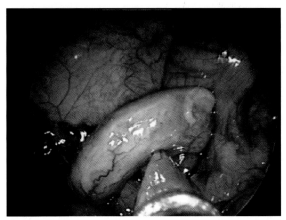

Fig. 4

- Urines analysis is useful to rule out pyelonephritis.
- Plain thoracic radiography is useful to rule out right lung infection.
- CT could be used if the appendix is not visualized by ultrasound.

This boy must be managed by prompt appendectomy using laparoscopy (Fig. 4).
We favor laparoscopic appendectomy especially in the following circumstances: girls, obese patients, suspected ectopic appendix, uncertain diagnosis.

Suggested Reading

1. Arca MJ Caniano DA (2003) In: Mattei P (eds). Paediatric Surgery. Lippincott Williams and Williams Philadelphia p. 395–398
2. Doria AS et al. US or CT for diagnosis of appendicitis in children and adults? A meta analysis. Radiology 2006; 10 1148/RADIO/2411050913
3. Valla JS. Evidence Based Surgery: Appendectomy by laparoscopy in children: better or not? Ped EndoSurg Inn Tech 2001; Vol 5 p 247–251

Q 184

Jean Stephane Valla

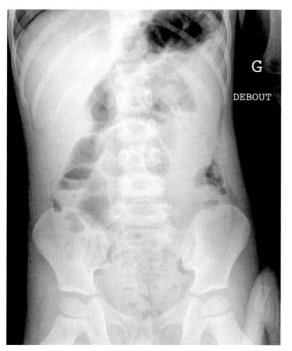

Fig. 1

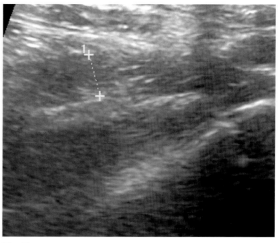

Fig. 2

A 3-year-old boy was referred to our department in emergency because of continuous periumbilical pain, fever (38.5°C), and anorexia that had started 18 h earlier. There was no vomiting, no constipation, and no diarrhea. Abdominal examination was difficult because the child felt poorly, was in pain, and was frightened. Assessing for true local tenderness or rebound tenderness was inconclusive; the abdomen was slightly distended. Rectal examination was refused by the family. The rest of the examination was normal.

• What are findings from the abdominal radiography (Fig. 1) and the ultrasonography (Figs. 2, 3)?
• How do you manage this young patient?

Fig. 3

A 184

In this case the diagnostic work-up is not clear. The clinical and radiological examinations are not conclusive: there is simple adynamic ileus on the abdominal radiograph (Fig. 1), pericecal fluid (Fig. 2), and hyperechogenicity of the right iliac fossa (Fig. 3), but the appendix is not visualized—a rather common situation in infants.

A period of observation and reexamination will often solve the problem. This boy was sedated and reexamined 1 h later. Diffuse periumbilical tenderness was evident at that time, which justified performing a CT scan in emergency, all the more so because of the blood sample results: white blood cell count (WBC), 29,400; polynuclear neutrophil (PNF), 89; C-reactive protein (CRP), 153.

The CT scan confirmed the presence of free fluid in the peritoneal cavity and showed a fecalith located on the left of the medial line because of the mesoceliac ectopic position of the appendix (Figs. 4, 5). The final diagnosis is appendicular generalized peritonitis.

The patient must be carefully treated with intravenous infusion, triple antibiotics, and analgesia. When stable, the child is taken to the operating room. The procedure can be conducted by laparoscopy. A peritoneal liquid sample must be taken. The fecalith must be removed (Fig. 6) as well as the appendix. The abdominal cavity must be copiously irrigated and aspirated dry. Antibiotics are continued for at least 5 days.

Suggested Reading

1. Paya K et al. Perforating appendicitis. An indication of laparoscopy? Surg. Endosc 2000; Vol 14 p 182–4
2. Peng YS et al. Clinical criteria for diagnosis perforated appendix in paediatric patients. Pediat Emerg Care 2006; Vol 22 p 475–9
3. Yakmurlu A et al. Laparoscopic appendectomy for perforated appendicitis: a comparison with open appendectomy. Surg Endosc 2006; Vol 20 p1051–4

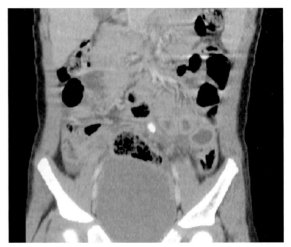

Fig. 4

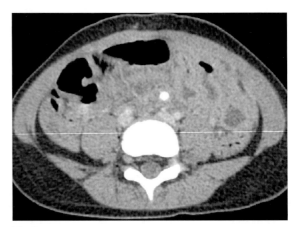

Fig. 5

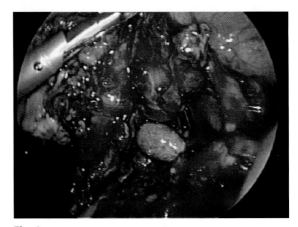

Fig. 6

Q 185

Salam Yazbeck

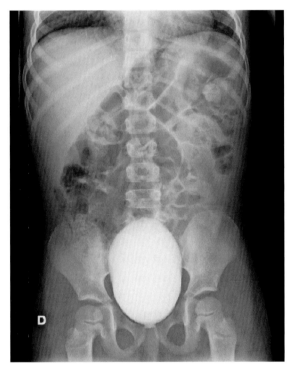

Fig. 1

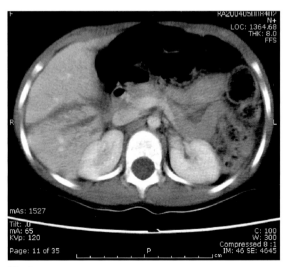

Fig. 2

An 8-year-old girl collided with a post while skiing. In the emergency room she was pale, anxious, and complained of diffuse abdominal pain. Physical examination confirmed the diffuse abdominal pain with peritoneal irritation signs. Her heart rate was 120 bpm and her blood pressure was 105/60. After initial resuscitation she underwent plain abdominal radiography (Fig. 1), abdominal ultrasound (Fig. 2), and CT of the abdomen (Fig. 3).

- Describe Figs. 1–3.
- What would your management plan be?
- What would be an indication for exploratory laparotomy in this case?
- What should your diagnosis and management be if this patient had a massive rectal bleeding episode after 4–5 days?

Fig. 3

A 185

Figure 1 shows a plain abdominal radiograph that is normal without intra-abdominal free air or bowel dilatation. On ultrasound, a deep laceration in segment 5 of the liver is noted. The CT scan confirms the isolated liver trauma in the same area.

Management should start immediately with IV fluids (20 cc/kg) on arrival in the emergency room before any imaging examination. Once vital signs are stable, imaging can be undertaken. The patient should be admitted to the intensive care unit for close monitoring of vital signs.

Most patients with liver trauma will not need surgery. However, laparotomy is mandatory if the vital signs cannot be stabilized or if the patient needs multiple transfusions (>40 cc/kg).

Massive rectal bleeding is a well-described complication of liver trauma, whereby an intrahepatic artery erodes in the biliary tree and the patient presents with massive GI bleeding, called hemobilia. This will necessitate urgent embolization of the involved artery, and if it is not possible a laparotomy with partial liver resection will be needed.

Suggested Reading

1. Landau A, Van As AB, Numanoglu A et al. Liver injuries in children: the role of selective non-operative treatment. Injury 2006; 37:66–71
2. Leone Re Jr, Hammond JS. Non-operative treatment of pediatric blunt hepatic trauma. Ann Surg 2001; 67:138–142

Q 186

Salam Yazbeck

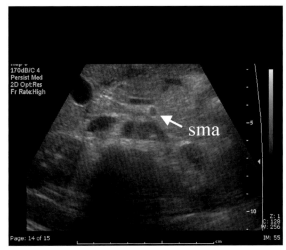

Fig. 1

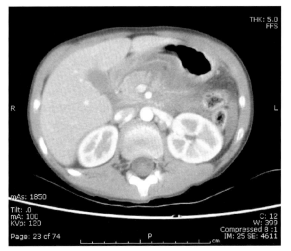

Fig. 2

A 10-year-old boy was brought to the emergency room 3 h after falling from his bicycle while going downhill. He hit the handle bar with his abdomen during the fall. On arrival, he complained of abdominal pain, which increased with walking. He had vomited twice.

On physical examination, his heart rate was 130 bpm, blood pressure was 120/80, and his oxygen saturation 100%. On abdominal examination, there was voluntary guarding, with a slight tenderness in the epigastrium where a superficial abrasion was noted.

Laboratory investigations showed a white blood cell (WBC) count of 22,000, a hemoglobin count of 135, and a normal platelet count as well as normal liver function tests. The serum amylase level was slightly elevated. The emergency room physician ordered an abdominal ultrasound and a CT scan of the abdomen (Figs. 1 and 2).

- What would your management plan be?
- What is your interpretation of Figs. 1 and 2?
- What would you recommend next?
- What is the most common complication that can be expected in this case?
- How would you manage this complication?

A 186

Initial management is to assure stabilization of the vital signs before any imaging is done.

The ultrasound shows a fracture line in the pancreas at the level of the superior mesenteric artery with a fluid collection anteriorly. The CT scan shows a fracture in the body of the pancreas.

The patient was kept NPO with parenteral nutrition. Oral feeding was initiated on day 8 but it was not tolerated and the patient received nasojejunal gavage. A follow-up ultrasound examination on day 11 showed a heterogeneous peripancreatic collection of 6×3×4 cm. Nasojejunal gavage was continued and the patient was sent home on day 19.

The boy was readmitted on day 25 with nausea; there was epigastric tenderness on physical examination. He tolerated the gavage. Ultrasound showed a pancreatic pseudocyst that was ready for drainage (Fig. 3).

Percutaneous drainage was done and the amount of drainage decreased rapidly in a few days. The patient was sent home on postprocedure day 4. The drain was removed 10 days later and the patient was followed up in the outpatient clinic. He resumed a normal oral diet and underwent a follow-up ultrasound examination 6 weeks post-trauma that showed only a slight scarring in the pancreas.

Other management possibilities of pancreatic injury are described in the literature; some are more surgically aggressive, others demand higher technology. The approach described here is neither surgically aggressive nor technologically demanding.

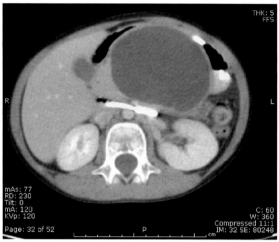

Fig. 3

Suggested Reading

1. Bass J, Di Lorenzo M, Desjardins JG et al. Blunt pancreatic injuries in children: the role of percutaneous external drainage in the treatment of pancreatic pseudocysts. J Pediatr Surg 1988; 23:721–724
2. Canty TG Sr, Weinman D. Management of major pancreatic duct injuries in children. J Trauma 2001; 50:1001–1007
3. Wales PW, Shuckett B, Kim PC. Long-term outcome after non-operative management of complete traumatic pancreatic transection in children. J Pediatr Surg 2001; 36:823–827

Q 187

Nancy Rollins and Korgun Koral

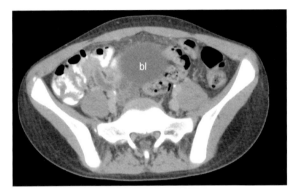

Fig. 1

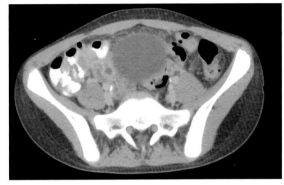

Fig. 2

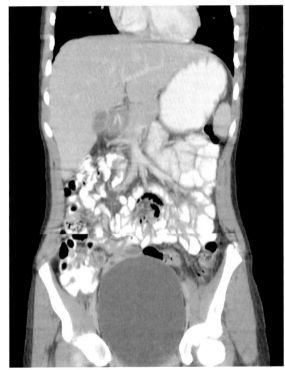

Fig. 3

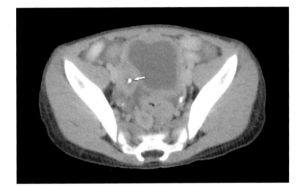

Fig. 4

A 12-year-old girl presented to the emergency room with a 3-day history of vomiting and a 2-day history of abdominal pain in the left lower quadrant. The white blood cell count was elevated (17,300/ml).

- What radiological study should be performed first?
- Which test should be performed next: ultrasonography or CT?
- What are the pros and cons for each?

CT of the abdomen was performed with coronal reformations (Figs. 1–3; *bl*, urinary bladder; *c*, cecum).

- What is the diagnosis?
- What does Fig. 4 show?
- What is the thickness threshold for appendicitis on ultrasonography?
- What are some complications of this condition and how are they treated?

A 187

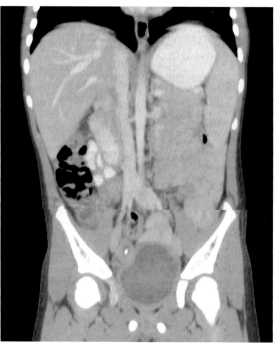

Fig. 5

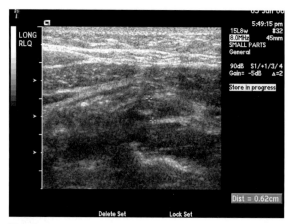

Fig. 6

At many institutions the first examination is supine and upright radiography of the abdomen. This helps identify other causes of abdominal pain such as gastrointestinal obstruction, bowel perforation, appendicolith, and lower lobe pneumonia/pleural effusion. In about two-thirds of the cases the presentation is convincing enough, and without further testing surgery is performed.

At many pediatric institutions ultrasonography is the test of preference. Lack of ionizing radiation, patient preparation, and portability are advantages of ultrasonography. Depending on the surgeon's preference CT may also be used, provided that the technical parameters related to radiation are adjusted for the pediatric population. CT provides the advantage of identifying appendicitis in children who have excess body fat, retrocecal appendix, or unrelated intra-abdominal pathology such as omental infarct, mesenteric adenitis, renal/ureteral stone, and hydronephrosis. Figures 1 and 2 show a blind-ending tubular structure with thickening and enhancement of the wall. This tubular structure cor-

responds to a fluid-filled structure and connects to the cecum from its medial aspect. The coronal reformation (Fig. 3) shows the same findings. Figures 4 and 5 are images of another patient showing an appendicolith (*arrow* in Fig. 4) in the fluid-filled appendix whose wall is thickened. There is some periappendiceal fluid. Figure 6 is an image from an ultrasonography examination of the right lower quadrant in another patient, showing a blind-ending tubular structure which is not compressible under manual pressure. The diameter of this tubular structure is 6 mm. The most commonly used threshold is 6 mm, although some use 7 mm.

The most common complication of appendicitis is perforation resulting in local inflammation and abscess formation. Abscesses can be subhepatic, pelvic (most commonly in cul-de-sac), or periappendiceal. In many instances surgeons prefer percutaneous drainage of the abscess and intravenous antibiotic therapy before appendectomy.

Suggested Reading

1. Kuhn JP, Slovis TL, Haller JO. Caffey's Pediatric Diagnostic Imaging. Elsevier Ed. 2004

2. Siegel MJ, Coley BD. Pediatric Imaging. Lippincott Williams & Wilkins Ed. 2006

Q 188

Nancy Rollins and Korgun Koral

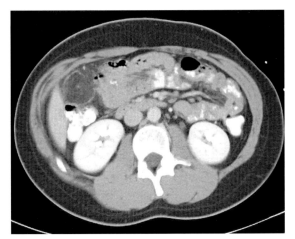

Fig. 1

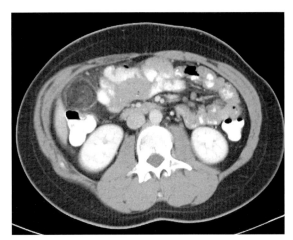

Fig. 2

A 15-year-old patient presented with a 4-day history of abdominal pain localized to the right lower quadrant. The white blood cell count was elevated to 12,500/ml. Plain radiographs of the abdomen were unremarkable. Contrast-enhanced CT of the abdomen was performed (Figs. 1, 2).

- What are the findings?
- Is there appendicitis? Can appendicitis be confidently excluded?
- What is differential diagnosis?
- What is the most likely diagnosis?
- What is the cause of this condition and how is it treated?

A 188

There is a localized focus of fatty stranding forming the shape of a mass in the right lower quadrant anterior to the descending colon. An enlarged appendix cannot be identified.

Acute appendicitis cannot be definitively excluded, because in appendicitis periappendiceal inflammatory changes may obscure the visualization of the appendix.

The differential diagnosis includes acute appendicitis, epiploic appendagitis, fibrosing sclerosing mesenteritis, and pancreatitis.

The most likely diagnosis is omental infarction.

The exact cause of omental infarction is not known but the mechanism involves interruption of arterial blood supply to the omentum. Definitive diagnosis and treatment are achieved by surgery. Conservative management is occasionally chosen; however, the similarity of the clinical presentation and sometimes the imaging findings to appendicitis makes surgery the usually preferred treatment.

Suggested Reading

1. Federle MP. Diagnostic Imaging: Abdomen. Amirsys Ed. 2005

Q 189

Alba Cruccetti and Luciano Mastroianni

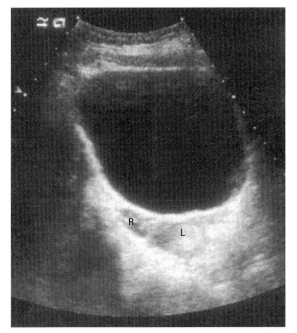

Fig. 1

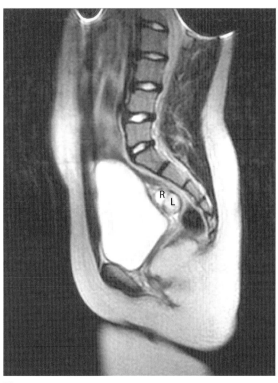

Fig. 2

A 10-year-old girl presented to our emergency department with a 2-day history of abdominal pain and fever.

On examination the abdomen was not distended and there was no guarding, only a mild tenderness in the inferior abdominal quadrant.

The white blood cell count was normal, with absence of left shift.

The first radiological investigation performed is shown in Fig. 1.

- What does Fig. 1 show?
- Why did the surgeon perform the second examination?
- What do Figs. 2 and 3 show?
- What pathological condition is affecting this child?
- What is the best way to manage this condition?

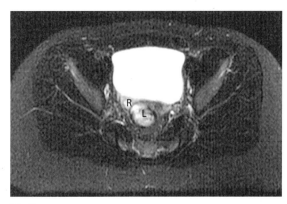

Fig. 3

A 189

This premenarchal girl is affected by a pelvic mass.

The abdominal ultrasound scan shows a pelvic mixed mass with an inhomogeneous structure (size 3×1.8 cm) located behind the uterus and attached to the right ovary (Fig. 1). No blood flow within the mass was detected with color and power Doppler sonography. The left ovary was not identified.

MR imaging shows a heterogeneous pelvic medial ovarian mass (size 3.5×4×2.5 cm) with a predominately hyperintense signal containing small areas with hypointense lesions on T1- and T2-weighted images; the right ovary and the uterus seem to be normal (Figs. 2–4).

Alpha-fetoprotein (αFP) and beta human chorionic gonadotropin (βHCG) levels were normal.

The diagnosis of left ovarian torsion precipitated by a large mass was suspected on the basis of the MR imaging and ultrasound scan.

A diagnostic laparoscopy showed the left ovarian mass to be twisted and attached to the right ovary and to the uterus (Fig. 5). The left ovarian mass appeared necrotic after it was untwisted: left oophorectomy and right oophoropexy were performed.

The final histology showed a mature teratoma with necrotic areas.

Ovarian pathology is uncommon in children, but it must be included in the differential diagnosis of all girls who present with abdominal pain. Ultrasound is usually the first-line examination performed in an emergency setting, but CT and MR imaging can be useful in cases of ambiguous ultrasound findings, especially in patients with subacute symptoms and a suspected adnexal mass.

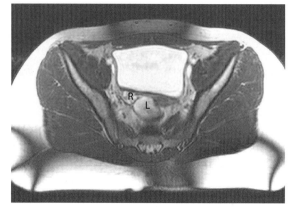

Fig. 4

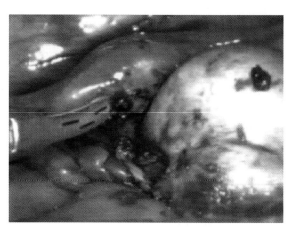

Fig. 5

Suggested Reading

1. Bader T, Ranner G, Haberlik A. Torsion of a normal adnexa in a premenarcheal girl: MRI findings. Eur Radiol 1996; 6:704–6
2. Cass DL. Ovarian torsion. Semin Pediatr Surg 2005; 14:86–92
3. Cass DL, Hawkins E, Brandt ML, Chintagumpala M, Bloss RS, Milewicz AL, Minifee PK, Wesson DE, Nuchtern JG. Surgery for ovarian masses in infants, children, and adolescents: 102 consecutive patients treated in a 15-year period. J Pediatr Surg 2001; 36:693–9
4. James S. Meyer, Carroll M. Harmon, M. Patricia Harty, Richard I. Markowitz, Anne M. Hubbard and Richard D. Bellah. Ovarian torsion: Clinical and imaging presentation in children. J Pediatr Surg 1995; 30:1433–1436

Q 190

Alba Cruccetti and Luciano Mastroianni

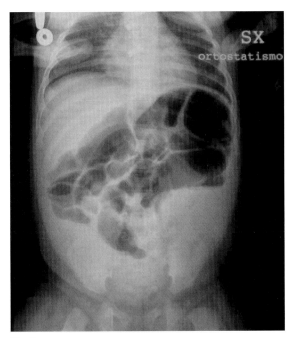

Fig. 1

Fig. 2

A 3-month-old girl presented to our emergency department with a 2-day history of irritability, abdominal pain, and vomiting.

On examination, her abdomen was distended with diffuse guarding and tenderness on the right lower quadrant, but no palpable mass.

The white blood cell count was 21,500/mm³, with a left shift.

The first radiological investigation performed is shown in Fig. 1.

- What does Fig. 1 show?
- Why did the surgeon perform the second examination?
- What does Fig. 2 show?
- What pathological condition is affecting this child?
- What is the best way to manage this condition?

Suggested Reading

1. Bakir B, Poyanli A, Yekeler E and Acunas G. Acute torsion of a wandering spleen: imaging findings. Abdom Imaging 2004; 29:707–709
2. Brown CV, Virgilio GR and Vazquez WD. Wandering spleen and its complications in children: a case series and review of the literature. J Pediatr Surg 2003; 38:1676–1679
3. Steinberg R, Karmazyn B, Dlugy E, Gelber E, Freud E, Horev G and Zer M. Clinical presentation of wandering spleen. J Pediatr Surg 2002; 37:E30

A 190

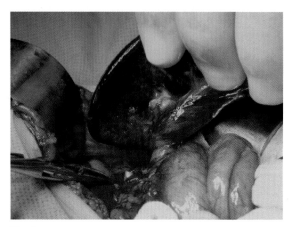

Fig. 3

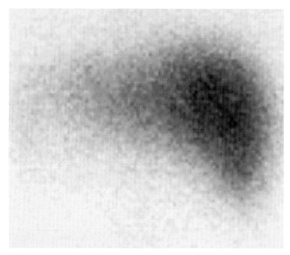

Fig. 4

This infant is affected by wandering spleen. Wandering spleen is a rare condition characterized by incomplete fixation of the spleen by its ligaments causing hypermobility with migration to the lower abdomen or pelvis. Wandering spleen involves a risk of torsion. Diagnosis is difficult because of the lack of symptoms until splenic torsion occurs. Patients may present with an asymptomatic abdominal mass, an acute abdomen, or pain associated with a mass. The most common clinical presentation is an acute, chronic, or intermittent abdominal pain due to splenic torsion.

Figure 1 shows a plain abdominal radiograph with several markedly distended loops of bowel and absence of gas in the rectum, in the right and left lower quadrant. Ultrasonography revealed a medially and lower displaced spleen. A barium enema was normal without signs of extrinsic compression of the intestinal loops.

The CT scan (Fig. 2) shows the enlarged spleen located in the left lower quadrant and pelvis.

The patient was taken to the operating room for exploration. At operation the spleen was torsed 360°

around its pedicle (Fig. 3), and it had no ligamentous attachments. The spleen appeared dusky, but after detorsion it returned to a more normal color. Extraperitoneal splenopexy was performed, returning the spleen to the left upper quadrant.

The postoperative period was uneventful. The patient recovered well, but because of a rising platelet count a liver–spleen scan was performed. This scan showed abnormal splenic uptake (Fig. 4), and the patient was treated as an asplenic patient with vaccines and prophylactic antibiotics. A repeat liver–spleen scan several months later showed return of splenic perfusion, and the patient's platelet count normalized.

Wandering spleen is rare, especially in the pediatric population, and diagnosis is difficult because of the lack of symptoms until splenic torsion occurs. Laboratory findings are nonspecific, but the diagnosis can be confirmed with imaging techniques.

Q 191

François Luks

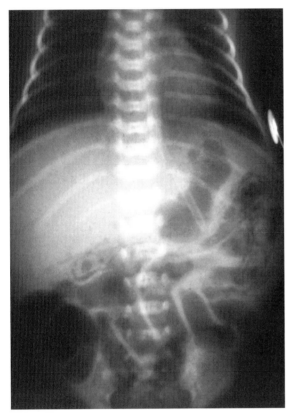

Fig. 1

Fig. 2

A 22-day-old infant, born prematurely at 27 weeks' gestation, was breathing spontaneously on supplemental oxygen via a nasal cannula, was on intravenous alimentation, and received trophic enteral feeding at 1 ml/h.

In the last 48 h, the infant had several episodes of apnea followed by bradycardia, and has passed one blood-streaked stool. His abdomen was noted to be distended. A nasogastric tube was inserted and an abdominal radiograph was obtained (Fig. 1).

- What is the differential diagnosis?
- What does the radiograph show?
- What should further work-up and treatment consist of?

The following morning, the infant was noted to be tachypneic (up to 70 breaths/min) and had a transient episode of hypotension. He was intubated and placed on assisted ventilation.

Physical examination revealed increased, diffuse abdominal tenderness, and abdominal wall changes were also noted (Fig. 2).

A repeat radiograph was obtained (Fig. 3). It was decided to proceed with surgical exploration of the abdomen.

- What does the physical examination of the abdomen suggest?
- Which finding on the repeat radiograph prompted surgical management?
- What are the therapeutic options?

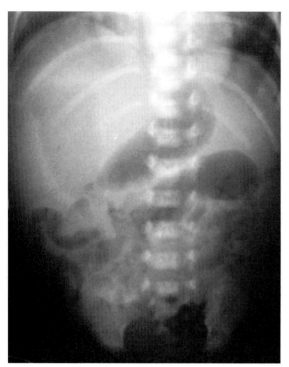

Fig. 3

A 191

Feeding intolerance, increased and/or bloody nasogastric aspirates, increased frequency of apnea and bradycardia episodes, bloody stools, and abdominal distension can all be signs of necrotizing enterocolitis (NEC). The differential diagnosis includes sepsis, colonic immaturity (causing abdominal distension, vomiting, and a pseudo-obstructive picture), and midgut volvulus (minimal abdominal distension initially, but the signs of intestinal ischemia seen with advanced volvulus may be mistaken for NEC). The initial radiograph (Fig. 1) shows evidence of intestinal pneumatosis, characterized by a stippled gas pattern within the intestinal wall (presumably the colon, although it is very difficult to differentiate the large from the small bowel in the neonate). At the hepatic flexure, a head-on view of the bowel shows a "target" pattern of gas: a central, luminal gas bubble, with concentric hyperdense mucosa/submucosa, a radiolucent layer of gas bubbles, and a hyperdense muscularis and serosa.

NEC is typically divided into: stage I, "suspected" NEC, without radiographic evidence of pneumatosis or perforation; stage II, "definite" NEC, characterized by pneumatosis intestinalis, a fixed, atonic bowel loop on serial examinations, or portal venous gas; and stage III ("advanced" NEC), when complications occur (perforation, abscess) or there is evidence of systemic deterioration (septic shock, leuko- and thrombocytopenia).

The appearance of the abdominal wall the next morning suggests significant distress or ischemia of the underlying bowel. The erythema, with its distribution along the colonic frame, suggests underlying large bowel necrosis.

The repeat supine radiograph shows a radiolucent shadow over the right aspect of the liver, suggesting free air accumulating to the right of the falciform ligament (Fig. 4, *arrows*). Detection of free air is difficult in newborns. An alternative is to obtain a cross-table lateral view of the supine infant: free air will be visible as a pocket of gas over the liver (Fig. 5, *arrows*).

Indications for surgical treatment of NEC include hard signs of intestinal perforation (free air on a radiograph) or evidence of intestinal ischemia or necrosis (abdominal wall erythema/abscess, persistence of an atonic loop on successive radiographs). Clinical deterioration *without* hard evidence of intestinal perforation may also require surgical exploration but, in these cases, the outcome is dismal regardless of the approach. In the present patient, necrosis of most of the colon was found (Fig. 6). The small bowel was normal. A subtotal colectomy was performed, leaving a Hartman's pouch and a terminal ileostomy.

Other therapeutic options include primary anastomosis (rarely used) and exteriorization of the diseased segment of bowel. The latter approach is used in cases of dire emergency when formal resection and the creation of one or more stomas would dangerously prolong operative time. It usually requires a second-look operation or bed-side resection of the exteriorized loop.

In the extreme low-birth-weight infant (less than 750 g), bed-side drainage of the peritoneal cavity has been advocated as temporizing or even definitive treatment. A recently published randomized study showed that, for extreme low-birth-weight infants, both approaches had similar results. The role of peritoneal drainage in larger infants is more controversial.

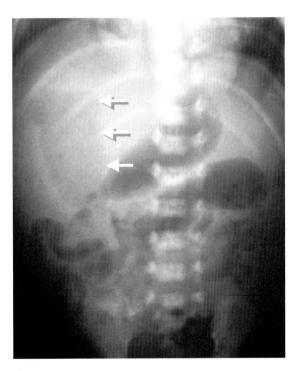

Fig. 4

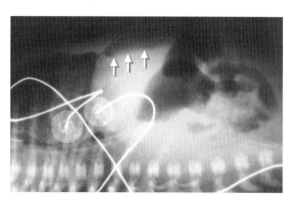

Fig. 5

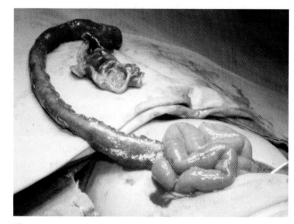

Fig. 6

Suggested Reading

1. Lessin MS, Luks FI, Wesselhoeft CW Jr et al. Peritoneal drainage as definitive treatment for intestinal perforation in infants with extremely low birth weight (<750 g). J Pediatr Surg 1998 Feb; 33(2):370–2

2. Moss RL, Dimmitt RA, Barnhart DC et al. Laparotomy versus peritoneal drainage for necrotizing enterocolitis and perforation. N Engl J Med 2006 May 25; 354(21):2275–6

3. Pierro A, Hall N. Surgical treatments of infants with necrotizing enterocolitis. Semin Neonatol 2003 Jun; 8(3):223–32

4. Schmolzer G, Urlesberger B, Haim M et al. Multi-modal approach to prophylaxis of necrotizing enterocolitis. J Perinatol 2006 Jun; 26(6):342–7

5. Sharma R, Hudak ML, Tepas JJ 3rd et al. Impact of gestational age on the clinical presentation and surgical outcome of necrotizing enterocolitis. Pediatr Surg Int 2006 Jul; 22(7):573–80

6. Singh M, Owen A, Gull S, Morabito A et al. Surgery for intestinal perforation in preterm neonates: anastomosis vs stoma. J Pediatr Surg 2006 Apr; 41(4):725–9

Q 192

Isabelle Vidal, Marc-David Leclair, and Yves Heloury

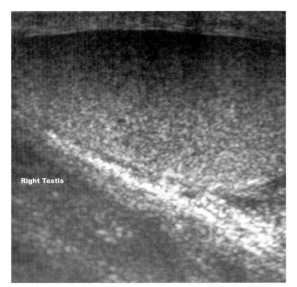

Fig. 1

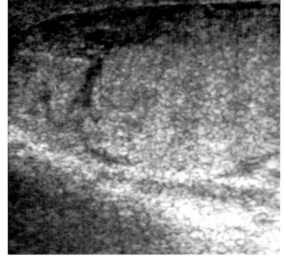

Fig. 2

A 15-year-old boy fell astride parallel bars during gymnastics training and sustained a blunt trauma of the left scrotum.

He had no pelvic injury, no dysuria, and no hematuria. The contralateral testis was normal.

On admission, he presented with extreme scrotal pain. Physical examination revealed a boy who had achieved puberty, and a swollen, severely tender scrotum with a visible hematoma. The testicle was not isolated or differentiated by palpation.

Scrotal ultrasound was performed for the right testis (Fig. 1) and the left testis (Fig. 2).

- How would you manage this young man?
- What should he be warned about concerning the evolution of his testis?

A 192

Surgical exploration found a ruptured albuginea, with partial necrosis of the exteriorized pulp. A minimal resection was performed, and the tunica albuginea was closed. Pathologic analysis of the pulp did not show any malignancy.

This boy may have severe blunt trauma of the testicle, after a perineal high-energy crash. In this context, we should not forget to check for the absence of pelvic fracture (examination of pelvis mobility) and the absence of urethral trauma that could be suspected if he had hematuria.

It is difficult to differentiate between hematocele (hematoma limited by the tunica vaginalis of the testis) and intratesticular hematoma contained in the tunica albuginea, the first inner layer of testicle. If there is a hematocele, on physical examination the testicle might not be palpated inside this collection, with an opaque transillumination, whereas in an intra-albuginea hematoma, the testicle and epididymis can be isolated or differentiated by palpation.

Ultrasound provides information for testicular trauma staging: testis contusion, rupture of the albuginea, or testicle fracture, with the testicular pulp outside of the albuginea, presenting a high risk of necrosis. Doppler study allows examination of the vascularization. This examination showed a heterogeneous echo pattern at the upper pole of the left testicular parenchyma with loss of contour definition, corresponding to a rupture of the tunica albuginea with protrusion of the testicular pulp.

Operative indications for blunt trauma include all situations where there is risk of necrosis of the testicular parenchyma. An explorative surgical procedure should be performed when there is suspicion of testicular rupture, suspicion of albugineal rupture, expanding hematomas, dislocation refractory to manual reduction, absent or abnormal vascular flow at Doppler sonography, and all serious trauma where clinical and radiological findings cannot confirm the absence of these injuries. This boy presenting with a rupture of the albuginea tunica and protrusion of the testicular pulp needs surgical exploration as soon as possible. It has been proven that early surgical management can reduce testicular infarction and increases the possibilities of conservative treatment.

Operative management involves evacuation of the hematocele, debridement of necrotic or devitalized tissue, copious irrigation, meticulous attention to hemostasis, and closure of the tunica albuginea. Total orchidectomy is rarely necessary, and conservative management can be performed for more than 50% of parenchyma loss. This surgical procedure should be accompanied by good analgesia and antibiotic prophylaxis. For this boy, surgical exploration confirmed the albugineal rupture. About half of his testicular parenchyma was externalized by this dysjunction, was partly necrotic, and had to be removed. There was no other injury of the testis or epididymis. Careful hemostasis was done, and the albuginea was sutured. Because there was no significant hematoma, no drainage was left.

Progressive testicular atrophy may occur despite a successful repair. A careful follow-up should include clinical examination and testicular ultrasound for the first year. If there is no testicular atrophy, most often neither endocrine nor exocrine testicular function is altered.

Suggested Reading

1. Buckley JC, McAninch JW. Use of ultrasonography for the diagnosis of testicular injuries in blunt scrotal trauma. J Urol 2006; 175:175–178
2. Hendry WF. Testicular, epididymal and vasal injuries. BJU International 2000; 86:344–348

Q 193

Isabelle Vidal, Marc-David Leclair, and Yves Heloury

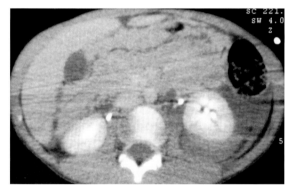

Fig. 1

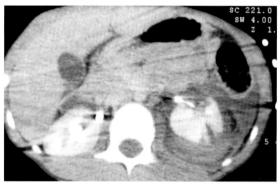

Fig. 2

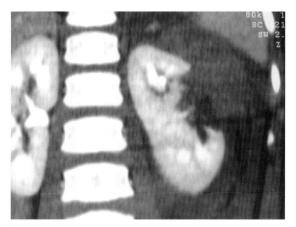

Fig. 3

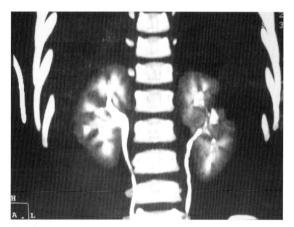

Fig. 4

A 7-year-old boy was admitted to hospital for left lumbar and flank trauma. Two hours earlier, he had fallen off his bicycle and landed flat on his back with high kinetic energy. He presented with pain in the lumbar region on palpation, and had massive hematuria. His abdomen was tender, without guarding, and was less painful than his back. He had stable hemodynamic parameters and had no vomiting.

The patient had normal biological hepatic and pancreatic values. The hemoglobin count was 10.7 g/dl 3 h after the shock and 9.4 g 6 h later. An abdominal CT scan was performed.

- What special slices should you ask for?
- The CT study is shown in Figs. 1–4; how would you analyze it?
- How would you manage this boy?

Twenty-four hours later, his hemoglobin rate dropped to 7.9 g/dl; he vomited, had abdominal distension, but no abdominal pain.

- Would you still continue with medical surveillance?

On day 5 after his accident, he had no fever, no ileus, and was carefully mobilized. He was discharged on day 7.

- What would your follow-up consist of?

A 193

This boy probably had a left retroperitoneal trauma, with at least renal contusion (macroscopic hematuria). One cannot rule out associated abdominal injuries.

Because renal trauma is suspected, you should ask for a contrast-enhanced CT examination. This allows one to view the intraperitoneal organs and renal vascularization, to check that the contralateral kidney is functional, and to check whether there is active bleeding. However, the most important aspect for renal injury is to scan the urinary tract later, after administration of contrast material, with excretory urography, which allows visualization of the urinary tract and shows extravasation of contrast material.

The CT examination showed a significant retroperitoneal perirenal hematoma (Fig. 1) and a renal fracture with cortical laceration (Fig. 2). There was no extravasation of contrast material, meaning that there was no urinary extravasation and that this parenchymal laceration did not extend into the collecting system (Figs. 3, 4).

Renal injuries were graded by the American Association for the Surgery of Trauma (AAST). Grade 1 corresponds to renal contusions, or nonexpanding subcapsular hematomas; grade 2 to nonexpanding perinephric hematomas confined to the retroperitoneum, or superficial cortical lacerations less than 1 cm in depth without collecting system injury; grade 3 to renal lacerations greater than 1 cm in depth that do not involve the collecting system; grade 4 to renal lacerations extending through the kidney into the collecting system, or injuries involving the main renal artery or vein with contained

hemorrhage, or segmental infarctions without associated lacerations, or expanding subcapsular hematomas compressing the kidney. Grade 5 is associated with shattered or devascularized kidney, complete laceration or thrombus of the main renal artery or vein, or ureteropelvic avulsions. Grades 1 and 2 are classified as minor traumas, and grades 3–5 as major traumas. This boy had a renal injury corresponding to grade 3.

The patient should be hospitalized, with bed rest. His hemodynamic parameters should be carefully monitored. The only need for surgical exploration on admission would be in the case of vascular injuries.

The patient presented with an intestinal ileus, consecutive to the significant hemoretroperitoneum. He had no hemodynamic trouble, and did not need surgical management. He had to remain fasting; if he had vomited, a nasogastric stent could have been helpful.

With this conservative management, his evolution was good: intestinal reflex ileus disappeared on the third day. Most kidney traumas do not require surgery, even in cases of deep parenchymal laceration, unless there are complications (persistent perirenal effusion of urine and blood, abscess, infection, secondary hypertension, renal atrophy).

The patient should undergo ultrasonography 1 month later so as to check the evolution of the trauma and to decide whether sports can be resumed. In severe trauma, a DMSA scan can be performed 1 year later to obtain a prognosis of renal function; blood pressure should be checked once a year.

Suggested Reading

1. Broghammer JA, Langenburg SE, Smith SJ, Santucci RA. Pediatric blunt renal trauma: Its conservative management and patterns of associated injuries. Urology 2006; 67:823–827

2. Buckley JC, McAninch JW. Pediatric renal injuries: management guidelines from a 25-year experience. J Urol 2004; 172:687–690

Q 194

Isabelle Vidal, Marc-David Leclair, and Yves Heloury

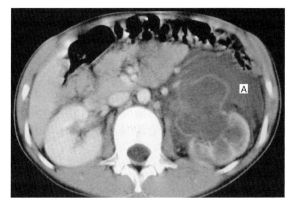

Fig. 1

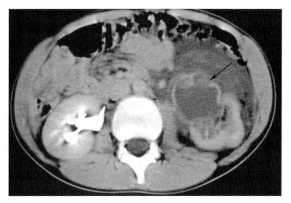

Fig. 2

A 9-year-old boy was brought to the emergency department after suffering abdominal trauma. He had fallen on his belly while walking 3 h earlier. He presented with left lumbar pain and left flank guarding. He had good hemodynamic constants. He had no medical history before this accident.

Before arriving at hospital, abdominal ultrasonography was performed. This examination showed a major perirenal effusion, with renal parenchyma contusion. There was no intraperitoneal injury.

- Would you ask for another radiological examination?
- Comment on Figs. 1 and 2.
- What management would you advise for this young boy?
- Figure 3 is a percutaneous contrast study of the left renal collecting system. Does it help you to define the exact nature of the renal trauma?

Renal DMSA scintigraphy was performed on the same day. The left kidney had no function.

- What would you propose?

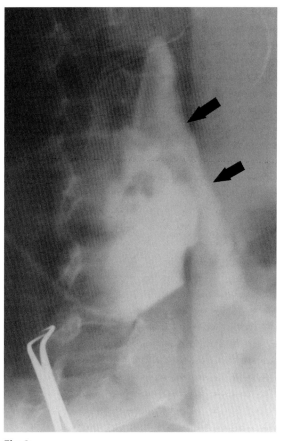

Fig. 3

A 194

It is surprising that this boy presented with blunt lumbar trauma after such a mild-energy collision. Usually, a fall from one's own height does not result in such severe pain. We should stay wary and suspect an underlying condition that could explain these clinical findings.

Ultrasonography is not precise enough for evaluation of kidney trauma. We should perform contrast-enhanced CT (paying special attention to later views) and urography. The American Association for the Surgery of Trauma (AAST) grading system of kidney injury is based on radiological features on CT: severity of parenchymal laceration, kidney vascularization, and existence of collecting system or renal pedicle injury.

Figure 1 is a CT scan with injection of contrast material. It is an early view after contrast medium injection (arterial time): it confirms left kidney trauma, with major retroperitoneal effusion. Both kidneys are well vascularized, and there is no pedicle injury. Figure 2 is a later study (urogram), to check the evacuation of contrast material by the kidneys. The right kidney has normal and well-opacified cavities, but the left one shows no excretion. Moreover, the limits of the left pelvis are well seen (*black arrow*): this pelvis is larger than the contralateral one. The boy had an undiagnosed left hydronephrosis that explains this severe trauma after such a mild

shock. Rupture of the occult hydronephrotic pelvis is suspected. You should keep in mind that this left kidney may be nonfunctional, as there is no contrast. There is no vascular dysfunction, since the parenchyma was well opacified on arterial time.

Because of this loss of function, we cannot assess whether the perirenal collection is only hematic or if there is urine leakage. It was decided to perform percutaneous nephrostomy, on day 1, to drain the injured pelvis and for opacification of the pelvis.

The contrast study confirms hydronephrosis, and on a later study (Fig. 3, *arrows*), there is significant contrast material leakage. You can conclude that there is rupture of the pelvis. Additionally, a puncture of the left perirenal effusion was made during this procedure to drain the hematuric fluid.

The diagnosis of ruptured hydronephrosis of a nonfunctional kidney was proposed. Conservative treatment is not logical, since there is no renal function to preserve. We performed left ureteronephrectomy, via a retroperitoneal approach. Intraoperative findings were the same as before: perirenal urinoma and fracture of the pelvis. A polar vessel was found, in front of a severe stenosis of the pyeloureteral junction. There was no postoperative complication.

Suggested Reading

1. Mulligan JM, Cagiannos I, Collins JP, Millward SF. Ureteropelvic junction disruption secondary to blunt trauma: excretory phase imaging (delayed films) should help prevent a missed diagnosis. J Urol 1998; 159:67–70

2. Rogers CG, Knight V, MacUra KJ, Ziegfield S, Paidas CN, Mathews RI. High-grade renal injuries in children—is conservative management possible? Urology 2004; 64:574–579

3. Sebastia MC, Rodriguez-Dobao M, Quiroga S, Pallisa E, Marinez-Rodriguez M, Alvarez-Castells A. Renal trauma in occult ureteropelvic junction obstruction: CT findings. Eur Radiol 1999; 9:611–615

Q 195

Isabelle Vidal, Guillaume Podevin, Etienne Suply, and Yves Heloury

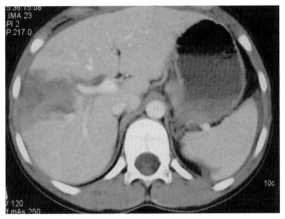

Fig. 1

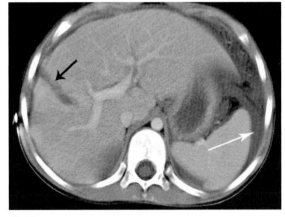

Fig. 2

A 9-year-old boy was brought to the emergency department after a bicycle accident. He presented with trauma of the right hemithorax. On clinical examination, he had a chest wall hematoma and abdominal pain in the right hypochondrium. There was hemodynamic stability.

- What explorations would you perform after this examination?
- What does Fig. 1 show?
- What could your approach be? In which conditions?
- What complications could occur in this type of abdominal trauma?

Ten days after this accident, the boy presented with acute abdominal pain and a fever of 39°C. Biological tests showed an inflammatory syndrome and an increased serum bilirubin rate. Ultrasonography findings showed significant abdominal effusion.

- Which complication can be evoked?
- CT was performed. What do Figs. 2 and 3 show?
- Which diagnosis could be proposed?
- How would you manage this complication?

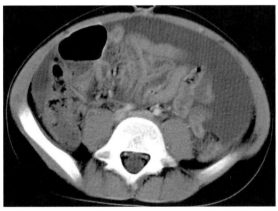

Fig. 3

A 195

This setting could correspond to blunt hepatic trauma. The liver is the second most frequently injured organ in children with blunt abdominal trauma, after the spleen.

The first thing to do is to evaluate trauma severity and look for associated thoracic, retroperitoneal, and other intraperitoneal injuries. Biological investigations (full blood count, liver function test, serum amylase, serum lipase, coagulation test, and pretransfusion test) and thoracoabdominal CT should be performed. CT is the investigation of choice in hemodynamically stable patients, to stage injuries and to make a complete abdominal evaluation.

Figure 1 is a CT scan showing liver laceration and contusion between the seventh and eighth segment of the liver and a mild peritoneal effusion which is probably a hemoperitoneum. There is no spleen injury.

For children, the most frequent approach is nonoperative management when there is no hemodynamic trouble or after successful resuscitation (hemodynamics stability obtained by transfusion inferior to 25–40 ml/kg/24 h). These patients should be monitored daily with clinical examinations (fever, pain, hemodynamics), biological tests (full blood count, liver function test), and radiological investigations if complications occur.

Possible complications are vascular injuries (such as massive hemorrhage, compressive subcapsular hematoma, arteriovenous fistula, superinfection of hematoma) and bile duct injuries leading to bilious collection (bilioma), or hemobilia.

All these findings are suggestive of bilious effusion. The CT scan shows a former liver fracture (Fig. 2) and massive peritoneal effusion (Fig. 3). Because the patient's hemodynamic parameters remained stable, this major intraperitoneal leakage is not hematic, but is more likely to be bilious. Bile duct injury is the most likely complication.

Antibiotics should be started, and this effusion should be drained: either by transcutaneous radiological target drainage or through a surgical approach (laparoscopy or laparotomy). Another approach could be endoscopic retrograde cholangiographic examination and biliary drainage, but in this case, the bile duct injury is far from the hepatic hilus and is not accessible to endoscopy. The third approach would be partial hepatectomy, to resect hepatic segments where there is bilious injury.

For this child, we made a US-guided puncture followed by CT drainage and, because drainage was not sufficient, a peritoneal washing was performed via laparotomy with drainage by a stent placed in front of the bile duct injury. This stent was removed 15 days later, and the boy had no other postoperative complications. A CT scan performed 1 month later showed cicatrization of the liver.

Suggested Reading

1. Almaramhi H, Al-Qahtani AR. Traumatic pediatric bile duct injury: nonoperative intervention as an alternative to surgical intervention. J Pediatr Surg 2006; 41:943–945
2. Hackam DJ, Potoka D, Meza M, Pollock A, Gardner M, Abrams P, Upperman J, Schall L, Ford H. Utility of radiographic hepatic injury grade in predicting outcome for children after blunt abdominal trauma. J Pediatr Surg 2002; 37:386–389
3. Landau A, van As AB, Numanoglu A, Millar AJ, Rode H. Liver injuries in children: the role of selective non-operative management. Injury 2006; 37:66–71
4. Pryor JP, Stafford PW, Nance ML. Severe blunt hepatic trauma in children. J Pediatr Surg 2001; 36:974–9

Q 196

Isabelle Vidal, Guillaume Podevin, Françoise Schmitt, and Yves Heloury

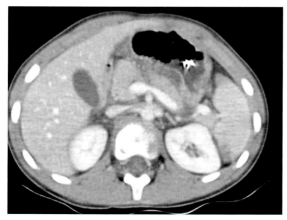

Fig. 1

An 8-year-old boy was brought to the emergency unit after a motor vehicle crash. He was secured in the car by a "two-point" seat belt.

On examination, there was abdominal pain, right hypochondrium guarding, abdominal wall hematoma, vomiting, and conjunctival paleness. His hemodynamic parameters stayed stable. There was no sign of trauma of the limbs or vertebrae.

- Which laboratory tests are needed immediately?
- Which radiological examination would you ask for first?
- What does Fig. 1 show?

The results of blood tests showed a hemoglobin level of 10.0 g/dl, normal liver function tests, and serum amylase and lipase rates increased 12-fold (335 UI/l and 1,909 UI/l, respectively).

- What is your diagnosis?
- Which treatment could you suggest?

A 196

This boy had a blunt abdominal trauma. There may be injuries of the intraperitoneal organs and intra-abdominal bleeding (suspected by the guarding associated with the pallor).

In these cases, laboratory tests are needed, including full blood count and the usual preoperative tests to perform good resuscitation, liver function tests (AST, ALT, gamma GT, alkaline phosphatase, and bilirubin), and pancreatic tests (serum amylase and lipase) in order to look for trauma of these organs.

In this emergency context, it is better to ask directly for a full-body CT scan, which is the most accurate examination for abdominal traumas. It can reveal more than 50% of pancreatic injuries. In addition, it simultaneously checks the chest, the vertebral spine, and the brain.

Figure 2 is an abdominal CT scan showing a transversal linear area of attenuation in the pancreatic isthmus that reveals a transection of the pancreas (*white arrow*); it is associated with a small collection under the liver and a traumatism of the lower part of the spleen (*black arrow*).

The boy suffered from a severe trauma of the pancreas with biological repercussions, although there was no correlation between the severity of the traumatism and the initial level of serum amylase and lipase. The CT scan shows a transection of the gland, which corresponds to a grade-III lesion in the pancreas injury scale of the American Association for the Surgery of Trauma (AAST).

CT is not accurate enough in the diagnosis of pancreatic injuries because it does not allow direct visualization of the pancreatic ducts, which is essential for the choice of treatment. The "gold standard" technique is endoscopic retrograde pancreatography (ERP), which accurately determines the type and location of duct injury and may allow direct endoscopic treatment by stenting. Magnetic resonance cholangiopancreatography (MRCP)

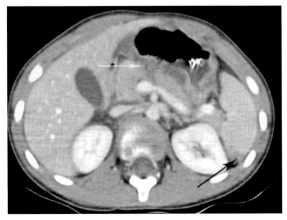

Fig. 2

is noninvasive and accurate for the detection of duct injuries; it could be a good examination to use, if available in emergency.

In pancreatic trauma with injury of the major duct, there are three possible approaches. First, initial medical treatment (diet, parenteral nutrition, antibiotics, analgesic, and possible drainage of pancreatic collection) may be initiated, with a secondary percutaneous or surgical drainage of pseudocysts if they develop, but this often implies a long hospital stay. Second, operative treatment includes two options: either drainage of pancreatic production through a Roux-en-Y loop applied on the pancreatic fracture, or partial distal pancreatectomy when the distal pancreatic segment is small. Third, ERP stenting could be a good alternative if it is achievable. This boy was treated surgically with a Roux-en-Y jejunostomy drainage. Medical treatment was then initiated comprising a combination of rest, diet, and octreotide for 12 days, after which the child recovered well, without any infection or complication.

Q 197

Isabelle Vidal, Guillaume Podevin, Anne Dariel, and Yves Heloury

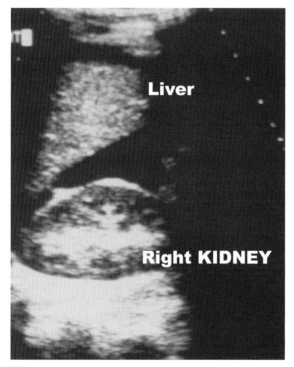

Fig. 1

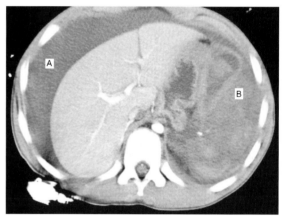

Fig. 2

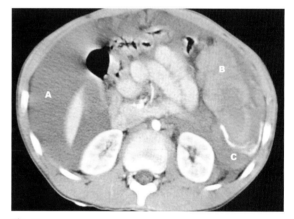

Fig. 3

An 11-year-old boy was involved in a motorbike accident. On admission, he had left hypochondrium pain without guarding and hematuria without any lumbar pain. There was no abdominal bruise or wound.

He was hemodynamically stable. Blood test results were normal (full blood count, liver and pancreatic function test). Abdominal US was performed (Fig. 1).

- Would you ask for another examination?
- What do Figs. 2 and 3 show?

Soon after his admission, his hemodynamic status became unstable: tachycardia (130 beats/min), low blood pressure (60 mmHg/30). Blood transfusion and macromolecule filling were required.

- What is the best way to manage this event?
- After successful management, what preventive measures should be taken?

A 197

This boy underwent splenectomy via laparotomy and his hemodynamic status became stable.

In general, hypochondrium pain is probably due to splenic trauma, and hematuria suggests kidney trauma. The hemodynamic status must be evaluated: paleness, tachycardia or bradycardia, low blood pressure, agitation, confusion.

The most important sign to look for is intraperitoneal effusion. The US (Fig. 1) shows intraperitoneal effusion between the liver and right kidney, which in this context is probably hematic.

An abdominal CT scan with and without contrast material should be performed to detect any abdominal or intestinal solid injuries. CT is more sensitive than US. US is not sensitive for abdominal solid trauma: it can detect subcapsular or intraparenchymal hematoma but not capsular tear or laceration.

The CT scan (Fig. 2) shows a massive hemoperitoneum (A), a devascularized and completely shattered spleen (B), and (Fig. 3) an active extravasation of contrast material in the splenic hilum and parenchyma (C), as well as a left renal laceration without urinary extravasa-tion or devascularization (not shown). There is no other abdominal injury. The injury is grade V according to the American Association for Surgery of Trauma grading scale: completely shattered spleen and hilar vascular injury, which devascularizes the spleen. This extravasation of contrast material corresponds to active bleeding.

The patient requires an immediate intervention for the hemodynamic instability and for the spleen injury with active bleeding. He should undergo urgent laparotomy for splenectomy to be performed. A total splenectomy is necessary because the spleen is totally shattered and devascularized. The renal injury is managed nonoperatively.

Close surveillance is required in an intensive care unit, followed by a stay in the children's surgical ward. Restricted activity after discharge is advised for the first few days. Prevention of infections is recommended to splenectomized patients: pneumococcal vaccine and antibiotic prophylaxis based on penicillin. The patient should always carry a special card for splenectomized patients with him. The parents' education is important: they have to consult a doctor when the child has fever.

Suggested Reading

1. Castagnola E, Fioredda F. Prevention of life-threatening infections due to encapsulated bacteria in children with hyposplenia or asplenia: a brief review of current recommendations for practical purposes. Eur J Haematol 2003; 71:319–326

2. Lutz N, Mahboubi S, Nance ML, Stafford PW. The significance of contrast blush on computed tomography in children with splenic injuries. J Pediatr Surg 2004; 39:491–494

3. Sato M, Yoshii H. Reevaluation of ultrasonography for solid-organ injury in blunt abdominal trauma. J Ultrasound Med 2004; 23:1583–1596

Q 198

Isabelle Vidal, Guillaume Podevin, Anne Dariel, and Yves Heloury

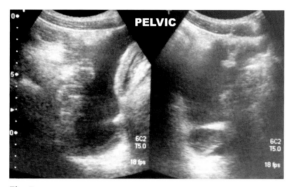

Fig. 1

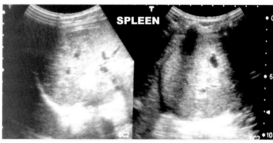

Fig. 2

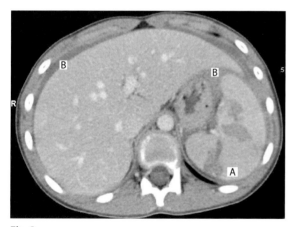

Fig. 3

Fig. 4

A 13-year-old boy was punched in the abdomen while playing with his brother. He immediately had abdominal pain, but did not vomit. On admission, he had left hypochondrium pain without guarding or rigidity. There was no abdominal excoriation, bruise or wound, and no hematuria. There was no other pertinent sign on initial examination.

He was hemodynamically stable. Blood test results were normal (full blood count, liver function test, serum lipase). Abdominal US was performed (Figs. 1, 2).

- Would you ask for another examination?
- What do Figs. 3 and 4 show?
- The patient remained hemodynamically stable. What is the best way to manage this abdominal trauma?
- Under certain circumstances this child could undergo urgent laparotomy—which ones?

A 198

The hypochondrium pain is probably due to splenic trauma, which is the most frequent abdominal trauma before liver or kidney injury. The hemodynamic status should be evaluated: paleness, tachycardia or bradycardia, low blood pressure, agitation, confusion.

The US study shows intraperitoneal effusion in the pelvis (Fig. 1) and a splenic subcapsular hematoma without any detection of laceration (Fig. 2). In this context, the intraperitoneal effusion is most probably a hemoperitoneum.

An abdominal CT scan with and without contrast material should be performed to detect abdominal solid injuries and to look for pneumoperitoneum. In addition, CT is used to stage solid organ injuries.

The CT scan shows a splenic subcapsular hematoma (probably ≥50% of surface area), two parenchymal lacerations (≥3 cm parenchymal depth) probably involving the trabecular vessels (Fig. 3, A), and a hemoperitoneum around the liver and spleen (Fig. 3, B) and in the pelvis (Fig. 4, A). There is no devascularization, no active extravasation of contrast material, and no other abdominal injury.

This is a grade-III injury according to the American Association for Surgery of Trauma grading scale: subscapular hematoma of ≥50% surface area, and laceration of ≥3 cm parenchymal depth involving the trabecular vessels. Grade I is a subcapsular hematoma of ≤10% sur-face area, or a laceration of ≤1 cm parenchymal depth. Grade II is a subcapsular hematoma of 10%–50% surface area, or an intraparenchymal hematoma ≤5 cm in diameter, or laceration of 1–3 cm parenchymal depth that does not involve a trabecular vessel. Grade IV is laceration involving the segmental or hilar vessels producing major devascularization (≥25% of spleen). Grade V is a completely shattered spleen or a hilar vascular injury which devascularizes the spleen.

This patient was managed nonoperatively. Conservative management of isolated blunt splenic injuries has become widely accepted for hemodynamically stable children. Treatment and management of children with splenic trauma can be more conservative than for adults. The child is often monitored in an intensive care unit and then in the children's surgical ward. Bed rest is imperative and the patient should remain lying down for a specified period depending on the severity of the spleen injury and on the clinical evolution.

This child could require immediate intervention for hemodynamic instability. Secondary hemorrhage is found in three situations: secondary splenic rupture, persistent active bleeding which is originally unknown, or hemorrhagic resurgence of hematoma. This situation is very rare in children, except when it concerns adolescents and older children.

Suggested Reading

1. Dobremez E, Lefevre Y, Harper L, Rebouissoux L, Lavrand F, Bondonny JM, Vergnes P. Complications occurring during conservative management of splenic trauma in children. Eur Pediatr Surg 2006; 16:166–170
2. Godbole P, Stringer MD. Splenectomy after paediatric trauma: could more spleens be saved? Ann R Coll Surg Engl 2002; 84:106–108
3. Ozturk H, Dokucu AI, Onen A, Otcu S, Gedik S, Azal OF. Non-operative management of isolated solid organ injuries due to blunt abdominal trauma in children: a fifteen-year experience. Eur J Pediatr Surg 2004; 14:29–34

Q 199

Deepika Nehra, Samuel Rice-Townsend, and Sanjeev Dutta

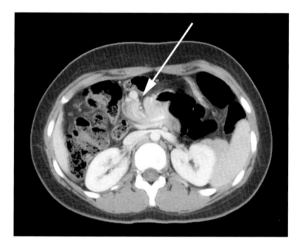

Fig. 1

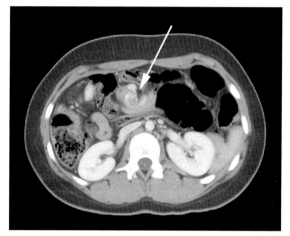

Fig. 2

An 18-year-old girl presented with intermittent abdominal pain, nonbilious emesis, anorexia, and malaise that had lasted several days.

Medical history revealed chronic difficulty with feeding and frequent emesis as a neonate, progressing to a pattern of intermittent recurrent episodes of diffuse abdominal pain associated with nonbilious emesis, characteristically resolving within days to a week.

She had a laparoscopic cholecystectomy 3 years earlier for presumed symptomatic cholelithiasis, with no report of intra-abdominal disease at that time.

The surgeon ordered a CT scan of the abdomen and pelvis, shown in Figs. 1 and 2.

- What is the most notable finding (indicated by the *arrows*) on the CT scan?
- Why is this a concerning finding and what pathological condition does it indicate?
- Describe how the suspected abnormality typically occurs.
- Why is the suspected condition considered a surgical emergency?
- How do patients with the suspected condition typically present?
- What are the treatment options for such an abnormality?
- Describe the typical surgical management.

A 199

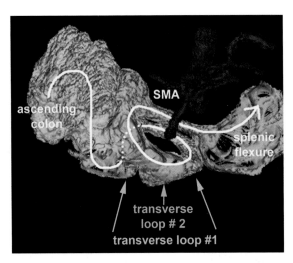

Fig. 3

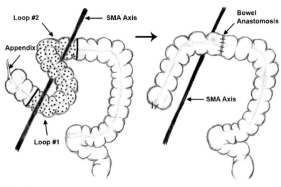

Fig. 4

A "whirlpool" pattern (*arrows*) involving a branch of the superior mesenteric artery (SMA) is seen on the CT scan. This pattern results from clockwise rotation of the bowel and the superior mesenteric vein (SMV) around the pedicle of the SMA and is a hallmark of midgut volvulus. In a case of suspected midgut volvulus, the CT scan should also be assessed for signs of bowel ischemia. These include bowel wall thickening, mesenteric edema with engorgement of mesenteric vessels, and intramural air. Free intraperitoneal air indicates bowel perforation. Upper gastrointestinal (UGI) series and US are other useful imaging modalities in the diagnosis of midgut volvulus.

Typically, volvulus occurs in the setting of malrotation. The abnormal positioning of the duodenojejunal junction and cecum with malrotation results in a short bowel mesentery and narrow SMA pedicle. The midgut has a propensity to twist around this narrow base, compressing the SMA and placing the entire midgut at risk for ischemia and eventual necrosis.

Midgut volvulus classically presents with vomiting and high intestinal obstruction in the neonate. Vomiting (classically bilious) occurs in more than 90% of all infants with volvulus. In older children, the symptoms are vaguer including failure to thrive, recurrent abdominal pain, and chronic diarrhea. Intermittent volvulus can re-

sult in episodes of abdominal pain and vomiting which may temporarily resolve only to precipitate a life-threatening crisis later. Older patients have higher complication rates due to delayed diagnosis.

Surgical intervention is the only treatment. All patients with volvulus or suspected volvulus should have an operation. During laparotomy, the volvulus is untwisted in a counterclockwise fashion. If the SMA pedicle appears narrow, the Ladd procedure is indicated. This involves division of the mesenteric (Ladd) bands, placement of the bowel in a position of nonrotation to widen the mesenteric base, and appendectomy.

This patient was taken for emergent laparotomy for suspected midgut volvulus. At laparotomy no volvulus was apparent, but a highly unusual rotational abnormality was found. The transverse colon appeared to encircle the mesenteric root in a spiral fashion (Fig. 3).

This is an extremely unusual finding. Typically a "whirlpool" pattern is highly specific for midgut volvulus. In this case, initial attempts at unspiraling the colon from around the root of the mesentery were unsuccessful, and a bowel resection with primary reanastomosis was performed (Fig. 4).

The patient had an uneventful recovery with no further symptoms.

Q 200

Deepika Nehra, Samuel Rice-Townsend, and Sanjeev Dutta

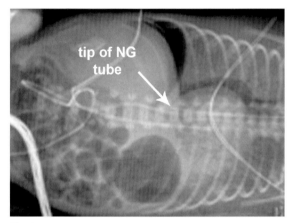

Fig. 1

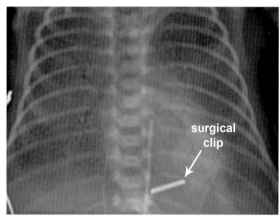

Fig. 2

A 25-week gestational age newborn appeared critically ill and was emergently intubated for severe respiratory distress. A nasogastric (NG) tube was passed with difficulty.

The patient decompensated further and bilious secretions were suctioned from the endotracheal (ET) tube. The abdomen became distended with ventilation.

Initial laboratory test results were remarkable for a white blood cell count (WBC) of 40×10^3 cells/μl with a left shift (12% bands).

Postintubation chest radiography was performed (Fig. 1).

- What are the salient findings on the radiograph (Fig. 1)?
- What are the most likely etiologies for the findings in Fig. 1?
- What is the most likely underlying etiology in this particular case?

The patient was taken emergently to the operating room.

- Based on the postoperative chest radiograph (Fig. 2) and the contrast study (Fig. 3), what procedure was performed on this child and why was this procedure deemed most appropriate?
- What are other management options of the acute condition?

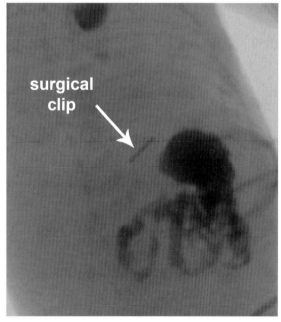

Fig. 3

- In the setting of this intervention, what important complication should be carefully ruled out at the time of definitive repair?

A 200

The left lateral decubitus film (Fig. 1) is useful in the evaluation of pneumothorax (PTX) when upright positioning is difficult. The lucency along the right chest base and right heart border represent PTX and pneumomediastinum, respectively. Note the grossly distended stomach. The NG tube is unusually positioned with the tip midline at T12; normally it should veer left toward the stomach.

Important causes of PTX in a newborn include parenchymal air leak and perforated viscus. Air leaks are common in premature newborns on mechanical ventilation for respiratory distress syndrome (RDS). Esophageal perforation typically occurs in premature neonates after repeat attempts at ET intubation or passage of naso/orogastric tubes. The treatment is typically medical with broad-spectrum antibiotics, parenteral or gastrostomy feedings, and tube thoracostomy for PTX or effusion. Risk factors for iatrogenic esophageal perforation are: prematurity, multiple attempts at intubation or passage of naso/orogastric tubes, bloody aspirate, and unusual positioning of naso/orogastric tube.

This boy was managed conservatively for suspected iatrogenic esophageal perforation with needle thoracotomy to evacuate the PTX and broad-spectrum antibiotics.

The ongoing bilious ET aspirate, gastric distention, and persistent infiltrate on chest radiographs are all clues to the underlying etiology. This boy was diagnosed with esophageal atresia (EA) with distal tracheoesophageal fistula (TEF). Contrast studies are neither indicated nor routinely performed to confirm the diagnosis.

The child required emergent occlusion of the TEF to improve respiratory status, but would probably not physiologically tolerate a thoracotomy for definitive repair. For this reason, he had emergent placement of a hemoclip at the GE junction to prevent further aspiration of gastric contents through the fistula. The clip is evident on the chest radiograph (Fig. 2). A contrast study (Fig. 3) was performed to assess the integrity of the GE junction clip and it confirmed the EA and functionality of the clip in preventing reflux through the fistula.

Other surgical options for the acute management of a patent fistula include: ligation of the fistula; placement of a gastrostomy tube to evacuate the gastric contents and prevent reflux; and inflation of a Fogarty catheter within the fistula which is a temporizing measure to help bridge toward definitive repair.

The child's status improved greatly. He underwent definitive repair with thoracotomy for ligation of the TEF and repair of the EA at 3 months of age. The clip was removed with careful inspection for stricture at the distal esophagus.

At the time of writing, the boy was 4 months old and had been doing well since discharge. The most likely long-term complication is gastroesophageal reflux disease.

Suggested Reading

1. Konkin DE, O'hali WA, Webber EM, Blair GK. Outcomes in esophageal atresia and tracheoesophageal fistula. Journal of Pediatric Surgery 2003; 38(12):1726–1729
2. Sapin E, Gumpert L, Bonnard A, Carricaburu E, Sava E, Contencin P, Helardot PG. Iatrogenic pharyngoesophageal perforation in premature infants. European Journal of Pediatric Surgery 2000; 10(2):83–87
3. Spitz L (2005) Esophageal Atresia and Thracheoesophageal Malformations. In: Ashcroft KW, Holcomb GW, Murphy JP (eds) Pediatric Surgery 4th edition. Elsevier Saunders, Philadelphia, pp 352–370

Q 201

Deepika Nehra, Samuel Rice-Townsend, and Sanjeev Dutta

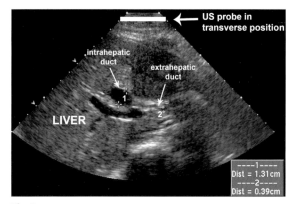

Fig. 1

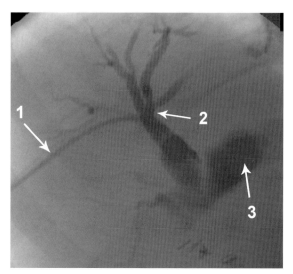

Fig. 2

A 14-year-old boy underwent laparoscopic cholecystectomy at an outside hospital for chronic cholecystitis. He presented 1 week later with a 2-day history of jaundice.

He denied any associated pain, nausea, vomiting, fever, and diarrhea. He also denied prior episodes of jaundice.

- What are important pathological conditions to consider when evaluating a patient with postoperative jaundice?
- What questions can you ask to narrow the differential diagnosis?

Liver function tests (LFTs) were ordered: total bilirubin 16.3 mg/dl, conjugated bilirubin 9.2 mg/dl, aspartate transaminase (AST) 127 U/l, alanine transaminase (ALT) 387 U/l, alkaline phosphatase (AP) 367 U/l.

- What do these results indicate?

US was performed to evaluate the biliary system. The probe was applied to the mid abdomen and angled toward the right side.

- What does the US image (Fig. 1) demonstrate?
- What are the common complications following laparoscopic cholecystectomy?

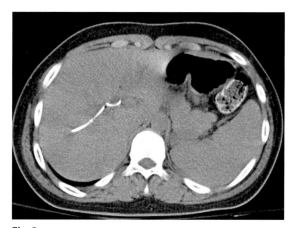

Fig. 3

- Based on the transhepatic cholangiogram (PTC) shown in Fig. 2, what complication does this child most likely have? What do the *arrows* correspond to?
- As evidenced by the finding on the CT scan (Fig. 3), how is this patient's condition initially managed?
- What are treatment principles and options in a patient with iatrogenic bile duct injury?

A 201

Important etiologies to consider in a postoperative patient with jaundice include increased bilirubin production, cholestasis, hepatocellular (HC) disease, and preexisting conditions. A resorbing hematoma, drug-induced hemolysis, or blood transfusions can increase bilirubin production. Benign postoperative cholestasis and sepsis can lead to intrahepatic cholestasis in a postoperative patient. In contrast, extrahepatic cholestasis is usually secondary to common bile duct stones, cholecystitis, pancreatitis, or bile duct stricture or injury. HC injury may result from ischemia, sepsis, anesthetics, TPN, or viral hepatitis. Preexisting conditions, like Gilbert's or Dubin–Johnson syndromes, should also be considered.

Urine color? When jaundice is due to elevated conjugated bilirubin, the urine turns a tea color as the water-soluble conjugated form is excreted. Unconjugated bilirubin is not water-soluble and does not affect urine color. *Stool color?* When jaundice is a result of complete biliary obstruction, the patient's stools are clay-colored or acholic.

The patient had a conjugated hyperbilirubinemia which is indicative of an obstructive pattern. The elevated transaminases suggest HC damage.

The ultrasound (Fig. 1) is remarkable for a dilated intrahepatic duct and normal-caliber extrahepatic duct.

Complications from laparoscopic cholecystectomy are rare. The most important are major bleeding, wound infection, bile leak, and bile duct injury (BDI). The most common pattern of BDI results from misidentification of the common bile duct (or right hepatic duct) for the cystic duct followed by deliberate clipping of the misidentified duct. Other complications include bowel perforation, liver laceration, and abscess formation from spillage.

This patient has postoperative cholestasis from iatrogenic injury to the biliary tree at the porta hepatis. The transhepatic cholangiogram shows a dilated anterior

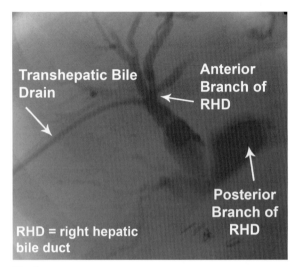

Fig. 4

and posterior branch of the right hepatic duct, suggesting injury to the right hepatic duct (Fig. 4).

Important principles in the treatment of a BDI injury are: (a) controlling sepsis and any ongoing bile leak, (b) relieving biliary obstruction, (c) delineating biliary anatomy with further imaging, and (d) planning surgery. In this case, the patient was not septic and there was no obvious biloma to drain. Initial imaging includes US and endoscopic retrograde cholangiopancreatography (ERCP). Bile leaks are usually amenable to endoscopic management with placement of a biliary stent. A percutaneous transhepatic drain can relieve biliary obstruction (Fig. 3). The US and PTC further delineate biliary anatomy and identify the specific location of the injury.

Definitive surgical repair usually necessitates a Roux-en-Y hepaticojejunostomy.

This boy underwent a Roux-en-Y repair with postoperative resolution of his jaundice and bile flow obstruction.

Suggested Reading

1. Connor S, Garden OJ. Bile duct injury in the era of laparoscopic cholecystectomy. The British journal of surgery 2006; 93(2):158–168
2. Faust TW, Reddy KR. Postoperative jaundice. Clinics in liver disease 2004; 8(1):151–166
3. Sicklick JK, Camp MS, Lillemoe KD, Melton GB, Yeo CJ, Campbell KA, Talamini MA, Pitt HA, Coleman J, Sauter PA, Cameron JL. Surgical management of bile duct injuries sustained during laparoscopic cholecystectomy: perioperative results in 200 patients. Annals of surgery 2005; 241(5):786–792
4. Way LW, Stewart L, Gantert W, Liu K, Lee CM, Whang K, Hunter JG. Causes and prevention of laparoscopic bile duct injuries: analysis of 252 cases from a human factors and cognitive psychology perspective. Annals of surgery 2003; 237(4):460–469

Q 202

Deepika Nehra, Samuel Rice-Townsend, and Sanjeev Dutta

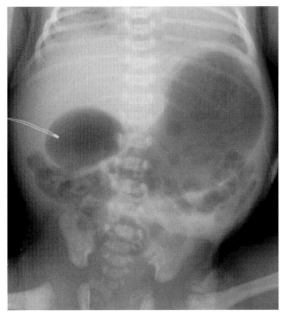

Fig. 1

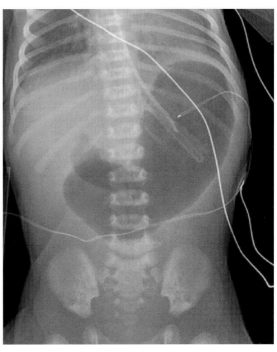

Fig. 2

Baby A was born by normal spontaneous vaginal delivery (NSVD) after an uncomplicated pregnancy. Shortly after delivery the child developed respiratory distress, requiring supplemental oxygen, and abdominal distention. An initial abdominal radiograph was acquired (Fig. 1).

Baby B was born by NSVD after an uncomplicated pregnancy. She had an uneventful stay in the nursery and was discharged on day-of-life 2 after she had passed meconium and was tolerating feeds. About 24 h later, she had considerable dark yellow emesis associated with feeding and had only a minimal green smear for stool. She presented to the emergency department and an abdominal radiograph was acquired (Fig. 2).

- What are the salient findings in Figs.1 and 2?
- What potential etiologies can explain these findings?
- What is the main difference between Fig. 1 and 2?
- What is the most likely diagnosis in each case?
- What imaging study can help confirm the diagnosis in each case?
- How would you manage Baby A? Baby B?

A 202

There is a "double bubble" sign with a distended gas-filled stomach and a grossly dilated proximal duodenum in both figures. The double bubble sign indicates duodenal obstruction.

The most common causes of duodenal obstruction are duodenal atresia, duodenal stenosis, annular pancreas, and rotational abnormalities. In the case of a rotational abnormality, the duodenal obstruction is secondary to either congenital peritoneal bands (Ladd's bands) or midgut volvulus.

In Fig. 1 there is clearly gas in the more distal small bowel/colon. In Fig. 2 there is no visible gas distal to the proximal duodenum.

The presence or absence of bowel gas distal to the proximal duodenum helps to determine the most likely etiology. In the case of an isolated double bubble with no distal gas, duodenal atresia is most likely. However, contrary to popular belief, an isolated double bubble does not entirely rule out malrotation, although the surgeon expects some distal gas in this situation. In the presence of distal gas, midgut volvulus must be highly suspected.

An upper gastrointestinal (UGI) series helps to further evaluate the case. In duodenal atresia, the duodenum has a club-shaped end. In malrotation with volvulus, the proximal duodenum terminates in a characteristic "corkscrew" or "birdbeak" fashion. Alternatively, ultrasonography can be used to rule out malrotation at risk for volvulus. Children with an abnormal ultrasound should either have a UGI series (to rule out volvulus) or have an exploratory laparotomy.

Baby A and B highlight the fact that the presence or absence of distal gas cannot be used to definitively diagnose the patient with either duodenal atresia or midgut volvulus.

In Fig. 1, the distal gas makes malrotation with volvulus highly suspected. Emergent operation is performed. At laparotomy, although there is malrotation there are no obvious Ladd's bands and there is no volvulus. The cause of the duodenal obstruction is found to be an annular pancreas. The malrotation is corrected and the annular pancreas is bypassed with a duodenoduodenostomy.

In Fig. 2, the absence of distal gas makes duodenal atresia highly likely and the patient is taken for elective operation. At laparotomy, there is obvious malrotation with midgut volvulus and a normal duodenum. The volvulus is reduced and a Ladd's procedure performed.

Any patient with a double bubble sign in the presence of distal gas should be taken for emergent operation. In the case of an isolated double bubble, if the patient is taken promptly to the operating room no further imaging is needed but, if surgery is to be delayed, it is prudent to obtain a UGI series to rule out malrotation with midgut volvulus.

Both patients did well postoperatively with no complications.

Suggested Reading

1. Hajivassiliou CA. Intestinal obstruction in neonatal/pediatric surgery. Seminars in Pediatric Surgery 2003; 12(4):241–253
2. Orzech N, Navarro OM, Langer JC. Is ultrasonography a good screening test for intestinal malrotation? Journal of Pediatric Surgery 2006; 41(5):1005–1009
3. Rathaus V, Grunebaum M, Ziv N, Kornreich L, Horev G. The bubble sign in the gasless abdomen of the newborn. Pediatric Radiology 1992; 22(2):106–109
4. Schmidt H, Abolmaali N, Vogl TJ. Double bubble sign. European Radiology 2002; 12(7):1849–1853

Q 203

Yves Aigrain and Pascale Philippe-Chomette

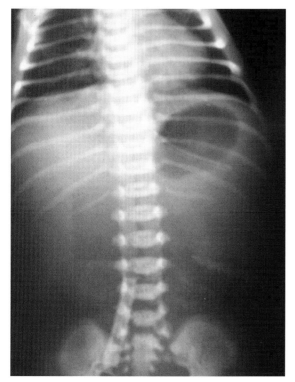

Fig. 1

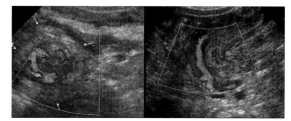

Fig. 2

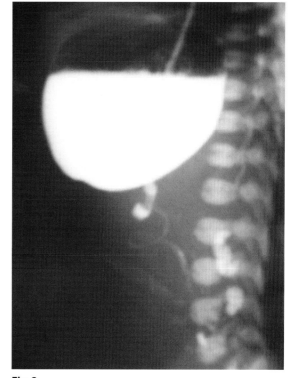

Fig. 3

A 5-day-old boy with bilious vomiting was referred to our department. Clinical examination showed bilious vomiting, no abdominal distension but a painful abdomen. A standard abdominal radiograph was acquired (Fig. 1).

- What is the main diagnosis?

- What other radiological examinations could be helpful in making the diagnosis?
- How do you interpret the US image (Fig. 2) and how do you interpret the examination shown in Fig. 3?
- Is a gastrointestinal tract examination needed?
- What is your approach?

A 203

This boy is affected by neonatal midgut volvulus with intestinal malrotation.

Clinically, the boy is 5 days old with bilious vomiting, no abdominal distension, and is in pain. The standard radiograph shows gastric distension without distal aeration.

Most patients who present with acute midgut volvulus are infants (30% present within the first week of life) and the most common symptom is vomiting (95%).

Pain and tenderness are constant.

After plain film radiography revealing either a gasless abdomen or upper intestinal distension (in 20% of cases a duodenal obstruction is identified by a double bubble sign), US color Doppler can help with the localization of mesenteric vessels to confirm the diagnosis of intestinal malrotation and the gastrointestinal tract examination can identify the malrotation or the total upper obstruction.

The US image shows the clockwise whirlpool sign on color Doppler US. It is the definite sign of midgut volvulus. We can see the wrapping of the superior mesenteric vein and the mesentery around the superior mesenteric artery.

The contrast image shows gastric distension with volvulus and duodenal obstruction.

Because of the whirlpool sign on the Doppler US image and all the clinical signs, we should operate on the child without performing any other examination.

The only thing to do before laparotomy is rehydration of the child. Intravenous fluids are administrated rapidly to correct hypovolemia with no further delay for intervention.

If the child is not in a life-threatening situation, a gastrointestinal tract examination should be done to define the malrotation. Without active volvulus, it can be rather difficult to identify the inversed position of the superior mesenteric vein and the superior mesenteric artery on US images.

We operated on the child, who had midgut acute volvulus and intestinal malrotation; the duodenum and jejunum lay to the right of the spine and the complete small bowel was on the right. The small bowel had to be rotated in a counterclockwise fashion to reduce the volvulus; dissection continued until the cecum and the ascending colon was moved to the left away from the duodenum widening the base of the mesentery.

Suggested Reading

1. Epelman M. The whirlpool sign. Radiology 2006 Sep; 240(3):910–1
2. Long FR, Kramer SS, Markowitz RI, Taylor GE. Radiographics patterns of intestinal malrotation in children. Radiographics 1996 May; 16(3):547–56
3. Orzech N, Navarro OM, Langer JC. Is ultrasonographic a good screening test for intestinal malrotation? J Pediatr Surg 2006 May; 41(5):1005–9

Q 204

Yves Aigrain and Pascale Philippe-Chomette

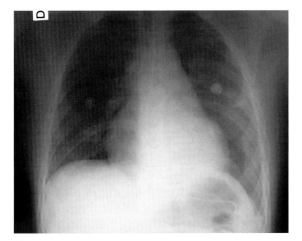

Fig. 1

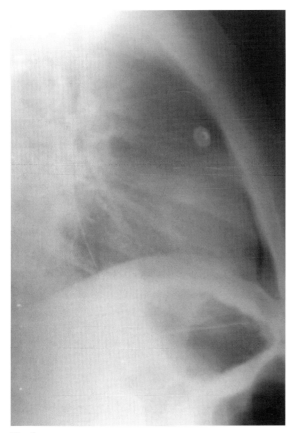

Fig. 2

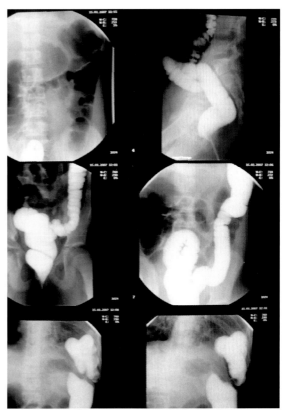

Fig. 3

An 11-year-old boy presented with painful abdominal distension and vomiting. Six years previously, he had suffered a thoracic penetrating injury without subsequent surgical exploration.

The pain was localized in the upper left quadrant of the abdomen.

- Comment on the standard chest (Figs. 1, 2).
- What is your hypothesis?
- Barium enema findings (Fig. 3) were conclusive; why?
- What is your approach?

A 204

On the standard chest radiograph, air is seen in the left diaphragmatic area; the abdominal radiograph shows colonic distension, and colonic splenic flexure is not visible.

The first hypothesis is colonic incarceration due to unrecognized traumatic diaphragmatic hernia.

The barium enema study shows opacification of the rectum, rectosigmoid, and a stop at the level of the splenic flexure without transverse opacification, confirming colonic incarceration.

The child was immediately operated on. The transverse colon and splenic flexure were incarcerated in the thoracic area with suffusion and colonic suffering. After complete reintegration of the colon, the child recovered fully.

Diaphragmatic repair was performed at the same time by laparotomy.

Blunt or penetrating injuries need complete investigations to confirm diaphragmatic integrity. The diagnosis of colonic incarceration could be missed with a high life-threatening risk for the patient. The diagnosis is suggested on plain film radiographs showing basilar opacification and obliteration of a clear diaphragmatic border. A nasogastric tube may help identify an intrathoracic position of the stomach. CT helps in identifying other intra-abdominal organs herniated into the chest.

If the diagnosis is made shortly after injury, the repair is best made via laparotomy because of the high incidence of associated intra-abdominal injuries.

Suggested Reading

1. Esme H, Solak O, Sahin DA, Sezer M. Blunt and penetrating traumatic ruptures of the diaphragm. Thorac Cardiovasc Surg 2006 Aug; 54(5):324–7
2. Von Hoppell, UO, Bautz P, De Groot M. Penetrating thoracic injuries: What we learnt. Thorac Cardiovasc Surg 2000; 48:55–61

Q 205

Felix Schier

A 10-year-old boy presented with right-sided lower abdominal pain for 1 day. He experienced nausea, but there was no vomiting and no diarrhea. There was no fever. The pain had an increasing tendency. The child did not want to drink or eat. He avoided any movement of the psoas muscle. There was a marked tenderness on palpation of the right lower abdomen. The Blumberg and Rovsing signs were both positive.

Among the laboratory test results, there was a normal leukocyte count and a slightly elevated C-reactive protein (CRP) level.

Ultrasound yielded the image shown in Fig. 1.

- What is the most likely diagnosis?
- Which treatment is indicated?
- Is a laparoscopic approach preferable or an open, conventional approach?

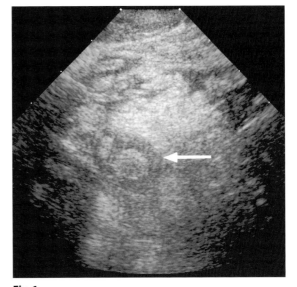

Fig. 1

A 205

The child has gangrenous appendicitis.

In general, laboratory values are not very useful in the differential diagnosis of acute appendicitis. It has been found that the change in total neutrophil count on the first day after onset of symptoms and the change in CRP level on the second and third days during in-hospital observation may serve as useful parameters in differentiating acute appendicitis from other acute abdominal diseases. Usually, however, there are no full 3 days for waiting. Appendicitis is either diagnosed within 1 day or another diagnosis is considered.

The white blood count is of little value in acute appendicitis. It seems that interleukin (IL)-6 or CRP levels are correlated with acute appendicitis, but not the leukocytes. There is no significant difference in diagnostic use between IL-6 and CRP. Therefore, in clinical practice, the CRP is a relatively reliable indicator.

Clinically, there is no big difference between appendicitis in children and adults. The typical, migrating pain is observed in all age groups. The negative appendectomy rate is higher in adults, possibly because the diagnosis is even easier to establish in children. Otherwise, statistically, mortality and morbidity, including wound infection rate and intra-abdominal abscess rate, are similar in adults and children. Contrary to traditional teaching, diagnosing acute appendicitis in children is similar to that in adults. The outcome of acute appendicitis in children is not associated with a delay in presentation or a delay in diagnosis.

The ultrasonographic picture (Fig. 1) is a transverse section of the right lower quadrant. Within hyperechoic mesenteric fat, a "bull's eye sign" is seen (*arrow*) with a diameter of 1.5 cm. Also, there is marked thickening of the bowel wall.

CT scans for the diagnosis of appendicitis are unusual in Europe. In the USA, they seem to be used more frequently, although their specificity largely depends on the experience of the radiologist attending and they require radiation.

There is no need to perform emergency appendectomy in the middle of the night. It has been shown repeatedly that the procedure may safely be performed within regular working hours.

The question remains open whether laparoscopic or open appendectomy is better. A Cochrane review supports the view that in those clinical settings where surgical expertise and equipment are available and used often, laparoscopy seems to have various advantages. In contrast, in settings where laparoscopy is not very common, a laparoscopic appendectomy may be an uncomfortable adventure. Still, in young female patients or in any other circumstances in which the diagnosis is not yet definitively established, laparoscopy is the superior technique. The intraoperative view and visualization are better with laparoscopy, and irrigation is also easier. Clinically, however, especially with respect to postoperative recovery, there is no obvious advantage of laparoscopy over the open approach. The degree of peritonitis and local inflammation or even perforation determines postoperative recovery, not the technical approach.

Suggested Reading

1. Ceydeli A, Lavotshkin S, Yu J, Wise L. When should we order a CT scan and when should we rely on the results to diagnose an acute appendicitis? Curr Surg 2006; 63:464–468,
2. Lee SL, Ho HS. Acute appendicitis: is there a difference between children and adults? Am Surg 2006; 72:409–413
3. Sack U, Biereder B, Elouahidi T, Bauer K, Keller T, Trobs RB. Diagnostic value of blood inflammatory markers for detection of acute appendicitis in children. BMC Surg 2006; 28:15
4. Sauerland S, Lefering R, Neugebauer EA. Laparoscopic versus open surgery for suspected appendicitis. Cochrane Database Syst Rev 2004; 18:CD001546
5. Taylor M, Emil S, Nguyen N, Ndiforchu F. Emergent vs urgent appendectomy in children: a study of outcomes. J Pediatr Surg 2005; 40:1912–1915
6. Wu HP, Huang CY, Chang YJ, Chou CC, Lin CY. Use of changes over time in serum inflammatory parameters in patients with equivocal appendicitis. Surgery 2006; 139:789–796

Q 206

Felix Schier

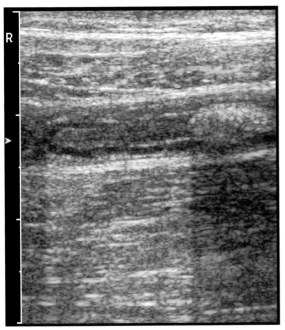

Fig. 1

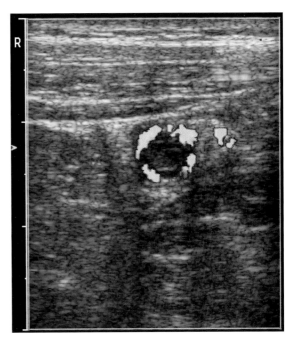

Fig. 2

A 12-year-old boy had recurrent, right-sided, lower abdominal pain for at least 2 weeks. He had no fever. There was tenderness on palpation of the right lower abdomen.

The laboratory values showed a normal leukocyte count and C-reactive protein (CRP) level.

Ultrasound yielded the images shown in Figs. 1 and 2.

- What is the most likely diagnosis?

A 206

Figure 1 is a sonogram of the right lower abdomen. The appendix appears extended, wall-thickened, and contains a hyperechoic oval structure at the tip, including a dorsal acoustic shadow.

Figure 2 is a color-coded Doppler sonogram demonstrating marked hypervascularity within the appendiceal wall.

The diagnosis is fecalith and appendicitis.

It has been found that a fecalith of the appendix may be a cause of chronic, right lower quadrant abdominal pain, at least in adult patients. This may well be the case also in children. In these patients, the classical signs of acute appendicitis may be absent, such as fever, localized pain on palpation, or leukocytosis. On CT, a fecalith and appendiceal thickening may be demonstrated, without mesenteric infiltration, abscess, or collection. Thus, the fecalith would serve as a marker rather than an actual cause of appendicitis. It was also shown that focused CT scans with additional lung and bone windows proved optimal in detecting fecaliths which were not visible on the scout localizer scans, despite windowing modifications. Surgery would cure the problem if the patient and parents are not ready to tolerate the finding and the symptoms.

When retained within the abdominal cavity, they may cause intra-abdominal or intrapelvic abscesses. Fecaliths missed during laparoscopic appendectomy have been published repeatedly as a cause of subsequent abscess formation. They definitely are a risk factor for the development of postoperative complications.

Retained fecaliths have been removed laparoscopically. It appears logical to attempt to localize and remove them laparoscopically after a previous laparoscopic intervention.

If a perforated appendicitis is treated nonoperatively, the presence of a fecalith on radiologic imaging is related to a recurrence rate of appendicitis of almost three times higher than if there is no fecalith. Thus, an abscess with fecalith has a far lower rate to heal—with antibiotics—than an abscess without a fecalith.

Suggested Reading

1. Ein SH, Langer JC, Daneman A. Nonoperative management of pediatric ruptured appendix with inflammatory mass or abscess: presence of an appendicolith predicts recurrent appendicitis. J Pediatr Surg 2005; 40:1612–1615
2. Giuliano V, Giuliano C, Pinto F, Scaglione M. Chronic appendicitis "syndrome" manifested by an appendicolith and thickened appendix presenting as chronic right lower abdominal pain in adults. Emerg Radiol 2006; 12:96–98
3. Guillem P, Mulliez E, Proye C, Pattou F. Retained appendicolith after laparoscopic appendectomy: the need for systematic double ligature of the appendiceal base. Surg Endosc 2004; 18:717–718
4. Nitecki S, Karmeli R, Sarr MG. Appendiceal calculi and fecaliths as indications for appendectomy. Surg Gynecol Obstet 1990; 171:185–188
5. Smith AG, Ripepi A, Stahlfeld KR. Retained fecalith: laparoscopic removal. Surg Laparosc Endosc Percutan Tech 2002; 12:441–442

Q 207

Felix Schier

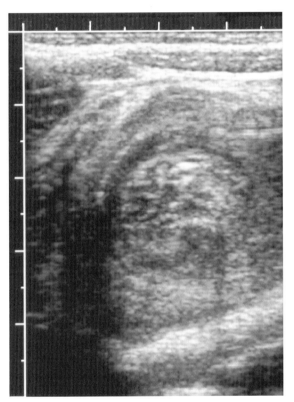

Fig. 1

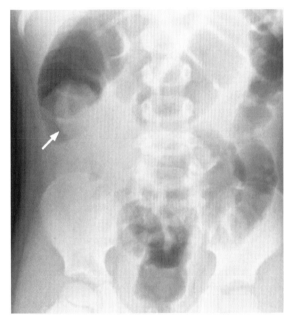

Fig. 2

A 2-year-old boy, previously healthy, suddenly displayed colicky attacks of abdominal pain. The child vomited several times and passed bloody stool 8 h later.

There was a mass palpable at the right lower abdomen.

Laboratory values were normal except for a slight leukopenia.

Imaging studies are shown in Figs. 1 and 2.

- What is the most likely diagnosis?

A 207

Figure 1 is a sonogram of the right lower abdomen. A target-shaped structure with a diameter of 3.3 cm is identified. The bowel walls are thickened.

During pneumatic reduction, the head of the intussusceptum is still visible within the cecum (Fig. 2, *arrow*).

The diagnosis is ileocolic intussusception.

In Europe, intussusception is the most common cause of acute intestinal obstruction in children younger than 5 years. The classic triad of symptoms (abdominal pain, abdominal mass, bloody stools) is present in 30% of patients. Etiologically, it has been linked to rotavirus vaccine, without proof so far. The peak incidence is in children of 3–9 months of age.

Is it commonly believed that in school-age children, intussusception is more commonly caused by some organic abnormality than in younger children. This is not uniformly confirmed, however.

Interestingly, the management of pediatric intussusception outside tertiary centers is not uniform or standardized. This probably applies to all European countries. Outside tertiary care centers the approach to intussusception varies widely. In England for example, pediatricians favor air or saline, surgeons prefer water-soluble contrast media, and radiologists still use barium. Today, possibly stimulated by the success rate of our Asian colleagues, air is far more frequently used than 25 years ago,

and the success rate has also risen from 45% to more than 80%.

Otherwise, the basic techniques in intussusception are uniform. An attempt is made to reduce the intussusceptum by air or liquid. Approaches vary with respect to the conventional "open" approach versus the laparoscopic approach.

Laparoscopy is indicated if the reduction is incomplete (as in this case) or uncertain. In a distended abdomen, however, an open approach may be safer. There is an approximately 10% chance that the intussusception has spontaneously reduced during induction of anesthesia. This is why Chinese pediatric surgeons perform a last reduction attempt with the patient on the table; with an overall success rate of more than 90%. These 10% spontaneous reductions are also an aspect which principally favors laparoscopy in intussusception.

It has been found that over the last 25 years, the duration of symptoms and signs prior to diagnosis is now three times longer than earlier. In contrast, however, the incidence of pain, vomiting, abdominal mass, and rectal blood has decreased. The classical symptoms seem less dramatic than they were 25 years ago. Furthermore, fewer lead points are found today than earlier. The reason for this is unclear.

Along the same lines, today fewer children require surgery than earlier, but more children need resections.

Suggested Reading

1. Calder FR, Tan S, Kitteringham L, Dykes EH. Patterns of management of intussusception outside tertiary centres. J Pediatr Surg 2001; 36:312–315

2. Grimprel E, de La Rocque F, Romain O, Minodier P, Dommergues MA, Laporte-Turpin E, Lorrot M, Parez N, Caulin E, Robert M, Lehors H, Cheron G, Levy C, Haas H; Groupe de Pathologie Infectieuse Pediatrique; Groupe Francophone d'Urgences et de Reanimation Pediatrique; Societe Francaise de Chirurgie Pediatrique: Management of intussusception in France in 2004: investigation of the Paediatric Infectious Diseases Group, the French Group of Paediatric Emergency and Reanimation, and the French Society of Paediatric Surgery Arch Pediatr 2006; 13:1581–1588

3. Huppertz HI, Soriano-Gabarro M, Grimprel E, Franco E, Mezner Z, Desselberger U, Smit Y, Wolleswinkel-van den Bosch J, De Vos B, Giaquinto C. Intussusception among young children in Europe. Pediatr Infect Dis J 25, Suppl 2006; S22–29

4. Ikeda T, Koshinaga T, Inoue M, Goto H, Sugitou K, Hagiwara N. Intussusception in children of school age. Pediatr Int 2007; 49:58–63

5. Schier F. Experience with laparoscopy in the treatment of intussusception. J Pediatr Surg 1997; 32:1713–1714

Q 208

Felix Schier

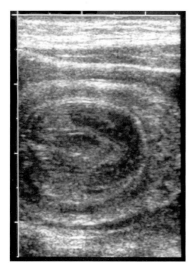

Fig. 1

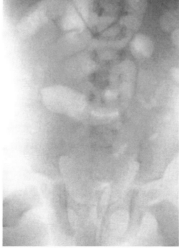

Fig. 2

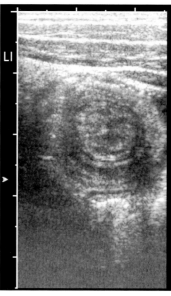

Fig. 3

A 2-year-old boy had abdominal pain, joint pain, a purpuric rash at the lower extremities, hematuria, and occult gastrointestinal blood loss. A nonspecific viral infection had preceded these symptoms several days earlier.

Laboratory values were normal except for a leukopenia.

Imaging studies are shown in Figs. 1,2.

- What is the most likely diagnosis?

A 208

Figure 1 is an ultrasonogram of the left upper abdomen. There is a "target sign" with a diameter of 2.2 cm. The bowel walls are enlarged.

Figure 2 shows a plain abdominal view. There is an irregular air distribution pattern in the proximal small bowel. Also, there is decreased gas within the distal bowel, a sign of incomplete obstruction.

The diagnosis is jejunojejunal intussusception with abdominal wall bleeding in Henoch–Schönlein purpura.

Figure 3 is shown for comparison: This is a target sign of 1.7 cm diameter at the left upper abdomen, caused by jejunojejunal intussusception in a 7-year old boy without Henoch–Schönlein. In contrast to the Henoch–Schönlein purpura intussusception there is no bowel wall thickening.

Enema reduction is considered ineffective in small bowel intussusception. There are, however, reports that enemas can be safely performed in intussusception from Henoch–Schönlein.

Literature reports differ on the rate of observed spontaneous reductions of small bowel intussusception. In contrast, others report a surgery rate of virtually 100% because of the presence of pathologic lead points and/or bowel complications. Some surgeons had the idea to wait for spontaneous reduction because they had seen cases of spontaneous reduction upon performing laparotomy. Today it would appear more appropriate to perform laparoscopy in these cases, with the option either to confirm a spontaneous reduction or to encounter an intussusception amenable to laparoscopic reduction (which is technically easier than an ileocolic intussusception) or to proceed to a laparoscopy-assisted procedure with exteriorizing the involved bowel segment via the umbilicus. A conventional "open" approach would appear exaggerated today.

Do all small bowel intussusceptions require surgery? There are no uniform observations. It has been found that an intussusception length greater than 3.5 cm during sonography is a strong independent predictor of the need for surgical intervention.

Intussusception from bowel wall hematoma may also be a consequence of trauma, not only from Henoch–Schönlein purpura.

Suggested Reading

1. Erichsen D, Sellstrom H, Andersson H. Small bowel intussusception after blunt abdominal trauma in a 6-year-old boy: case report and review of 6 cases reported in the literature. J Pediatr Surg 2006; 41:1930–1932
2. Koh EP, Chua JH, Chui CH, Jacobsen AS. A report of 6 children with small bowel intussusception that required surgical intervention. J Pediatr Surg 2006; 41:817–820
3. Munden MM, Bruzzi JF, Coley BD, Munden RF. Sonography of pediatric small-bowel intussusception: differentiating surgical from nonsurgical cases. AJR Am J Roentgenol 2007; 188:275–279
4. Schwab J, Benya E, Lin R, Majd K. Contrast enema in children with Henoch-Schonlein purpura. J Pediatr Surg 2005; 40:1221–1223
5. Sonmez K, Turkyilmaz Z, Demirogullari B, Karabulut R, Aral YZ, Konus O, Basaklar AC, Kale N. Conservative treatment for small intestinal intussusception associated with Henoch-Schonlein's purpura. Surg Today 2002; 32:1031–1034

Q 209

Felix Schier

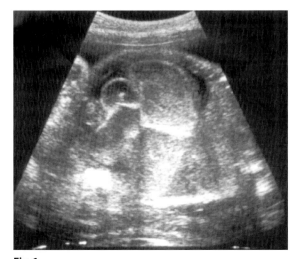

Fig. 1

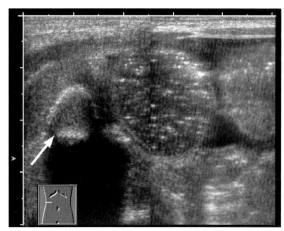

Fig. 3

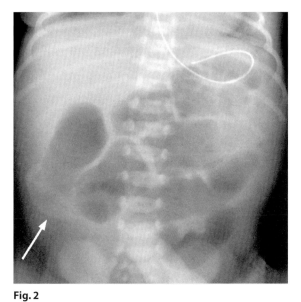

Fig. 2

Fig. 4

During a routine interuterine screening, distended bowel loops and intra-abdominal calcifications were seen. Shortly after birth, the newborn had a distended abdomen and vomited bile. Both scrota appeared moderately inflamed, were edematous, and had a slightly brownish discoloration.

Laboratory values showed signs of infection. Imaging studies are shown in Figs. 1–4.

- What is the most likely diagnosis?

A 209

Figure 1 is a prenatal ultrasound showing distended bowel loops and signs of calcification.

Figure 2 is a plain abdominal radiograph taken on the first day of life. The bowel loops are distended as in ileus. The *arrow* points to an oval-shaped grainy calcification.

Figure 3 is a transsection of the right lower abdomen. Again, dilated bowel loops are seen as in ileus. There is ascites between the bowel loops. The *arrow* points to a hyperechoic structure like a calcification (with acoustic shadow).

Figure 4 is a radiograph of the scrotum demonstrating calcifications of the scrotum.

The diagnosis is intrauterine meconium peritonitis after bowel perforation.

The perforation is caused by distal obstruction. Meconium acts as an aseptic chemical.

Prenatal ultrasonography allows one to suspect meconium peritonitis. This in turn allows transfer of mother and child to a tertiary center for delivery and appropriate management. It has been found that the chances of survival of these babies then are excellent if they are not associated with cystic fibrosis.

Prenatal MR imaging has recently been described as an add-on in order to improve the low diagnostic yield of prenatal ultrasound for meconium peritonitis. It has been suggested to also perform a postnatal contrast CT scan in order to define persistent intestinal perforation invisible with prenatal ultrasound.

Meconium periorchitis is a rarity. Clinically, a soft swelling of the scrota is seen. The swelling may be associated with bluish discoloration of the scrotum. There is a risk of unnecessary surgery of this condition. It has been stated that the "mass" and the calcifications will resolve spontaneously without compromising the testicle. Sonographic features together with an abdominal plain film radiograph are diagnostic, and visualization of the normal testicle may be helpful in differentiating this tumor-like lesion from scrotal tumors.

Even meconium thorax has been reported. In these cases, meconium peritonitis extends through muscular defects in the diaphragm up into the thorax. Meconium thorax has also been identified with prenatal ultrasound.

Not all intra-abdominal calcifications are caused by meconium peritonitis. Patients with anorectal anomalies and rectourethral fistulae are also reported to show intraluminal calcified meconium. It has been postulated that intestinal stasis and mixing of urine and meconium may be predisposing factors for the calcification of meconium. In these cases, intraluminal calcifications may appear as discrete punctate flecks within the distribution of the bowel, in contrast to meconium peritonitis, where the calcifications are linear and plaque-like, occurring anywhere in the abdominal cavity and scrotum.

Suggested Reading

1. Chan KL, Tang MH, Tse HY, Tang RY, Tam PK. Meconium peritonitis: prenatal diagnosis, postnatal management and outcome. Prenat Diagn 2005; 25:676–682
2. Miller JP, Smith SD, Newman B, Sukarochana K. Neonatal abdominal calcification: is it always meconium peritonitis? J Pediatr Surg 1988; 23:555–556
3. Patole S, Whitehall J, Almonte R, Stalewski H, Lee-Tannock A, Murphy A. Meconium thorax: a case report and review of literature. Am J Perinatol 1998; 15:53–56
4. Simonovsky V, Lisy J. Meconium pseudocyst secondary to ileal atresia complicated by volvulus: antenatal MR demonstration. Pediatr Radiol 6, 2007
5. Varkonyi I, Fliegel C, Rosslein R, Jenny P, Ohnacker H. Meconium periorchitis: case report and literature review. Eur J Pediatr Surg 2000; 10:404–407

Q 210

Felix Schier

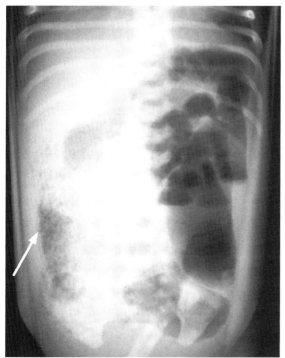

Fig. 1

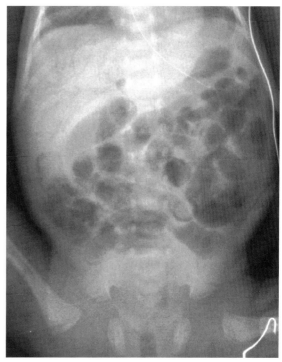

Fig. 2

A premature infant weighing 1,500 g developed a distended abdomen and feeding intolerance. Biliary vomiting set in and the child became septic within a few hours. Eventually, the child was close to shock. The right lower abdomen was distended, reddened, and tender. Blood was passed perianally. Laboratory values yield a septic picture.

Imaging studies yielded the figures shown here (Figs. 1, 2).

- What is the most likely diagnosis?

A 210

Figure 1 is an abdominal plain film radiograph in upright position. Gas is distributed unequally within the abdomen. Bowel loops in the middle and left upper abdomen are massively dilated. Some air–fluid levels are identified. The *arrow* points to a dilated bowel loop with foamy stool/gas content in the right abdomen. In addition there is a double contour of the bowel wall, the so-called pneumatosis intestinalis.

Figure 2 is an abdominal plain film radiograph of a different patient with the child supine. On the right liver lobe a radial "pneumoportogram" is seen, demonstrating air-filled portal veins. Bowel loops are massively dilated as in ileus.

The diagnosis is necrotizing enterocolitis with pneumatosis intestinalis and pneumoportogram.

Portal venous gas is usually associated with extensive bowel gangrene and high mortality.

With respect to radiologic signs of necrotizing enterocolitis, it may be stated that most patients have pneumatosis intestinalis, mild to severe, and one-third of patients have pneumoperitoneum. In approximately 15% of patients portal venous gas can be demonstrated; 10% have both, portal venous gas and pneumatosis intestinalis.

Radiologists seem to find it difficult to establish a reliable diagnosis when evaluating radiologic signs of necrotizing enterocolitis. It has repeatedly been shown that there is a relatively high observer variability. The indication for surgery thus cannot rely solely on radiology.

Diffuse distention and asymmetric bowel gas pattern are early signs. Pneumatosis intestinalis and portal venous gas are remarkable signs. Subserosal air makes linear pneumatosis, submucosal air demonstrates a bubbly appearance. In premature infants younger than 2 weeks the radiographic appearance of colonic stool is rare.

As in the above case, neonates most commonly present with feeding intolerance, delayed gastric emptying, abdominal distention or tenderness (or both), occult or gross blood in the stool, lethargy, apnea, respiratory distress, or poor perfusion.

Some indications for surgery are obvious: pneumoperitoneum, paracentesis positive for brown fluid or bacteria, portal venous gas, severe pneumatosis intestinalis; numerous others are less evident, such as erythema, dilated loops on serial radiographs, fixed abdominal mass etc.

Approximately 30% of all children with necrotizing enterocolitis will undergo surgery. About 50% of the operated children die. The smaller and the sicker the child, the higher the mortality rate.

Postoperative complications of surgery are wound dehiscences, intra-abdominal abscesses, and intestinal strictures. In dramatic cases short bowel syndrome may ensue.

Virtually no progress has been made in the last 30 years with respect to the pathophysiology of necrotizing enterocolitis. Several mechanisms are still under discussion—immature intestinal motility and digestion, immature intestinal circulatory regulation, immature intestinal barrier function, abnormal bacterial colonization, immature intestinal innate immunity—without an answer so far. No wonder that surgery does not achieve better results.

Suggested Reading

1. Caplan MS, Jilling T. New concepts in necrotizing enterocolitis. Curr Opin Pediatr 2001; 13:111–115
2. Kosloske AM, Musemeche CA, Ball WS Jr, Ablin DS, Bhattacharyya N. Necrotizing enterocolitis: value of radiographic findings to predict outcome. AJR Am J Roentgenol 1988; 151:771–774
3. Kosloske AM, Necrotizing enterocolitis In: Surgery of Infants and Children: Scientific principles and practice. Keith T. Oldham, Paul M. Colombani, and Robert P. Foglia (eds). Lippincott-Raven Publishers, Philadelphia, p 1201–1213, 1997
4. Lin PW, Stoll BJ. Necrotising enterocolitis. Lancet 2006; 368:1271–1283
5. Di Napoli A, Di Lallo D, Perucci CA, Schifano P, Orzalesi M, Franco F, De Carolis MP. Inter-observer reliability of radiological signs of necrotising enterocolitis in a population of high-risk newborns. Paediatr Perinat Epidemiol 2004; 18:80–87

Q 211

Felix Schier

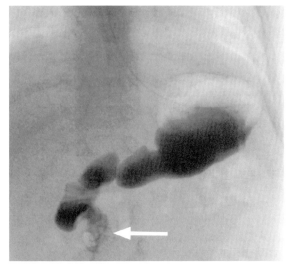

Fig. 1

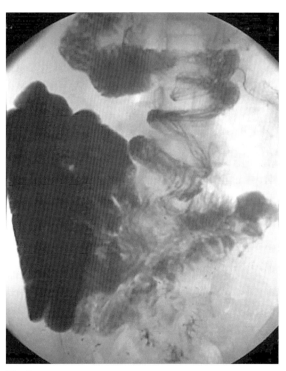

Fig. 2

A 3-week-old girl presented with frequent vomiting after feedings. The physical examination was normal. Laboratory values were also normal. Imaging studies yield the figures shown here (Figs. 1–2).

- What is the most likely diagnosis?

A 211

The contrast medium remains for an unusually long period of time within the pars descendens of the duodenum. Next, the contrast medium passes into a short segment of the duodenum running immediately to the right of the vertebral column (*arrow*) and not proceeding to the left upper abdomen as normally. Eventually, the contrast medium passes into small bowel segments more distally.

On the sonogram (Fig. 1), a "target sign" with a central vessel is identified within the left abdomen and prevertebrally.

A color-coded Doppler sonogram demonstrates that the blood vessels run in a spiral in this same area ("whirlpool sign"). The Doppler flow pattern demonstrates that barely the end diastolic blood flow is maintained.

Figure 2, for comparison, shows volvulus in a different patient: a 5-year old girl with recurrent abdominal pain. Note the typical "corkscrew sign" of the proximal jejunum.

The diagnosis is malrotation with incomplete volvulus.

Midgut volvulus is provoked by intestinal malrotation, a congenital abnormal position of the duodenojejunal junction, and is a potentially life-threatening condition, although chronic conditions have occasionally been seen (see Fig. 2). Radiologically, the diagnosis is considered straightforward. However, there seems to be a remaining approximately 15% of upper GI tract examinations which are equivocal and lead to a false-positive or false-negative interpretation. This difficulty seems to increase with increasing patient age.

In ultrasonography, abnormal orientation of the superior mesenteric artery and vein has been described in malrotation. Ultrasonography alone was found to be false positive in 21% and false negative in 2%. Among abnormal ultrasounds, inversion of the superior mesenteric

vein and artery and the "whirlpool sign" were more predictive for malrotation and volvulus than anterior/posterior orientation. Therefore, ultrasonography seems a good screening tool that effectively rules out malrotation at risk for volvulus. The conclusion was that children with an abnormal ultrasound should have an upper GI study or go to the operating room, depending on clinical findings.

Studies of patients up to adulthood have demonstrated that identification of the clockwise whirlpool sign on sonography is an accurate way of diagnosing volvulus, precluding the need for further investigations and allowing for prompt surgical intervention.

Should a patient with asymptomatic malrotation undergo a prophylactic Ladd's procedure? It has been shown that the gain in life expectancy was highest when asymptomatic malrotation was treated at 1 year of age and steadily declined until asymptomatic malrotation was treated at 20 years of age. An increasing advantage of observation over prophylactic surgery on life expectancy was observed after the second decade of life. A twofold increase in mortality risk for an elective Ladd's procedure decreased the age threshold to 14 years, whereas a fourfold increase decreased the threshold to 7 years. The conclusion was that Ladd's procedure should be considered for children diagnosed with asymptomatic malrotation, particularly those who are younger and with a low risk of postoperative mortality.

Surgically, we have perhaps been too aggressive in the past when encountering seemingly nonviable small bowel in volvulus. A case of a newborn has been described in whom the complete small bowel appeared ischemic and nonviable during surgery for volvulus. The abdomen was closed and the child left alone. Weeks later, subsequent relaparotomy showed that 40 cm of bowel had unexpectedly survived. And so did the child.

Suggested Reading

1. Applegate KE, Anderson JM, Klatte EC. Intestinal malrotation in children: a problem-solving approach to the upper gastrointestinal series. Radiographics 2006; 26:1485–1500
2. Houben CH, Mitton S, Capps S. Malrotation volvulus in a neonate: a novel surgical approach.Pediatr Surg Int 2006; 222:393–394
3. Orzech N, Navarro OM, Langer JC. Is ultrasonography a good screening test for intestinal malrotation? J Pediatr Surg 2006; 41:1005–1009
4. Taori K, Sanyal R, Attarde V, Bhagat M, Sheorain VS, Jawale R, Rathod J. Unusual presentations of midgut volvulus with the whirlpool sign. J Ultrasound Med 2006; 25:99–103

Q 212

Felix Schier

A newborn presented with anal atresia. The abdomen was markedly distended and the child displayed progressive circulatory decompensation.

Laboratory values showed signs of the beginning of sepsis. Imaging studies yield the picture shown here (Fig. 1).

• What is the most likely diagnosis?

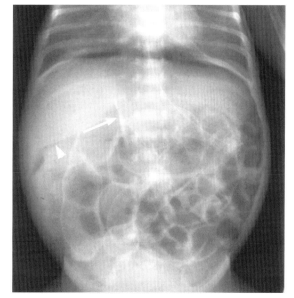

Fig. 1

A 212

Figure 1 is an abdominal plain film radiograph in reclining position. The abdomen is distended and bowel loops are dilated. There is tent-shaped intraperitoneal, subdiaphragmatic free air. A linear shadow (*arrow*) is created by air around the falciform ligament (the so-called football sign). In addition, there is free air below the liver (*arrowhead*).

The diagnosis is pneumoperitoneum after bowel perforation.

Spontaneous perforation of the colon in newborns is occasionally reported. Also, a few cases of spontaneous colonic perforations in children with anal atresia are known. Practically all recover completely after surgery. The cause mostly remains unknown.

Other parts of the GI tract may also perforate spontaneously without signs of necrotizing enterocolitis (NEC). Focal GI perforations occurring in the very-low-birth weight infant represent a clinically distinct phenomenon. Very likely, the traditionally accepted diagnostic criteria for bowel perforation due to NEC are unreliable in this condition.

Spontaneous perforations of the small bowel in small children have also been reported. A pathogenetic mechanism is unknown so far. Again, the prognosis was good after surgery. Typical of isolated intestinal perforations without signs of NEC are isolated perforations on healthy bowel, in contrast to NEC. Interestingly the survival after NEC perforation and after isolated perforation of the small bowel is equally bad (60% and 50%, respectively).

In surgery for perforation a decision has to be made between resection and anastomosis and stoma. It has been found that in preterm neonates, resection and anastomosis is an acceptable option in spontaneous idiopathic intestinal perforation as well as in NEC.

Suggested Reading

1. Calisti A, Perrelli L, Nanni L, Vallasciani S, D'Urzo C, Molle P, Briganti V, Assumma M, De Carolis MP, Maragliano G. Surgical approach to neonatal intestinal perforation. An analysis on 85 cases (1991–2001). Minerva Pediatr 2004; 56:335–339
2. Harms K, Ludtke FE, Lepsien G, Speer CP. Idiopathic intestinal perforations in premature infants without evidence of necrotizing enterocolitis. Eur J Pediatr Surg 1995; 5:30–33
3. Komuro H, Urita Y, Hori T, Hirai M, Kudou S, Gotoh C, Kawakami H, Kaneko M. Perforation of the colon in neonates. J Pediatr Surg 2005; 40:1916–1919
4. Mintz AC, Applebaum H: Focal gastrointestinal perforations not associated with necrotizing enterocolitis in very low birth weight neonates. J Pediatr Surg 1993; 28:857–860
5. Singh M, Owen A, Gull S, Morabito A, Bianchi A. Surgery for intestinal perforation in preterm neonates: anastomosis vs stoma. J Pediatr Surg 2006; 41:725–729

Q 213

Felix Schier

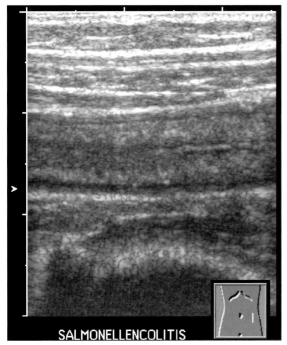

Fig. 1

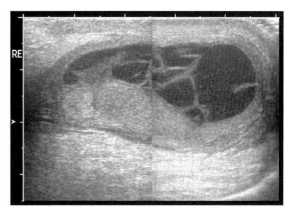

Fig. 2

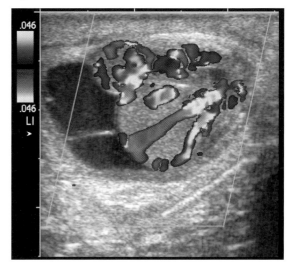

Fig. 3

A 4-year-old boy presented with an acutely painful, reddened, and enlarged scrotum. The child also suffered from severe diarrhea and had fever.

Laboratory values pointed to an infectious process. Imaging studies yield the pictures shown here (Figs. 1–3).

- What is the most likely diagnosis?

A 213

Figure 1 is a longitudinal section of the left colon. The submucosa is enlarged, the mesenterial fat tissue is not enlarged. The bowel lumen is massively narrowed.

Figure 2 is a longitudinal section of the scrotum. The wall of the scrotum is massively thickened. There is a hydrocele with hyperechoic septae, indicating infection of the hydrocele. The testicle is found at the back of the scrotum, with the epididymis on top, also enlarged and hyperechoic.

Color-coded Doppler sonography (Fig. 3) demonstrates good perfusion in the testicle and also the epididymis, thus ruling out testicular torsion. This is reactive hyperemia, a consequence of infection.

Salmonellae were eventually identified in the hydrocele of the same species as in the feces.

The diagnosis is acute scrotum in septic salmonellosis.

Extraintestinal manifestations of salmonellosis in pediatric patients are found predominantly in infants less than 3 months of age. Genital involvement is a complication which has been described in a few isolated cases. The children may erroneously undergo surgery on suspicion of testicular torsion, while orchitis is the correct diagnosis. *Salmonella enteritidis* will be cultured from the intraoperative swab. All other cultures from blood, CSF, and urine may prove sterile. The risk of extraintestinal manifestations is the reason why it has been suggested that children less than 3 months of age with suspected or proven salmonellosis should receive early antibiotic treatment.

In adult patients, apparently, the most notable echographic finding is an enlarged and heterogeneous epididymis, predominantly in its body and tail. Testicular involvement consisted of a diffusely hypoechoic testis or focal intratesticular areas. Thickening of the scrotal wall and tunica albuginea and moderate hydrocele were also noted occasionally. Follow-up scans occasionally revealed intratesticular abscesses.

Ultrasonography is not significantly better than the merely clinical diagnosis of orchitis. Statistically it has been found that the presence of dysuria and micturition disorders points to orchitis. There seems to be a considerable risk of misdiagnosis. Clinical parameters are still of importance in surgical decision making when orchitis is a possibility.

Suggested Reading

1. Berner R, Schumacher RF, Zimmerhackl LB, Frankenschmidt A, Brandis M. Salmonella enteritidis orchitis in a 10-week-old boy. Acta Paediatr 1994; 83:992–993
2. Ciftci AO, Senocak ME, Tanyel FC, Buyukpamukcu N. Clinical predictors for differential diagnosis of acute scrotum. Eur J Pediatr Surg 2004; 14:333–338
3. Foster R, Weber TR, Kleiman M, Grosfeld JL. Salmonella enteritidis: testicular abscess in a newborn. J Urol 1983; 130:790–791
4. Huang CB, Chuang JH. Acute scrotal inflammation caused by Salmonella in young infants. Pediatr Infect Dis J 1997; 16:1091–1092
5. Salmeron I, Ramirez-Escobar MA, Puertas F, Marcos R, Garcia-Marcos F, Sanchez R. Granulomatous epididymo-orchitis: sonographic features and clinical outcome in brucellosis, tuberculosis and idiopathic granulomatous epididymo-orchitis. J Urol 1998; 159:1954–1957

Q 214

Brice Antao and Azad Najmaldin

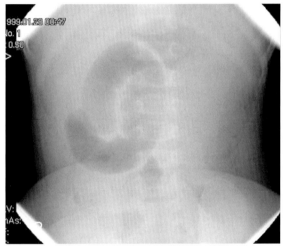

Fig. 1

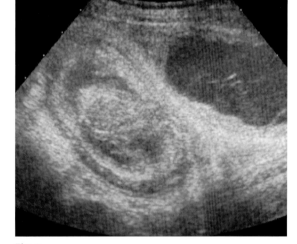

Fig. 2

A 6-month-old infant presented with severe abdominal pain, vomiting, and bleeding per rectum.
- What is the possible diagnosis?
- What signs might you find on clinical examination?
- What is the initial management of this condition?
- What features in Fig. 1 are suggestive of this condition?
- What do Figs. 2 and 3 show?
- What other investigations may be useful in this condition?
- What is the definitive management for this condition?
- What is the final outcome of this condition?

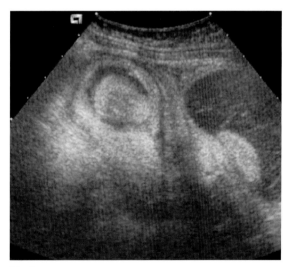

Fig. 3

A 214

The suspected diagnosis is intussusception. It is a full thickness invagination of one portion of intestine into another. The most common intussusception is ileocolic. It commonly presents between 3 months and 3 years of age with the peak being between 5 and 9 months. The classical triad (abdominal pain, vomiting, and bleeding per rectum) occurs in only one-third of cases. Profound lethargy, diarrhea, and abdominal distension are also present, not uncommonly. Bleeding per rectum is often described as red currant jelly stool.

In early stages, the child usually appears lethargic between attacks of abdominal pain. As the disease progresses, signs of dehydration, hypotension, or even septic shock may set in. The hallmark findings are a right hypochondrium sausage-shaped mass with emptiness in the right lower quadrant (Dance sign). In advanced cases, there may be abdominal distension and signs of peritonitis. In rare cases, the intussusception may prolapse through the rectum.

Initial management is appropriate intravenous fluid resuscitation, nasogastric decompression, and antibiotic cover.

Figure 1 is an abdominal radiograph which shows features of small-bowel obstruction (dilated small-bowel loops and air–fluid level). The other features suggestive of intussusception are an abdominal mass in the upper quadrant, abnormal distribution of bowel gas, and sparse or absent large-bowel gas.

Figures 2 and 3 demonstrate ultrasonographic features of intussusception. Ultrasonography is a useful noninvasive diagnostic investigation. The characteristic findings are of a target lesion as seen in transverse section (Fig, 2) and a pseudokidney sign on longitudinal section (Fig. 3). A target lesion consists of two rings of low echogenicity separated by a hyperechoic ring. Similarly, a pseudokidney sign appears as superimposed hypoechoic and hyperechoic layers.

A CT scan of the abdomen gives a high diagnostic yield. The classical ying-yang sign of an intussusceptum inside an intussuscipiens is not very consistent and when present is almost diagnostic of intussusception. Laparoscopy and capsule endoscopy are useful diagnostic tools and can provide information regarding the cause in cases of recurrent intussusception.

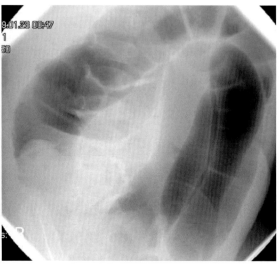

Fig. 4

Contrast or air enema (Fig. 4) is diagnostic and therapeutic. In the absence of hemodynamic instability and/or peritonitis, pneumatic or hydrostatic reduction is the first line of treatment. This is done through a catheter placed inside the rectum with the buttocks taped to prevent leak. The maximum pressure of air insufflation should not exceed 150 mmHg and the barium column should not be higher than 1 m. In cases of perforation and peritonitis and in critically ill patients, air and hydrostatic enema reduction are contraindicated. In these situations, and if pneumatic or hydrostatic reduction has failed, operative reduction is indicated. In cases of perforation, gangrene/necrosis of the bowel, and in the presence of a lead point, intestinal resection and anastomosis are necessary. The patient presented here underwent successful pneumatic reduction of the intussusception and was discharged home 24 h later.

Recurrences can occur in 2%–20% of cases and usually within 6 months of initial presentation. An underlying pathological condition (lead point) such as Meckel's diverticulum or polyps should be suspected in all recurrent cases.

Q 215

Brice Antao and Azad Najmaldin

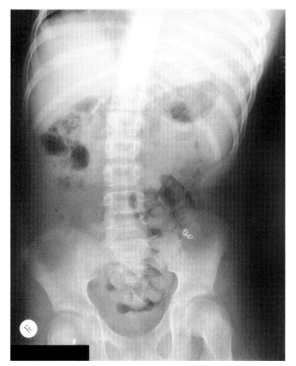

Fig. 1

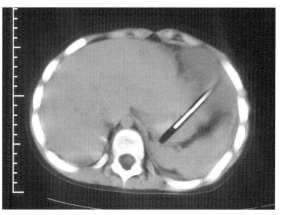

Fig. 2

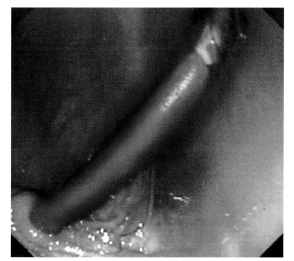

Fig. 3

A 12-year-old boy with learning difficulties presented with sudden-onset left-sided chest pain and respiratory distress. Four weeks prior to this, he had complained of vague abdominal pains.

- What features are seen in Fig. 1, suggestive of the diagnosis?
- What other investigation is useful in assessment of this child?

- Why did the surgeon perform the examination as shown in Fig. 3
- What is the underlying pathophysiological condition relating to the child's current symptoms?
- What is the best line of treatment of this child?
- What was the outcome of treatment?

A 215

On clinical examination, the child was very distressed and there was decreased air entry on the left side of chest. There was a past history of ingestion of various foreign bodies.

Figure 1 is a radiograph of the chest and abdomen. It shows a linear foreign body in the left side of the chest with pleural effusion and collapse of the lung around it.

A CT scan of the chest as outlined in Fig. 2 is a useful examination in order to assess the extent of damage to the underlying structures. It delineated the foreign body which looked like a pencil lodged within the left lung and a surrounding empyema, collapsed lung, and mediastinal shift.

From the CT scan, it was assumed that the pencil had perforated the esophagus and lodged in the left thoracic cavity. Prior to surgery, an upper gastrointestinal (GI) endoscopy was carried out to assess the status of the upper GI tract. At endoscopy (Fig. 3) the blunt end of the pencil was seen lodged in the lateral wall of the stomach.

The foreign body had perforated through the stomach and diaphragm into the chest, causing empyema and collapse of the lung. The child had probably ingested the foreign body at the time of the original complaints of abdominal pain 4 weeks prior to admission. The reason for there not being any evidence of pneumoperitoneum and/or generalized peritonitis is the close proximity of the stomach to the left hemidiaphragm aided by the child's scoliotic posture, gradual migration of the foreign body, and omental adhesions.

Most foreign bodies lodged in the upper GI tract can be removed endoscopically. It is generally recommended that foreign bodies greater than 3 cm in length are removed because they are likely to perforate the intestinal tract. The foreign body in this case was not removed endoscopically because it had already migrated into the chest, there was an advanced empyema, and the site of the perforation in both the stomach and diaphragm required formal repair. Thoracoscopy may be considered in similar circumstances. Through a left lateral thoracotomy, an eyeliner pencil, 4 cm long, was removed. The surrounding lung and chest wall was decorticated and the perforation in the stomach and diaphragm was repaired. An intercostal drain was left in situ.

The intercostal drain was removed on the second postoperative day and the child was allowed home 2 days later. At 1-year follow-up, the child remained well.

Suggested Reading

1. Antao B, Foxall G, Guzik I, Vaughan R, Roberts JP. Foreign body ingestion causing gastric and diaphragmatic perforation in a child. Pediatr Surg Int 2005; 21:326–328
2. Arana A, Hauser B, Hachimi-Idrissi S, et al. Management of ingested foreign bodies in childhood and review of the literature. Eur J Pediatr 2001; 160:468–472
3. Lam PY, Marks MK, Fink AM, et al. Delayed presentation of an ingested foreign body causing gastric perforation. J Paediatr Child Health 2001; 37:303–304

Q 216

Brice Antao and Azad Najmaldin

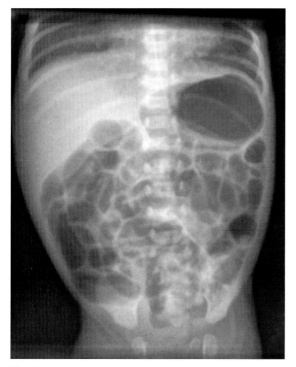

Fig. 1

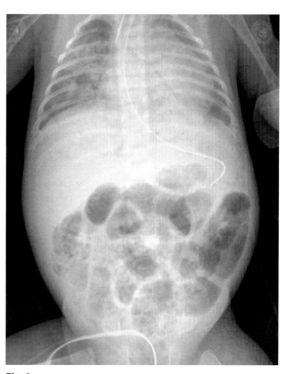

Fig. 2

A newborn baby who was delivered at 31 weeks' gestation and weighed 1.8 kg developed abdominal distension and bloody stools following introduction of enteral feeds at 3 days of age.

- What changes are seen in Fig. 1, suggestive of the diagnosis?
- What is the management of this condition?

Two days later, the patient's general condition deteriorated, and there was increased ventilatory requirement, gross abdominal distension, and bilious nasogastric aspirates. A repeat abdominal radiograph was acquired (Fig. 2).

- Why was additional imaging (Fig. 3) performed?

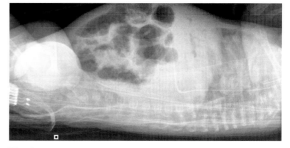

Fig. 3

This baby underwent laparotomy the following day.

- How else could this condition be managed?
- What are the most common long-term complications of this condition?

A 216

This is a case of necrotizing enterocolitis (NEC). It typically affects premature infants with a low birth weight following oral feeds. Neonates with NEC usually present with abdominal distension and/or signs of sepsis (apnea, bradycardia, unstable temperature, hypotension, or hypoglycemia). As the disease progresses the abdominal distension increases and the abdominal wall becomes edematous and erythematous. Other features include bilious vomiting, hematemesis, and rectal bleeding.

Figure 1 is an abdominal radiograph, which shows dilated loops of bowel. There is evidence of intramural gas (pneumatosis intestinalis), which is characteristic of NEC.

Uncomplicated cases are managed conservatively with broad-spectrum antibiotics, nasogastric decompression, and parenteral nutrition and the outcome is usually good.

Deterioration is likely to be due to progression of the disease. Progress can be monitored by daily measure of inflammatory markers (leukopenia and thrombocytopenia) and abdominal radiographs. A repeat abdominal radiograph (Fig. 2) shows increased bowel distension, extensive pneumatosis intestinalis, presence of portal venous gas, and possibly a pneumoperitoneum. A single loop or multiple loops of bowel that retain the same position and shape on serial abdominal films for 24–36 h (the so-called fixed loop sign) are usually suggestive of full-thickness bowel necrosis.

The presence of free intra-abdominal gas may be excluded by a lateral decubitus plain abdominal radiograph (Fig. 3).

The indications for surgical intervention are: deterioration of clinical condition and/or the presence of an abdominal mass, a fixed loop sign, or free intraperitoneal gas. This patient underwent laparotomy and a mass was identified in the right side of abdomen. A stoma was created proximal to the mass and the distal end of bowel was brought out as a mucous fistula. Extreme premature and low-birth-weight neonates and those that are critically ill may be managed with an intraperitoneal drain in the first instance and definitive surgery at a later date.

In this case, the neonate made a good recovery and the stoma was closed 8 weeks later. Full enteral feeds were commenced and he was thriving at the 3-month follow-up. Single or multiple strictures and short gut syndrome are not uncommon long-term complications of advanced NEC.

Suggested Reading

1. DeCurtis M, Paone C, Vetrano G, et al. A case control study of necrotizing enterocolitis occurring over 8 years in a neonatal intensive care unit. Eur J Pediatr 1987; 146:398–400
2. Fotter R, Sorantin E. Diagnostic imaging in necrotizing enterocolitis. Acta Pediatr Suppl 1994; 396:41–44
3. Horwitz JR, Lally KP, Cheu HW, et al. Complications after surgical intervention for necrotizing enterocolitis: A multicenter review. J Pediatr Surg 1995; 30:994–999
4. Morgan LJ, Shochat SJ, Hartman GE. Peritoneal drainage as primary management of perforated NEC in the very low birth weight infant. J Pediatr Surg 1994; 29:30–34

Q 217

Craig T. Albanese

A pregnant woman was noted to be large for her stage of pregnancy. An fetal abdominal ultrasound at 23 weeks' gestation was performed (Fig. 1).

- What are the findings?
- What are the differential diagnoses?
- Are there any other prenatal imaging studies or tests to be performed?

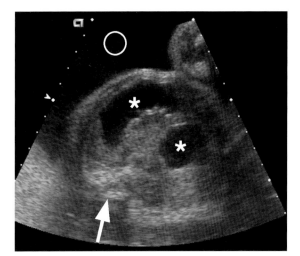

Fig. 1

A 217

The ultrasound (Fig. 1) reveals polyhydramnios (*circle*) and the double-bubble sign (*asterisks*) corresponding to the dilated stomach and duodenal bulb (spine, *arrow*). The double-bubble sign comes from fluid distention (prenatally) or gaseous distention (postnatally) of the stomach (one "bubble") and the proximal duodenum (the second "bubble"), with the pylorus separating the bubbles.

The differential diagnoses include all causes of complete duodenal obstruction such as duodenal atresia, duodenal stenosis, duodenal web, annular pancreas, preduodenal portal vein, and Ladd's bands associated with incomplete intestinal rotation.

A fetal echocardiogram should be obtained to assess for congenital heart disease. It should also be repeated postnatally. Fetal karyotyping should be offered to the family since this is associated with chromosomal abnormalities, most commonly trisomy 21 in 30% of cases.

Figure 2 is a postnatal plain abdominal radiograph demonstrating the double-bubble sign (*asterisks*).

This baby had an annular pancreas and trisomy 21. Figure 3 is showing an associated common atrioventricular canal (*arrowheads*) (common atria, *A*; fetal spine, *arrow*). He underwent an uneventful duodenoduodenostomy (*IVS*, interventricular septum).

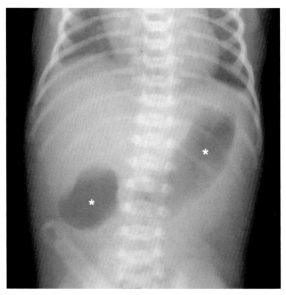

Fig. 2

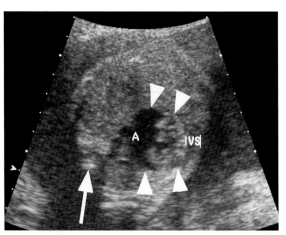

Fig. 3

Suggested Reading

1. Bailey PV, Tracy TF Jr, Connors RH, Mooney DP, Lewis JE, Weber TR. J Congenital duodenal obstruction: a 32-year review. Pediatr Surg 1993 Jan; 28(1):92–5
2. Bittencourt DG, Barini R, Marba S, Sbragia L. Congenital duodenal obstruction: does prenatal diagnosis improve the outcome? Pediatr Surg Int 2004 Aug; 20(8):582–5
3. Jimenez JC, Emil S, Podnos Y, Nguyen N. Annular pancreas in children: a recent decade's experience. J Pediatr Surg 2004 Nov; 39(11):1654–7

Q 218

Craig T. Albanese

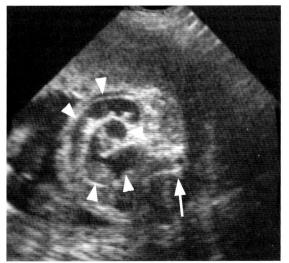

Fig. 1

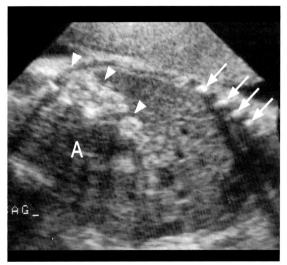

Fig. 2

A screening ultrasound at 18 weeks' gestation was normal. A follow-up examination of the fetal abdomen at 22 weeks (Fig. 1) revealed dilated loops of small bowel (*arrowheads*) with intraluminal meconium filling defects (spine, *arrow*). An ultrasound examination at 24 weeks (Fig. 2) demonstrated intra-abdominal calcifications (*arrowheads*) (fetal abdomen, *A*; fetal ribs, *arrows*). A subsequent examination at 26 weeks (Fig. 3) showed formation of a calcified meconium cyst (*arrowheads*).

- What anatomic/physiologic process led to these findings?
- What systemic disease is associated with these findings?

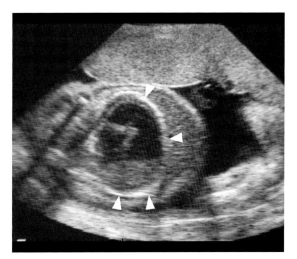

Fig. 3

A 218

A prenatal bowel perforation has occurred. Fatty acids in the meconium are saponified, resulting in calcifications. A pseudocyst can form and peritonitis may be evident at birth. This may be associated with cystic fibrosis.

At birth, the baby had a distended, erythematous abdomen with peritonitis. An abdominal radiograph (Fig. 4) at birth demonstrated a calcified meconium cyst (*arrowheads*). A subsequent water-soluble contrast enema (Fig. 5) demonstrated a microcolon (*arrowheads*) with filling defects in the distal ileum diagnostic for meconium ileus. At surgery, there was a meconium pseudocyst with a segmental volvulus and perforation of the terminal ileum. The pseudocyst was removed, the bowel irrigated free of meconium (using saline and *N*-acetyl-cysteine), and an ileostomy fashioned. The baby tested positive for cystic fibrosis.

Suggested Reading

1. Chan KL, Tang MH, Tse HY, Tang RY, Tam PK. Meconium peritonitis: prenatal diagnosis, postnatal management and outcome. Prenat Diagn 2005 Aug; 25(8):676–82
2. Dirkes K, Crombleholme TM, Craigo SD, Latchaw LA, Jacir NN, Harris BH, D'Alton ME. The natural history of meconium peritonitis diagnosed in utero. J Pediatr Surg 1995 Jul; 30(7):979–82
3. Eckoldt F, Heling KS, Woderich R, Kraft S, Bollmann R, Mau H. Meconium peritonitis and pseudo-cyst formation: prenatal diagnosis and post-natal course Prenat Diagn 2003 Nov; 23(11):904–8

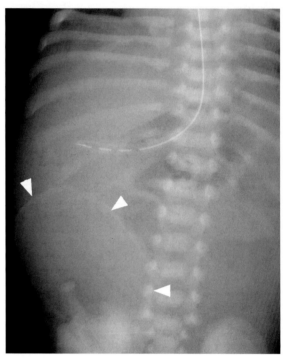

Fig. 4

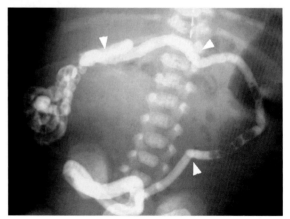

Fig. 5

Q 219

Craig T. Albanese

A routine prenatal ultrasound at 19 weeks' gestation revealed an abdominal wall defect.

- What are the findings on this ultrasound (Fig. 1)?
- What other prenatal tests should be done?
- What are some of the associated anomalies?
- What are the two main types of abdominal wall defects?

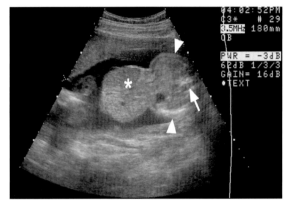

Fig. 1

A 219

There is a central abdominal wall defect (Fig. 1) in which the liver (*asterisk*) is outside the abdominal cavity (fetal abdomen, *arrowheads*; spine, *arrow*). Fetal MR imaging (Fig. 2) shows the herniated liver (*asterisk*) and small bowel (*arrowheads*) surrounded by the peritoneal membrane (*arrows*).

This lesion is associated with chromosomal abnormalities, cardiac defects, Beckwith–Wiedemann syndrome (macroglossia, hemihypertrophy, hyperinsulinism), cloacal exstrophy, and Pentalogy of Cantrell (epigastric omphalocele, sternal defect, pericardial defect, congenital heart disease, anterior diaphragmatic hernia). A fetal echocardiogram and karyotyping should be offered. An omphalocele should be distinguished from a gastroschisis. Gastroschisis is a smaller defect, located to the right of the umbilical cord, and has no investing membrane. Unlike an omphalocele, the liver is virtually never a part of the hernia, and the only associated anomaly is an approximately 7% incidence of intestinal atresia.

This child had a solitary omphalocele with no associated anomalies. It was closed primarily and she recovered uneventfully.

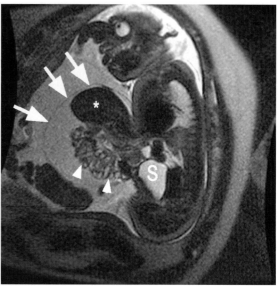

Fig. 2

Suggested Reading

1. Kitchanan S, Patole SK, Muller R, Whitehall JS. Neonatal outcome of gastroschisis and exomphalos: a 10-year review. J Paediatr Child Health 2000 Oct; 36(5):428–30

2. Ledbetter DJ. Gastroschisis and omphalocele. Surg Clin North Am 2006 Apr; 86(2):249–60

3. Maksoud-Filho JG, Tannuri U, da Silva MM, Maksoud JG. The outcome of newborns with abdominal wall defects according to the method of abdominal closure: the experience of a single center. Pediatr Surg Int 2006 Jun; 22(6):503–7

Q 220

François Becmeur

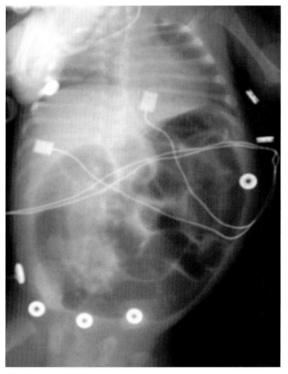

Fig. 1

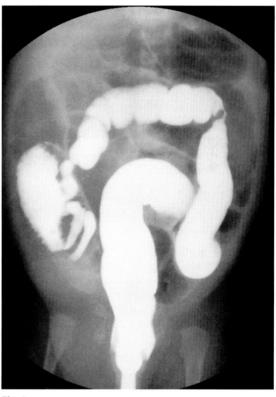

Fig. 2

A premature boy, born at 31 weeks of amenorrhea, presented with frankly bloody stools and abdominal distension at 8 days of life. An abdominal radiograph showed intestinal pneumatosis.

- Which diagnosis do you suspect?
- Which treatment do you choose?

The patient's evolution under treatment was favorable. One month later, the infant presented with severe abdominal distension associated with bile-stained vomiting and cessation of intestinal peristalsis. There were no clinical or biological infectious signs.

The doctors carried out a radiological study shown in Fig. 1.

- What is your assessment of this study?
- Which complementary examination would you require?
- How would you describe Fig. 2 and what do you deduce for the diagnosis and treatment?

A 220

Necrotizing enterocolitis is suspected. The treatment consists in placing the patient on bowel rest, parenteral nutrition is administered, and intravenous broad-spectrum antibiotics are given.

The premature infant presented with an intestinal occlusive syndrome.

Figure 1 is a radiograph of the abdomen without preparation. The radiograph shows a diffuse intestinal distension due to the occlusion.

To supplement the investigation, a rectal injection of water-soluble medium is made. On this radiograph (Fig. 2) we note the existence of a stenosis of the left colic angle, right colic narrowing, and dilation of the ileocecal loop.

The diagnosis of a postenterocolitis scar stenosis is suggested.

Surgical exploration is performed by laparotomy. A stenosis of the left colic angle and a bridle of the epiploon on the level of the ileocecal loop are found. A section of the adherence and a resection of the colic stenosis with end-to-end colic anastomosis are performed.

Suggested Reading

1. Chan KL, Ng SP, Chan KW, Wo YH, Tam PK. Pathogenesis of neonatal necrotizing enterocolitis: a study of the role of intraluminal pressure, age and bacterial concentration. Pediatr Surg Int 2003 Oct; 19(8):573–7
2. Chardot C, Rochet JS, Lezeau H, Sen N, Brouillard V, Caeymaex L, Verellen G, Otte JB, Gauthier F, Reding R. Surgical necrotizing enterocolitis: are intestinal lesions more severe in infants with low birth weight? J Pediatr Surg 2003 Feb; 38(2):167–72
3. Hallstrom M, Koivisto AM, Janas M, Tammela O. Laboratory parameters predictive of developing necrotizing enterocolitis in infants born before 33 weeks of gestation. J Pediatr Surg 2006 Apr; 41(4):792–8
4. Henry MC, Lawrence Moss R. Surgical therapy for necrotizing enterocolitis: bringing evidence to the bedside. Semin Pediatr Surg 2005 Aug; 14(3):181–9
5. Hofman FN, Bax NM, van der Zee DC, Kramer WL. Surgery for necrotising enterocolitis: primary anastomosis or enterostomy? Pediatr Surg Int 2004 Jul; 20(7):481–3

Q 221

Alessandro Settimi and Ciro Esposito

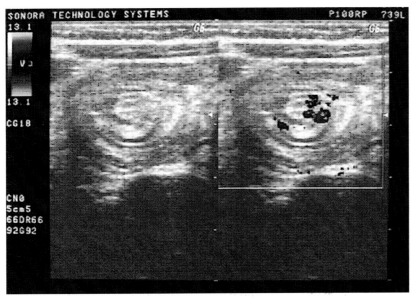

Fig. 1

A 7-month-old boy born after an uncomplicated pregnancy and delivery had normal growth without any pathological condition until a few hours before his hospitalization because of alimentary vomiting accompanied by mucous vomiting; the child was transferred to our institute.

On physical examination, an abdominal mass was found at the epigastric region. On rectal exploration, a small quantity of dark blood was found.

An abdominal color Doppler US (Fig. 1) was performed that indicated the need for other procedures to define the diagnosis and establish the treatment.

- What did the abdominal US show?
- Which other procedures were performed and what was their result?
- What was the diagnosis?
- What was the treatment?
- What was the follow-up?

A 221

The abdominal color Doppler US (Fig. 1) shows the typical feature of an intestinal intussusception with its characteristic aspects.

To define the site of the intestinal invaginated loops, a barium enema was performed, which also aimed to obtain bloodless reduction of the intussusception (Fig. 2).

The barium enema demonstrated the presence of an ileocecal invagination, with the minus sign corresponding to the colon.

During the procedure, reduction of the invagination was obtained and surgical disinvagination was therefore unnecessary.

Twenty-four hours after the disinvagination, the infant was doing well and was discharged.

In general, after a radiological resolution of the intussusception it is preferable to keep the patient hospitalized for about 24 h, and after two defecations of normal stools the patient can be discharged without any particular therapy.

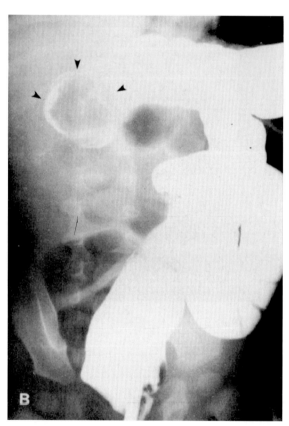

Fig. 2

Suggested Reading

1. Boehm R, Till H. Recurrent intussusceptions in an infant that were terminated by laparoscopic ileocolonic pexie. Surg Endosc 2003 May; 17(5):831–2

2. Crystal P, Barki Y. Using color Doppler sonography-guided reduction of intussusception to differentiate edematous ileocecal valve and residual intussusception. AJR Am J Roentgenol 2004 May; 182(5):1345

3. Poll LW, Lackmann GM, May P, Willnow U, Braunstein S, Engelbrecht V, Kemperdick H. Follicular lymphoid hyperplasia simulating intussusception in a 6-year-old boy: clinical, radiological and histopathological findings. Australas Radiol 2003 Dec; 47(4):453–6

4. Sonmez K, Turkyilmaz Z, Demirogullari B, Karabulut R, Aral YZ, Konus O, Basaklar AC, Kale N. Conservative treatment for small intestinal intussusception associated with Henoch-Schonlein's purpura. Surg Today 2002; 32(12):1031–4

5. van der Laan M, Bax NM, van der Zee DC, Ure BM. The role of laparoscopy in the management of childhood intussusception. Surg Endosc 2001 Apr; 15(4):373–6

8

Oncology

Introduction

Imaging studies are today the most important tool in the diagnosis, initial assessment of the extent, evaluation of the response to treatment, and follow-up of pediatric malignancies.

Modern advances in technology have allowed the development of sophisticated imaging modalities such as proton magnetic resonance spectroscopy (MRS) or positron emission tomography (PET). However, these new techniques entail a greater cost and increased difficulty in diagnostic procedures.

At the present time it can be accepted that conventional CT and MR imaging—for their sensitivity, anatomic delineation, and cost—are the best choice for the detection of central nervous system (CNS), abdominal, and pelvic lesions. Moreover, plain film radiographs must be considered of value as a first screening modality in patients with suspected thoracic or skeletal abnormalities.

However, it is to be noted that in the diagnosis of pediatric tumors, conventional CT and MR imaging should be performed with contiguous cuts of 10 mm or less in slice thickness in order to completely detect lesions of at least 20 mm in longest diameter. As a rule, we can correctly evaluate lesions no less than double the slice thickness applied.

Moreover, pulmonary lesions can be evaluated with chest radiography only when they are clearly defined and surrounded by aerated lung.

The above observations concern the baseline evaluation of a child with a suspected diagnosis of malignancy, but the evaluation of the extent of most solid tumors needs more accurate staging procedures. In the case of CNS location, MR imaging is considered to be more accurate and to offer better resolutions than CT. CT with and without contrast represents a far more valuable imaging modality than plain film radiographs for staging lesions in the lungs or mediastinum. In such cases, even more useful are spiral CT scan, also known as volumetric acquisition CT, and high-resolution CT; with both techniques there is little chance of missing small lesions falling between slices, as can happen with conventional CT. For bone lesions, radionuclide studies and MR imaging have proven to be more sensitive than plain films or CT in detecting early metastatic disease.

Assessment of tumor response to treatment, as a prospective end point in clinical trials or as a guide for the clinician in decisions regarding a single patient, is another important step in the management of pediatric solid tumors.

Criteria to measure tumor lesions were defined by the World Health Organisation in 1979. Recently, they have been revised by a large cooperative group in order to provide a simplified and reproducible response evaluation method based on the use of unidimensional measurements. This work has led to the publication of the Response Evaluation Criteria in Solid Tumors (RECIST) Guidelines, to which we refer.

At diagnosis, tumor lesions should be identified and defined as measurable if they can be accurately measured in at least one dimension, turning out equal to or greater than 20 mm with conventional techniques or to 10 mm with spiral CT scan. These lesions, up to a maximum of five per organ and ten in total, should be recorded at initial staging as "target lesions." Bone lesions, leptomeningeal disease, ascites, pleural and pericardial effusions, and cystic lesions are considered a priori nonmeasurable.

Correct evaluation of response requires that the same method of assessment and the same technique be used at baseline and during follow-up. It is particularly important, when using MR imaging, that lesions are measured by the same imaging sequences on subsequent examinations.

RECIST criteria of response are as follows: complete response is the disappearance of all target lesions; partial response is at least a 30% decrease in the sum of the longest diameter of target lesions, taking as reference the baseline sum longest diameter; progressive disease is at least a 20% increase in the sum of the longest diameter of target lesions, taking as reference the smallest sum longest diameter recorded since the treatment started or the appearance of one or more new lesions; stable disease is neither sufficient shrinkage to qualify for partial response nor sufficient increase to qualify for progressive disease, taking as reference the smallest sum longest diameter since the treatment started.

We now believe that we already have optimal tools in pediatric tumor imaging, provided that we use them correctly.

Q 222

Sabine Sarnacki

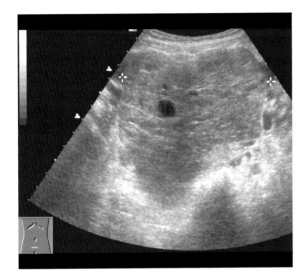
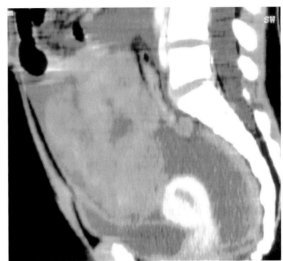

Fig. 1   **Fig. 2**

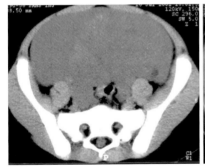
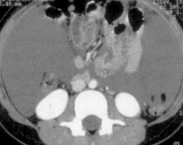
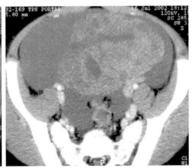

Fig. 3

A 4-year-old girl presented with vaginal bleeding. Clinical examination revealed a solid pelvic abdominal mass. The mother noticed the appearance of pubic hair and breast enlargement 2 months earlier.

A US examination was performed (Fig. 1).

- What complementary radiological examinations should be performed?

The abdominal CT scan (Figs. 2, 3) shows a heterogeneous ovoid lesion with ascites.

- What is the important sign to observe on Fig. 2?
- How do you interpret the ascites?

Measurements of alpha-fetoprotein and human chorionic gonadotropin (HCG) levels were performed, which were within normal ranges.

- Which additional biological examinations should be done?
- What treatment should be proposed?
- What is the follow-up?

A 222

This 4-year-old girl presented with an abdominal mass and signs of precocious pseudopuberty: vaginal bleeding, abnormal pubic hair development, and breast enlargement. This presentation suggests the presence of a secreting ovarian tumor. Juvenile ovarian granulosa cell tumor (JGCT) and malignant germinal tumor with a choriocarcinoma component are the most frequently encountered lesions, but embryonal carcinoma and Sertoli–Leydig cell tumors may also be revealed by precocious pseudopuberty signs.

The US exam shows a heterogeneous mass with solid and cystic components. The ovarian origin of the lesion may be difficult to confirm on this examination, but is suggested by the clinical presentation. An abdominal and thoracic CT scan should be performed to evaluate the local extension of the lesion and eliminate the presence of distant metastasis. JGCT almost always presents as stage-I disease; 3% of these tumors are bilateral and only 2% have extraovarian spread (peritoneum, lymph nodes, liver, and more rarely bone, lungs, CNS).

Figure 2 shows an enlargement of the uterus with endometrial hyperplasia linked to the estrogen secretion.

Because of high estrogen secretion, these tumors are rather vascular and bloody ascites and peritonitis may occur in ruptured forms. Ascites without any rupture, which is ascribed to pseudo-Meigs' syndrome, is present in 10% of cases. There is no prognostic value attached to the ascites.

The normal HCG level rules out the diagnosis of a malignant germ cell tumor comprising choriocarcinoma or embryonal carcinoma components. Thus, the diagnosis to retain is JGCT. This tumor usually synthesizes estrogen, but an elevation of testosterone and/or dehydroepiandrosterone (DHEA) may be observed, probably linked to a thecal testosterone-secreting area. These hormonal levels should be measured and be used as tumor markers for the follow-up. Inhibin B and antimüllerian hormone levels are elevated in about 100% of cases and return to normal after removal of the tumor. They are good markers for follow-up, as they seem to increase several months before recurrence.

If the tumor is localized, as in the present case and in the majority of JGCT observed during childhood and infancy (FIGO stage Ia), treatment consists of an ovariectomy with ascites analysis. Omentectomy is not indicated in localized lesions. Laparoscopy is not recommended because of the risk of tumoral spillage during extraction and thus of relapse.

Suggested Reading

1. Kalfa N, Patte C, Orbach D, Lecointre C, Pienkowski C, Philippe F, Thibault E, Plantaz D, Brauner R, Rubie H, Guedj AM, Ecochard A, Paris F, Jeandel C, Baldet P, Sultan C. A nationwide study of granulosa cell tumors in pre- and postpubertal girls: missed diagnosis of endocrine manifestations worsens prognosis. J Pediatr Endocrinol Metab 2005; 18:25–31

2. Lane AH, Lee MM, Fuller AF Jr, Kehas DJ, Donahoe PK, MacLaughlin DT. Diagnostic utility of Mullerian inhibiting substance determination in patients with primary and recurrent granulosa cell tumors. Gynecol Oncol 1999; 73:51–55

3. Schmitt R, Weichert W, Schneider W, Luft FC, Kettritz R. Pseudo-pseudo Meigs' syndrome. Lancet 2005; 366:1672

4. Schneider DT, Calaminus G, Harms D, Gobel U; German Maligne Keimzelltumoren Study Group. Ovarian sex cord-stromal tumors in children and adolescents. J Reprod Med 2005; 50:439–446

Q 223

Sabine Sarnacki

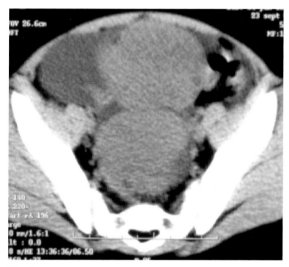

Fig. 1

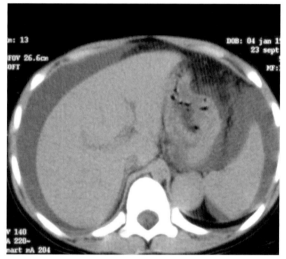

Fig. 2

A 7-year-old girl presented with abdominal distension. Clinical examination revealed a solid abdominal mass, and a pelvic CT scan showed bilateral ovarian masses (Figs. 1, 2) with ascites.

• How would you proceed to make a diagnosis?
• What do you see on the abdominal CT scan that directs the diagnosis?
• As a surgeon, how would you manage this situation?

A 223

All pediatric ovarian tumors may potentially be bilateral, but this is very rare except in pure mature teratoma where the bilaterality is about 8%–15% depending on the series. In contrast, the ovaries may be the secondary site of a primary neoplasm such as leukemia, non-Hodgkin's lymphoma (mainly Burkitt's lymphoma), neuroblastoma, alveolar rhabdomyosarcoma, Wilms' tumor, mucinous colon adenocarcinoma, and rhabdoid tumors. This hypothesis should be raised in the present case. The best way to make the diagnosis is to perform ultrasonography-guided percutaneous fine-needle aspiration of the ascites and, if negative, ultrasonography-guided percutaneous fine-needle aspiration or biopsy of the ovarian masses.

The CT scan shows abundant ascites and a tumoral syndrome of the left adrenal gland. Because of the presence of ascites, the diagnosis of lymphoma is more likely than the diagnosis of metastatic neuroblastoma. Other locations such as peripheral, abdominal, or mediastinal lymph nodes have to be searched for.

The treatment of a lymphoma is an emergency. The suspicion of this diagnosis in a department of surgery should lead to contact being made with a team of pediatric oncologists to find out how to proceed. If the patient has to be anesthetized for the fine-needle aspiration and/or needle biopsy of the masses, it is better to take advantage of the anesthesia to complete the evaluation of the disease (medullar biopsies, myelogram, lumbar puncture). The question of a central catheter or of a port-a-catheter should be raised because the treatment will begin as soon as possible.

Suggested Reading

1. McCarville MB, Hill DA, Miller BE, Pratt CB. Secondary ovarian neoplasms in children: imaging features with histopathologic correlation. Pediatr Radiol 2001; 31:358–364

2. Somjee S, Kurkure PA, Chinoy RF, Deshpande RK, Advani SH. Metastatic ovarian neuroblastoma: a case report. Pediatr Hematol Oncol 1999; 16:459–462

3. Young RH, Kozakewich HP, Scully RE. Metastatic ovarian tumors in children: a report of 14 cases and review of the literature. Int J Gynecol Pathol 1993; 12:8–19

Q 224

Sabine Sarnacki

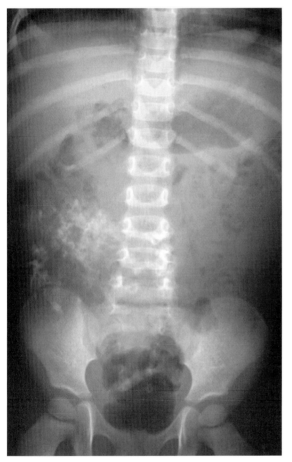

Fig. 1

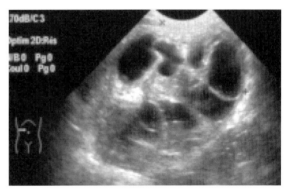

Fig. 2

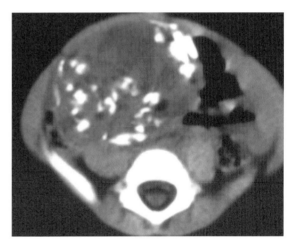

Fig. 3

A 26-month-old girl presented with a fever (38.5°C) without abdominal pain. Clinical examination revealed a solid abdominal mass.

- What is the key sign of the clinical examination that could be helpful in delineating the origin of the mass?

A standard abdominal radiograph was acquired (Fig. 1).
- How do you interpret this examination?
- At this stage of the observation, what should you do?

Abdominal and pelvic US examinations and a CT scan were performed (Figs. 2, 3).
- What information is provided by these examinations?
- What biological examinations should be performed before surgery? Why?
- What type of surgery would you propose for this patient?

A 224

The mobility of the mass must be checked, as it clearly indicates its mesenteric or ovarian origin. Because of the higher frequency of ovarian masses in girls, the mobility of the mass in this case suggests an ovarian origin. Fever in this situation is confusing but can be ascribed to an ordinary infection, and the discovery of the mass is incidental.

The abdominal radiograph shows multiple calcifications in the right part of the abdomen. Although calcifications are classically found in neuroblastoma and some Wilms' tumors, the presence of calcifications in a mobile mass leads to the diagnosis of ovarian tumor.

Considering the aspect of the calcifications, the first diagnosis to propose is a mature teratoma of the ovary. Clinical examination does not show any sign of precocious pseudopuberty and thus eliminates the diagnosis of ovarian granulosa cell tumor. Surgery may be proposed without any further investigation except for the measurement of alpha-fetoprotein and human chorionic gonadotropin (HCG) levels in order to eliminate the possibility of a malignant germinal tumor component.

The imaging pattern of ovarian teratomas is a complex mass in two-thirds of cases. Typical tooth-like or rim calcifications or ossifications are seen in 56% of cases. The characteristic sonographic appearance is that of a hypoechoic mass with an echogenic mural nodule frequently associated with acoustic shadowing linked to either calcification or a matted mixture of sebum and hair. In all, 10%–15% of benign teratomas appear as purely anechoic masses. Another 10%–15% contain primarily hair and fat and a sparse amount of fluid or sebaceous material, and they are predominantly echogenic. Figures 2 and 3 show a very heterogeneous lesion with solid and cystic components as well as the calcifications previously found on the standard abdominal radiograph. These images do not provide any additional information in the present case because: the mobility of the mass attests the ovarian origin, the presence of calcifications suggests a diagnosis of mature teratoma, and the negativity of the markers eliminates a malignant germ cell tumor. This will lead to primary surgery. The side of the lesion could not be identified on these examinations (in this case it was a left ovarian teratoma). US and CT scan may be helpful to ensure the normality of the opposite ovary and to evaluate the importance of the remaining ovarian parenchyma when conservative surgery can be attempted.

Beside the usual examinations required for any operation, it is preferable to obtain a blood sample for measurement of alpha-fetoprotein and HCG markers. The elevation of one of these markers shows a malignant component of the lesion and additional chemotherapy may be required. This information is also crucial for the follow-up, which includes measurement of the initially elevated marker.

If the markers are negative, conservative surgery (tumorectomy sparing the normal ovarian tissue) should be attempted, because the risk of onset of a contralateral tumor is about 10% in cases of teratoma. In the present case, the volume of the tumor probably precludes the feasibility of a tumorectomy. Although this tumor is certainly a mature benign teratoma (markers negative, numerous calcifications), laparoscopy is not recommended because a malignant nonsecreting component could not be formally eliminated as well as the risk of tumoral spillage during extraction.

Suggested Reading

1. Baranzelli MC, Bouffet E, Quintana E, Portas M, Thyss A, Patte C. Non-seminomatous ovarian germ cell tumours in children. Eur J Cancer 2000; 36:376–383
2. de Silva KS, Kanumakala S, Grover SR, Chow CW, Warne GL. Ovarian lesions in children and adolescents—an 11-year review. J Pediatr Endocrinol Metab 2004; 17:951–957
3. Garel L, Dubois J, Grignon A, Filiatrault D, Van Vliet G. US of the pediatric female pelvis: a clinical perspective. Radiographics 2001; 21:1393–1407
4. Templeman CL, Fallat ME, Lam AM, Perlman SE, Hertweck SP, O'Connor DM. Managing mature cystic teratomas of the ovary. Obstet Gynecol Surv 2000; 55:738–745

Q 225

Nancy Rollins and Korgun Koral

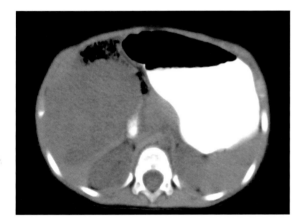

Fig. 1

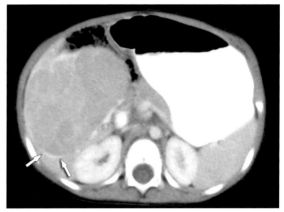

Fig. 2

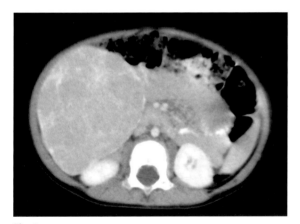

Fig. 3

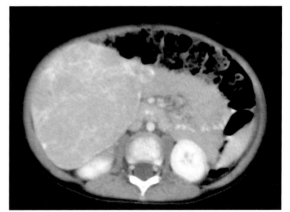

Fig. 4

A 5-month-old boy presented with an abdominal mass that was detected by his parents. Abdominal ultrasound showed a large mass in the liver. Abdominal CT without and with intravenous contrast material was performed (Figs. 1–4). The alpha-fetoprotein level was elevated.

- What are the findings?
- What is the differential diagnosis?
- What is the most likely diagnosis?

A 225

Noncontrast CT of the abdomen shows a large, round, hypodense mass occupying much of the liver. No calcifications are present. Contrast-enhanced images show the solid nature of the mass, which demonstrates heterogenous enhancement. The interface with the normal liver parenchyma is well delineated (Fig. 2, *arrows*). The right kidney is displaced by the mass.

The differential diagnosis includes hepatoblastoma, hemangioendothelioma, neuroblastoma metastasis, mesenchymal hamartoma, and hepatocellular carcinoma.

Hepatoblastoma is the most likely diagnosis given the patient's age and the elevated alpha-fetoprotein level. Hepatoblastoma is the most common hepatic malignancy in children. The role of imaging is to define the anatomy for preoperative planning and to monitor response to chemotherapy.

Suggested Reading

1.   Donnelly LF. Pocket Radiologist: Pediatrics. Amirsys Ed. 2002

Q 226

Nancy Rollins and Korgun Koral

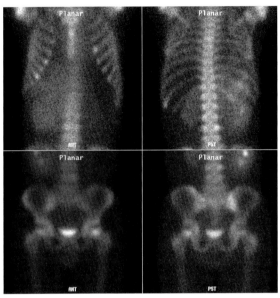

Fig. 1

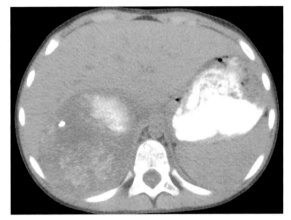

Fig. 2

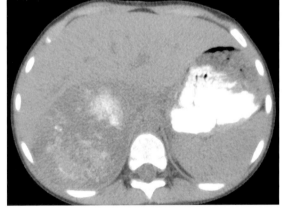

Fig. 3

A 5-year-old boy with bone pain underwent a whole-body bone scan following administration of 5 mCi of technetium 99m.

- What does the bone scan show (Fig. 1)?
- What are the findings on the CT scan (Figs. 2–4)?
- What is the differential diagnosis?
- What is the most likely diagnosis?
- What is the role of imaging in the staging of the disease?

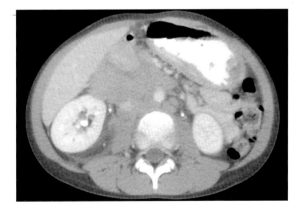

Fig. 4

A 226

A large area of abnormal uptake is seen in the right side of the abdomen.

There is a large, round, solid lesion with multiple foci of calcifications. The lesion is primarily retroperitoneal with encasement of the retroperitoneal vessels. The right kidney is displaced, but not infiltrated.

Wilms' tumor is the main differential diagnosis, but the extrarenal location of the lesion is helpful in excluding this possibility. In newborns, adrenal hemorrhage is a consideration. Other rare tumors of the adrenal glands, such as paraganglioma and adrenal carcinoma, are also in the differential diagnosis.

The most likely diagnosis is neuroblastoma.

Imaging is helpful in distinguishing stage-1 disease (confined to organ of origin) from stage 2 (outside the confines of organ of origin). Stage 3 (tumor crossing midline) and stage 4 (distant metastasis) can also be distinguished with imaging. For a particular subset of patients (stage 4S, age <1 year, metastatic disease confined to skin, liver, and bone marrow) there is an excellent prognosis.

Suggested Reading

1. Donnelly LF. Pocket Radiologist: Pediatrics. Amirsys Ed. 2002.
2. Kuhn JP, Slovis TL, Haller JO. Caffey's Pediatric Diagnostic Imaging. Kuhn JP, Slovis TL, Haller JO. Elsevier Ed. 2004
3. Siegel MJ, Coley BD. Pediatric Imaging. Lippincott Williams & Wilkins Ed. 2006

Q 227

Nancy Rollins and Korgun Koral

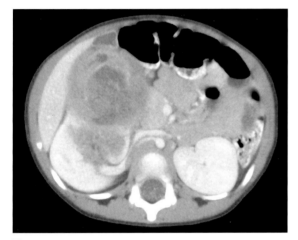

Fig. 1

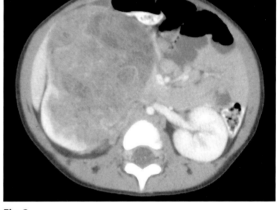

Fig. 2

A 3-year-old girl was found to have an abdominal mass during routine physical examination at her pediatrician. CT of the abdomen was performed (Figs. 1–3).

- What is the differential diagnosis prior to the CT examination?
- What does the scan show?
- What is the most likely diagnosis?
- What is the differential diagnosis?
- Why was a CT scan of the chest performed?
- What is the role of imaging in staging this disease?

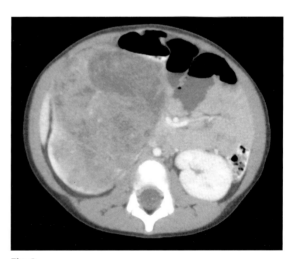

Fig. 3

A 227

In a child, the most common abdominal mass is hydronephrosis. Neoplasms such as neuroblastoma, Wilms' tumor, and lymphoma are in the differential diagnosis. An ultrasound examination of the abdomen should be the first step to distinguish between hydronephrosis and solid abdominal masses.

The CT scan (Figs. 1–3) shows a large mass arising from the right kidney. Unlike extrarenal masses, the kidney is not only displaced but is also infiltrated. In Fig. 2, the right renal vein does not opacify normally and tumor thrombus is visible in the displaced inferior vena cava. There is normal opacification of the left renal vein.

The differential diagnosis includes neuroblastoma, multilocular cystic nephroma, clear cell sarcoma, and rhabdoid tumor of the kidney.

The CT of the chest was performed to exclude lung metastasis. Several nodules were identified, the largest of which is in the superior segment of the right lower lobe (Fig. 4).

Staging of Wilms' tumor is surgical. Imaging is helpful in surgical planning and identifying distant metastasis (stage IV). Bilateral disease (stage V) can also be diagnosed with imaging. An abdominal ultrasound examination (Fig. 5) of another child shows bilateral large, solid masses in the lumbar regions. CT of the abdomen (Fig. 6) shows the solid, heterogenous masses arising from the kidneys. In the left-sided mass, foci of fat are present (*arrow*) representing entrapment of perirenal fat in the tumor.

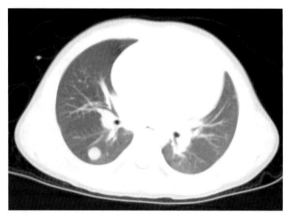

Fig. 4

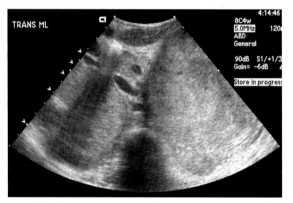

Fig. 5

Suggested Reading

1. Beckwith JB. National Wilms' Tumor Study: an update for pathologists. Pediatr Dev Pathol 1998; 1:79
2. Breslow NE et al. Clinicopathologic features and prognosis for Wilms' tumor patients with metastases at diagnosis. Cancer 1986; 58: 2501
3. Ritchey ML et al. Management and outcome of inoperable Wilms' tumor. A report of National Wilms' Tumor Study-3. Ann Surg 1994; 220:683

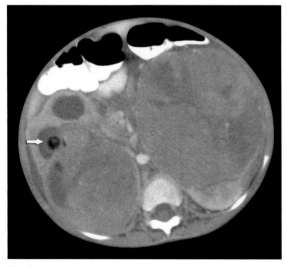

Fig. 6

Q 228

Alfonso Papparella, Mercedes Romano, and Pio Parmeggiani

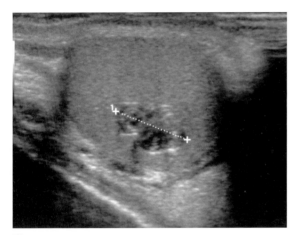

Fig. 1

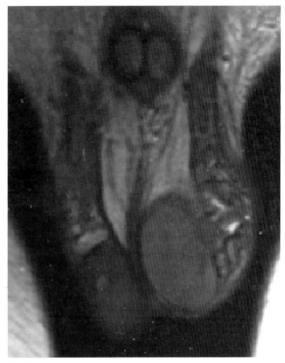

Fig. 2

A 10-year-old patient was affected by bilateral gynecomastia: Tanner stage P2, with sparse pubic hair and normal penis size for his age. No symptoms were reported.

The mother consulted an endocrinologist, who performed standard hormone screening, as well as mammary and testicular ultrasound tests.

- What are the (expected) results of the standard hormone screening?
- What does Fig. 1 (ultrasound) show?
- What is the most likely diagnosis?
- What is the differential diagnosis?

An NMR scan was requested.
- What does Fig. 2 show?
- What additional diagnostic tests would you suggest to reach a diagnosis?
- What is the most appropriate surgical treatment?

A 228

The diagnostic suspicion is that of testicular Leydigioma. Gynecomastia is detected in 20%–30% of these patients. In most cases, this benign tumor is sometimes diagnosed by chance, given its small size, and often in pediatric age (the peak incidence is in 4–5-year-old children).

In this case, on palpation of the right testis, there was a small intraparenchymal mass with a hard consistency, closely connected to the surrounding parenchyma, with no alterations of the epididymis and hydrocele.

Routine hormonal screening showed an increase in serum testosterone levels (2.0 ng/ml), whereas the levels of serum alpha-fetoprotein (1.3 ng/ml), carcinoembryonic antigen (CEA; 5.2 ng/ml), and beta-human chorionic gonadotropin (HCG; 0.1 mIU/ml) were within normal ranges.

The ultrasound image of the right side shows a small hypoechoic polylobular lesion with a small area of colliquation and calcifications (1 cm×1 cm; Fig. 1). The color Doppler showed a richly vascularized didymus, although the mass was poorly vascularized; no abnormalities involving the left didymus were detected.

The differential diagnosis includes early puberty due to a pituitary lesion, Leydig's cell hyperplasia, and nodular testicular hyperplasia associated with pediatric untreated congenital adrenal hyperplasia.

When dealing with a patient affected by testicular Leydigioma, a full hormonal screening is warranted, including urinary 17-ketosteroids, abdominal ultrasound, and MR imaging (Fig. 2). In this case, the NMR scan confirmed the presence of the small area in the right testis and no involvement of the satellite lymph node stations and of other abdominal organs such as the adrenal glands.

The surgical treatment of choice is orchifunicolectomy (Fig. 3), even though tumor enucleation has been reported. From the histopathological perspective, the macroscopic appearance of the testicular tissue is yellowish-brown in color (Fig. 4), given its role in the production of hormones.

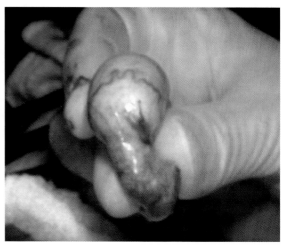

Fig. 3

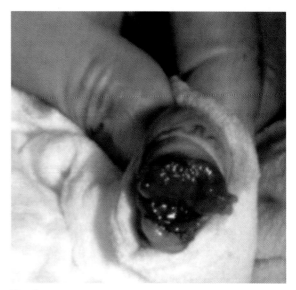

Fig. 4

Suggested Reading

1. Ciftci AO et al. Testicular tumors in children. J Pediatr Surg 2001; 36(12):1796–801
2. Carmignani L et al. High incidence of benign testicular neoplasms diagnosed by ultrasound. J Urol 2003; 170(5):1783–6
3. Henderson CG et al. Enucleation for prepubertal Leydig cell tumor. J Urol 2006; 176(2):703–5

Q 229

Masayuki Fujioka, Carl Muroi, Nadia Khan, and Yasuhiro Yonekawa

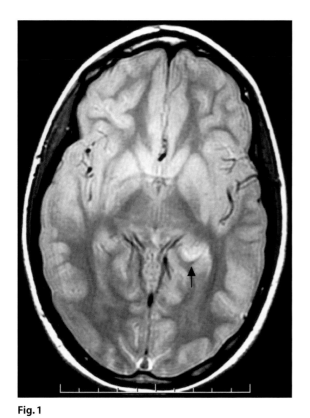

Fig. 1

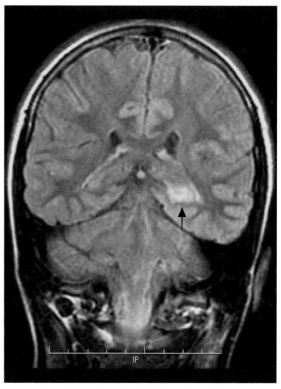

Fig. 2

A 14-year-old girl presented with seizures accompanied by loss of consciousness that had started 1 year earlier.

A head CT scan revealed no marked findings at that time and she was diagnosed as having juvenile myoclonic epilepsy (Janz syndrome).

The girl visited our hospital for further investigations because the epilepsy became intractable.

MR imaging was performed.

● What do Figs. 1 (T2-weighted image) and 2 (FLAIR) show?

The brain lesion did not appear on T1-weighted MR imaging.

● What kind of MR imaging examination should be considered next?

Electroencephalography showed epileptiform activity in the bilateral frontal cerebral regions (more active in the left). [(18)F]-fluorodeoxyglucose positron emission tomography (FDG-PET) showed the mild uptake of [(18)F]-FDG in the hippocampal lesion observed on MR imaging.

● What is the possible diagnosis of the lesion?
● How should the lesion be treated?

A 229

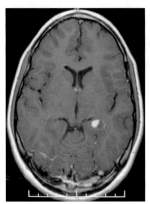

Fig. 3

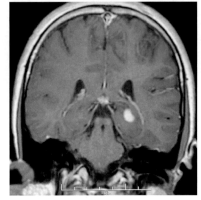

Fig. 4

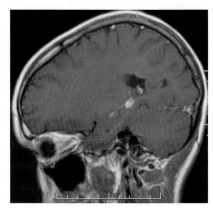

Fig. 5

The MR imaging study reveals a lesion of hyperintensity in the posterior portion of the left hippocampus on both T2-weighted and FLAIR images (Figs. 1, 2). The tumoral lesion appears to be located mainly in the cerebral cortex. A tumor derived from neuronal cells, therefore, should be considered as a possible etiology.

A gadolinium-diethylenetriamine pentaacetic acid (Gd-DTPA)-enhanced T1-weighted MR imaging study was performed (Figs. 3–5). These images show homogeneous enhancement of the tumor.

The MR imaging demonstrated no marked mass effect and no surrounding edema of the tumor. The homogeneous enhancement with Gd-DTPA on T1-weighted MR imaging and the slight uptake of 18F-FDG on the PET study suggest the tumor is relatively benign.

The tumor that led to the intractable epilepsy was surgically removed without any perioperative complications (in the sitting position, left paramedian suboccipital skin

incision, supracerebellar transtentorial approach). The tumor was removed completely. The histological study showed that the tumor was a ganglioglioma.

Gangliogliomas are glioneuronal tumors of children and young adults, and occur more frequently in the supratentorial region, especially the temporal lobe. Ganglioglioma is a basically benign tumor composed of neoplastic astrocytes (rarely oligodendrocytes) and ganglion cells. Solid gangliogliomas may be missed on CT scanning but revealed on MR images. Gangliogliomas tend to exhibit increased signal intensity on T2-weighted images, whereas they may be difficult to recognize on T1-weighted images. The solid portion is usually enhanced on Gd-DTPA T1-weighted MR images.

After 6 months, the epilepsy was well controlled with an anti-epilepsy drug and the follow-up MR imaging showed no recurrence of the tumor. At the time of writing, the girl was going to school without any sequelae.

Suggested Reading

1. Castillo M, Davis PC, Takei Y, Hoffman JC Jr. Intracranial ganglioglioma: MR, CT, and clinical findings in 18 patients. AJR Am J Roentgenol 1990; 155: 899–900.

2. Haddad SF, Moore SA, Menezes AH, VanGilder JC. Ganglioglioma: 13 years of experience. Neurosurgery. 1992; 31:171–178

Q 230

Masayuki Fujioka, Carl Muroi, Nadia Khan, and Yasuhiro Yonekawa

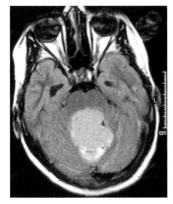
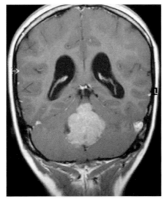
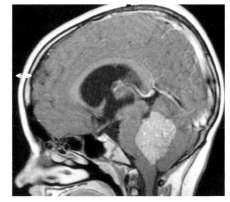

Fig. 1   **Fig. 2**   **Fig. 3**

A 12-year-old girl had difficulty in walking (unstable gait) for 2 weeks and had been complaining of a headache, vomiting, and visual disturbance (weak eyesight) for 1 week.

On admission to hospital, she had truncal ataxia, staggering gait, bilateral abducens nerve palsy, intermittent vertical and horizontal nystagmus, oral dyskinesia, incomplete palsy of the bilateral oculomotor nerves and of the bilateral facial nerves, and weak response of the right pharyngeal reflex.

CT scans showed a space-occupying lesion of isodensity in the intracranial posterior fossa.

The tumoral lesion appeared hypointense on T1-weighted MR images and hyperintense on T2-weighted imaging. Gd-DTPA T1-weighted MR imaging was performed.

- What do Figs. 1–3 (axial, coronal, and sagittal views) show?
- What is a possible diagnosis based on the clinical and radiological data?
- Which treatment should be considered?

A 230

The tumor occupies the fourth ventricle entirely and has Gd enhancement effects on T1-weighted MR images. The MR imaging study shows dilatation of the lateral ventricle, which suggests obstructive hydrocephalus.

The differential diagnosis for pediatric brain tumors in the posterior fossa includes medulloblastoma, ependymoma, and astrocytoma.

The tumor was totally removed surgically without any complication (sitting position, occipital midline skin incision, suboccipital approach). The pathological study revealed medulloblastoma. Medulloblastoma is the most common malignant pediatric brain tumor and usually arises within the cerebellar vermis, in the apex of the roof of the fourth ventricle (fastigium). It is composed of densely packed cells with round to oval or carrot-shaped nuclei and scanty cytoplasm. The neuroblastic Homer Wright rosette is one of the characteristic histological features.

The patient underwent postoperative chemotherapy and radiation therapy.

At the time of writing, the girl was doing very well and studying at school 1 year after the operation. Gd-DTPA T1-weighted MR imaging (Figs. 4, 5) shows no evidence of recurrence of the tumor.

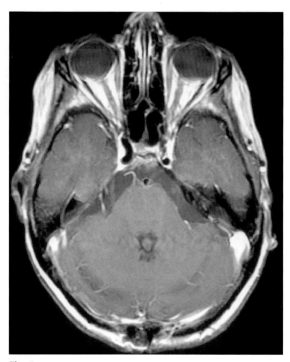

Fig. 4

Suggested Reading

1. Chawla A, Emmanuel JV, Seow WT, Lou J, Teo HE, Lim CC. Paediatric PNET: pre-surgical MRI features. Clin Radiol 2007; 62:43–52

2. Han JS, Benson JE, Kaufman B, Rekate HL, Alfidi RJ, Huss RG, Sacco D, Yoon YS, Morrison SC. MR imaging of pediatric cerebral abnormalities. J Comput Assist Tomogr 1985; 9:103–114

3. Packer RJ, Batnitzky S, Cohen ME. Magnetic resonance imaging in the evaluation of intracranial tumors of childhood. Cancer 1985; 56:1767–1772

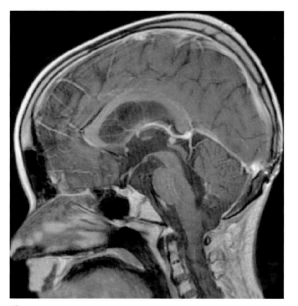

Fig. 5

Q 231

Masayuki Fujioka, Carl Muroi, Nadia Khan, and Yasuhiro Yonekawa

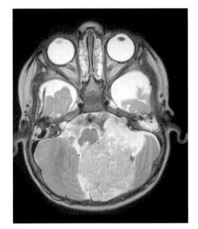
Fig. 1

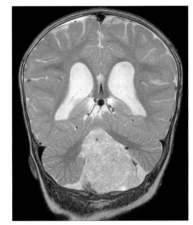
Fig. 2

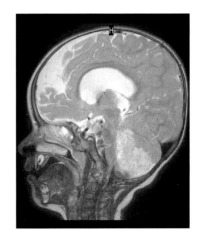
Fig. 3

A 6-month old boy was found to be hypoactive for his age. He was not able to sit by himself at 11 months.

The family doctor diagnosed the child with truncal ataxia and muscle hypotonia.

A CT study revealed a brain tumor in the posterior cranial fossa as an isodense space-occupying lesion, and the boy was referred to a neurosurgical unit.

- What do Figs. 1–3 (T2-weighted MR imaging) show?

This tumor appeared isointense on T1-weighted imaging and was homogeneously enhanced with Gd-DTPA on T1-weighted images.

- What pathological condition is affecting this child?
- What is the best way to manage this condition?

A 231

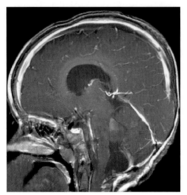

Fig. 4

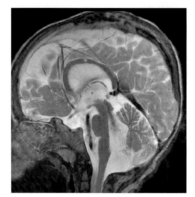

Fig. 5

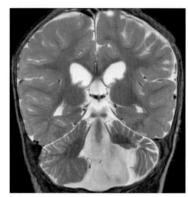

Fig. 6

The T2-weighted MR imaging demonstrates that the large hyperintense tumor occupies the space from the left lateral recess of the fourth ventricle through to the fourth ventricle, resulting in obstructive hydrocephalus.

This 1-year-old boy has a posterior fossa tumor in the fourth ventricle. The possible diagnosis of the tumor includes choroid plexus papilloma, medulloblastoma, and ependymoma.

The tumor compresses the brainstem from the left posterior side. Emergent removal of the tumor is considered necessary.

Total removal of the tumor was performed on the day after admission (sitting position, occipital midline skin incision, suboccipital craniotomy) without any surgical complication.

The histological study revealed a choroid plexus papilloma.

The tumor-removal operation resulted in no additional neurological deficits. An MR imaging study showed no apparent residual tumor 3 months after the operation (Figs. 4–6). At the time of writing, the boy's motor activity was improving and he was able to sit by himself.

Suggested Reading

1. Aksoy FG, Gomori JM. Choroid plexus papilloma of foramen of Luschka with multiple recurrences and cystic features. Neuroradiology 1999; 41:654–656
2. Martin N, Pierot L, Sterkers O, Mompoint D, Nahum H. Primary choroid plexus papilloma of the cerebellopontine angle: MR imaging. Neuroradiology 1990; 31:541–543
3. Sarkar C, Sharma MC, Gaikwad S, Sharma C, Singh VP. Choroid plexus papilloma: a clinicopathological study of 23 cases. Surg Neurol 1999; 52:37–39
4. Shin JH, Lee HK, Jeong AK, Park SH, Choi CG, Suh DC. Choroid plexus papilloma in the posterior cranial fossa: MR, CT, and angiographic findings. Clin Imaging 2001; 25:154–162
5. Tasdemiroglu E, Awh MH, Walsh JW. MRI of cerebellopontine angle choroid plexus papilloma. Neuroradiology 1996; 38:38–40

Q 232

Masayuki Fujioka, Carl Muroi, Nadia Khan, and Yasuhiro Yonekawa

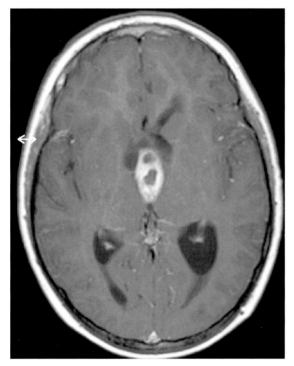

Fig. 1

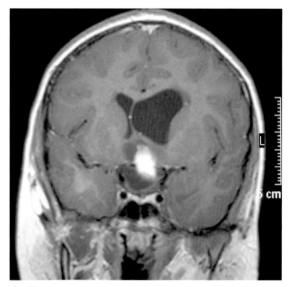

Fig. 2

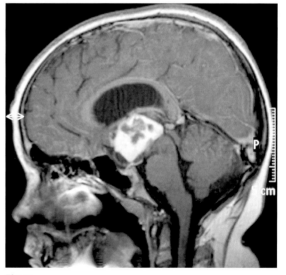

Fig. 3

An 11-year-old boy presented with obesity, increased appetite (hyperphasia), and growth failure (short stature) that had started when he was 7 years old.

He had been suffering from dizziness, general fatigue, and headache for 2 weeks, and from decreased visual acuity and diplopia for 1 week. He also suffered from downward ocular conjugate deviation for 2 days.

Gd-DTPA-enhanced T1-weighted MR imaging was performed on admission (shown in Figs. 1–3).

- What do these figures reveal?

With Gd enhancement, the lesion appeared hypointense on T1-weighted images and hyperintense on T2-weighted images.

- What does the differential diagnosis include?
- What is the best way to manage this condition?

A 232

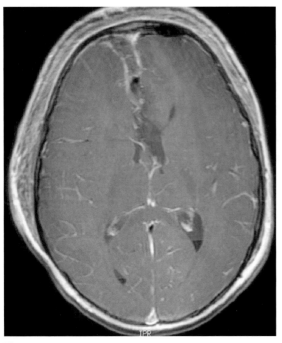

Fig. 4

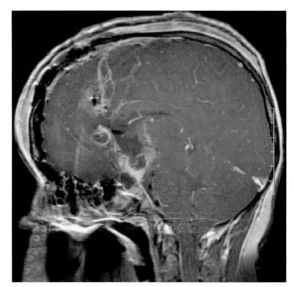

Fig. 5

The long-term presence of obesity, hyperphasia, and growth failure indicates hypothalamus-pituitary grand system dysfunction.

The Gd-T1-weighted MR imaging shows the tumor consisting of solid and cystic portions with the wall enhanced in the third ventricle. The optic chiasm and pituitary stalk are pressed from the top and deviated toward the bottom. The left lateral ventricle is remarkably dilated compared with the right.

The differential diagnosis for a pediatric suprasellar tumor that occupies the third ventricle includes cranio-pharyngioma, glioma, and germ cell tumor.

The tumor was surgically removed (supine position, frontal craniotomy, interhemispheric trans rostrum corporis callosi/lamina terminalis approach). The tumor was arising from the left hypothalamus. The histo-pathological study revealed a pilocytic astrocytoma. MR imaging after the operation (Figs. 4, 5) showed that the tumor was removed subtotally.

At the time of writing, the boy was doing well and going to school everyday without apparent regrowth of the tumor.

Suggested Reading

1. Bernaerts A, Vanhoenacker F, Debois V, Parizel PM. Juve-nile pilocytic astrocytoma. JBR-BTR 2003; 86:142–143
2. Fernandez C Figarella-Branger D, Girard N, Bouvier-Labit C, Gouvernet J, Paz Paredes A, Lena G. Pilocytic astrocyto-mas in children: prognostic factors—a retrospective study of 80 cases. Neurosurgery 2003; 53:544–553
3. Kayama T, Tominaga T, Yoshimoto T. Management of pilo-cytic astrocytoma. Neurosurg Rev 1996; 19:217–220

Q 233

Masayuki Fujioka, Carl Muroi, Nadia Khan, and Yasuhiro Yonekawa

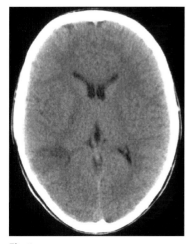
Fig. 1

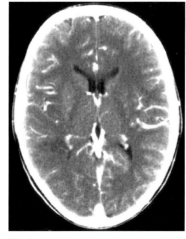
Fig. 2

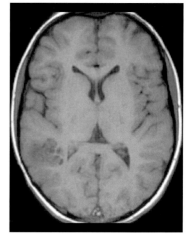
Fig. 3

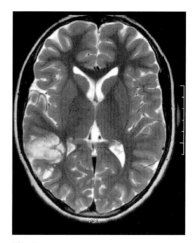
Fig. 4

A 9-year-old boy presented with partial epileptic seizure and secondary generalization leading to unconsciousness.
- What do the pre- and postcontrast CT scans (Figs. 1, 2) show?

Figures 3 and 4 represent T1-weighted and T2-weighted MR images, respectively.
- What are the findings from Figs. 3 and 4?

The boy was treated conservatively with carbamazepine, and periodical follow-up imaging studies were performed with CT and MR imaging.

After the initiation of medication, the attacks of unconsciousness disappeared. However, 2 years later, the patient developed olfactory hallucinations (once every several months), and consequently developed absence attacks.

In addition, auditory hallucinations occurred, and these partial complex seizures became tractable only with medication.
- What is a possible diagnosis of the lesion on the MR imaging study?
- What is the best way to manage this condition?

A 233

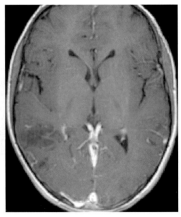

Fig. 5

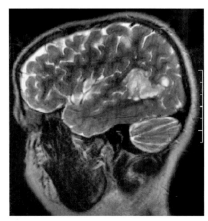

Fig. 6

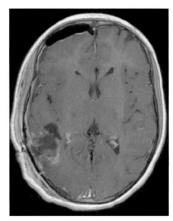

Fig. 7

The precontrast CT scan (Fig. 1) shows a cortical lesion of low density in the right posterior temporal lobe. The lesion extends toward the trigone of the lateral ventricle. The lesion has no mass effect and no enhanced portions on the postcontrast CT scan (Fig. 2).

The lesion appears hypointense on T1-weighted MR imaging and hyperintense on T2-weighted imaging (Figs. 3, 4). The MR images show a wedge-shaped, multicystic (bubbly) mass lesion in the temporal cortex without apparent surrounding edema.

The Gd-enhanced T1-weighted MR image (Fig. 5) shows no marked enhancement of the lesion. The T2-weighted MR image (sagittal view, Fig. 6) shows the bubbly mass extending from the posterior temporal lobe (superior and middle temporal gyrus) through the angular gyrus.

The lesion is considered very slow growing because the patient has a long history of partial complex seizures and imaging does not show any edema and/or mass effects of the lesion. For cortically based tumors with cystic components in children, the differential diagnosis includes ganglioglioma, dysembryoplastic neuroepithelial tumor, and pleomorphic xanthoastrocytoma.

The seizures were uncontrollable with medication. Electroencephalography revealed that the tumor was of epileptogenic focus. Therefore, total removal of the tumor was performed without any intra- or postoperative complications (Fig. 7, Gd-T1-weighted, axial view). Histology revealed a dysembryoplastic neuroepithelial tumor.

After the operation, the seizures subsided and disappeared. At the time of writing, the boy was going to school without any sequelae.

Suggested Reading

1. Fernandez C, Girard N, Paz Paredes A, Bouvier-Labit C, Lena G, Figarella-Branger D. The usefulness of MR imaging in the diagnosis of dysembryoplastic neuroepithelial tumor in children: a study of 14 cases. AJNR Am J Neuroradiol 2003; 24:829–834

2. Lee DY et al. Dysembryoplastic neuroepithelial tumor: Radiological findings (including PET, SPECT, and MRS) and surgical strategy. J Neurooncol 2000; 47:167–174

3. Ostertun B et al. Dysembryoplastic neuroepithelial tumors: MR and CT evaluation. AJNR 1996; 17:419–430

4. Stanescu Cosson R, Varlet P, Beuvon F, Daumas Duport C, Devaux B, Chassoux F, Fredy D, Meder JF. Dysembryoplastic neuroepithelial tumors: CT, MR findings and imaging follow-up: a study of 53 cases. J Neuoradiol 2001; 28:230–240

Q 234

Masayuki Fujioka, Carl Muroi, Nadia Khan, and Yasuhiro Yonekawa

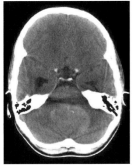
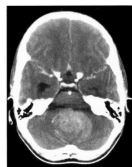
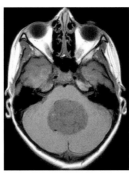
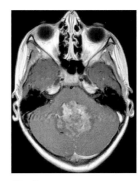

Fig. 1   **Fig. 2**   **Fig. 3**   **Fig. 4**

An 8-year-old girl had been suffering from vomiting in the morning for 2 months. In addition, she had a 2-week history of headache, unstable gait, and frequent falling down. She complained of difficulties in studying at school due to attention deficit.

On admission, a neurological study showed bilateral abducens nerve palsy, ataxic gait, abnormal finger-to-nose test results, and dysphagia.

- What do the pre- and postcontrast CT scans show (Figs. 1, 2)?
- What do the T1-weighted MR images with and without Gd-DTPA show (Figs. 3, 4)?
- What pathological condition is affecting this child?
- What is the best way to manage this condition?

A 234

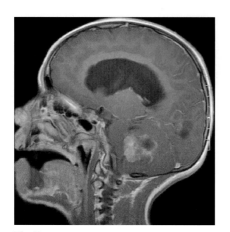

Fig. 5

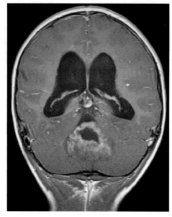

Fig. 6

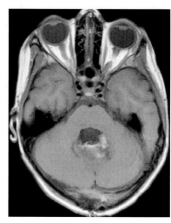

Fig. 7

Figure 1 shows a fourth-ventricle solid tumor of relatively high density on the precontrast CT scan. The dilatation of the inferior horns of the bilateral lateral ventricles indicates the presence of obstructive hydrocephalus. Figure 2 shows slight heterogeneous enhancement of the tumor on the postcontrast CT scan.

The spherical tumor appears relatively hypointense to brain matter on T1-weighted MR imaging (Fig. 3) and occupies the space of the fourth ventricle and mid-cerebellar area. The signal on the T1-weighted image is slightly heterogeneous, which is considered to be due to the presence of small cysts and clefts inside the tumor. The Gd-T1-weighted image (Fig. 4) shows heterogeneous enhancement of the tumor without surrounding brain edema.

Figures 5 and 6 (Gd-T1-weighted sagittal and coronal views, respectively) show a fourth-ventricle tumor with a cystic portion associated with the hydrocephalus. The solid portion of the tumor shows an enhancement effect. The tumor pushes the brainstem forward and the cerebellum backward.

The differential diagnosis for pediatric mid-posterior fossa tumor includes medulloblastoma, ependymoma, glioma (cerebellar pilocytic astrocytoma and dorsally exophytic brainstem glioma), choroid plexus papilloma, and atypical teratoid/rhabdoid tumor (usually off-midline).

For the diagnosis and the cure, the tumor was totally removed (sitting position, middle suboccipital craniotomy, infra-vermis approach) (Fig. 7, postoperative Gd-T1-weighted MR image). The histological diagnosis was medulloblastoma.

After the operation, no additional neurological deficits developed. The patient underwent postoperative chemotherapy and radiation therapy. The patient's ataxia improved and her gait returned to normal 3 months after the operation. The bilateral abducens palsy also improved. However, at the time of writing, the patient's dysphagia continued and she was undergoing rehabilitation therapy.

Q 235

Masayuki Fujioka, Carl Muroi, Nadia Khan, and Yasuhiro Yonekawa

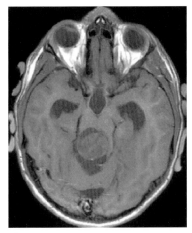

Fig. 1

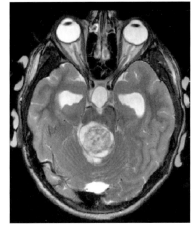

Fig. 2

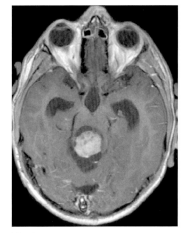

Fig. 3

A 15-year-old boy complained of deterioration in his visual acuity, which had started 1 week earlier. His family consulted an ophthalmologist. The ophthalmologic study revealed papilledema in the bilateral ocular fundus and right papillary dilatation.

A CT study was performed immediately afterward, revealing an intracranial tumor, and the boy was referred to our neurosurgical unit.

The neurological examination showed right oculomotor nerve palsy, right facial nerve palsy, and right hy-

poglossal nerve palsy; however, there was no apparent motor weakness of the upper and lower extremities. His consciousness level was clear and alert.

- What do Figs. 1 and 2 (T1- and T2-weighted MR images, axial views) show?
- What does Fig. 3 (Gd-T1-weighted MR images, axial and sagittal views, respectively) show?
- What pathological condition is affecting this child?
- What is the best way to manage this condition?

A 235

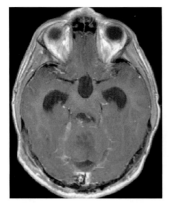 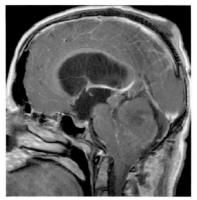 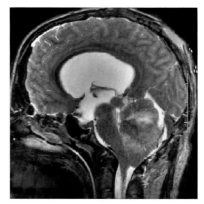

Fig. 4   **Fig. 5**   **Fig. 6**

Figures 1 and 2 show a dorsal brainstem tumor with solid and cystic portions. The solid portion of the tumor appears iso- to hypointense on T1-weighted images and moderately to heterogeneously hyperintense on T2-weighted images. There seems to be no apparent evidence of edema in the brain matter. The dilatations of the inferior horns (lateral ventricles) and of the third ventricle (sagging/extending downward) suggest obstructive hydrocephalus.

The solid portion—but not the cyst wall—of the tumor is heterogeneously enhanced on the Gd-T1-weighted images (Fig. 3). The tumor is located in the dorsal brainstem (from the midbrain to the pons levels) and the supracerebellar space. The roof of the fourth ventricle and the cerebellum is pushed downward by the tumor. Compression of the sylvian aqueduct by the tumor results in obstructive hydrocephalus.

The clinical symptoms of this boy are relatively mild compared to the size of the tumor and there is no marked edematous change in the peritumoral brain tissue on the neuroimaging study. Therefore, this tumor seems to be a slow-growing cystic brainstem tumor with mural nodules such as a low-grade astrocytoma that extends in an extra-axial direction.

This tectal tumor was removed subtotally (sitting position, occipital and suboccipital craniotomy, supracerebellar paraculmen approach, and occipital transtentorial approach). The histopathological study showed a pilocytic astrocytoma (WHO grade1) characterized by a biphasic pattern with a dense fibrillary matrix composed of bipolar cells and Rosenthal fibers and with loosely structured microcystic areas of cells resembling protoplasmic astrocytes.

Figures 4–6 (Gd-T1-weighted axial, Gd-T1-weighted sagittal, and T2-weighted sagittal, respectively) show that the solid portion of the tumor was totally removed and the cyst wall subtotally removed. The boy had no operative complications and no additional neurological deficits postoperatively. At the 6-month follow-up, he was in good condition, doing well, and going to school.

Suggested Reading

1. Bovdston WR, Sanford RA, Muhlbauer MS, Kun LE, Kirk E, Dohan FC Jr, Schweitzer JB. Gliomas of the tectum and periaqueductal region of the mesencephalon. Pediatr Neurosurg 1991–1992; 17:234–238

2. Bowers DC et al. Tectal gliomas: Natural history of an indolent lesion in pediatric patients. Pediatr Neurosurg 2000; 32:24–29

3. Daglioglu E et al. Tectal gliomas in children: The implications for natural history and management strategy. Pediatr Neurosurg 2003; 38:223–231

4. Fernandez C Figarella-Branger D, Girard N, Bouvier-Labit C, Gouvernet J, Paz Paredes A, Lena G. Pilocytic astrocytomas in children: prognostic factors—a retrospective study of 80 cases. Neurosurgery 2003; 53:544–553

5. Kestle J, Townsend JJ, Brockmeyer DL, Walker ML. Juvenile pilocytic astrocytoma of the brainstem in children. J Neurosurg 2004; 101(1 Suppl):1–6

Q 236

Masayuki Fujioka, Carl Muroi, Nadia Khan, and Yasuhiro Yonekawa

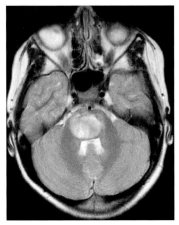

Fig. 1

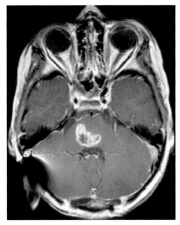

Fig. 2

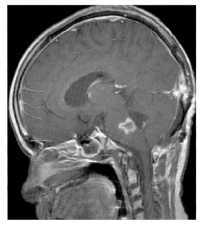

Fig. 3

An 8-year-old girl's right eye deviated medially for 1 week, according to her mother.

CT scans obtained by an ophthalmologist revealed a low to isodense change mainly in the lower pons. The girl was referred to a neurological department.

An MR imaging study showed a pontine–tegmentum lesion as a hypointense change of irregular shape on T1-weighted images and as a larger area of hyperintense change on T2-weighted imaging compared to the area on the T1-weighted image (Fig. 1).

On admission, the patient's neurological deficits comprised right abducens nerve palsy, left hemi-dysesthesia, left incomplete hemiparesis, cerebellar ataxia, and right auditory disturbance.

- What do Figs. 2, 3 (Gd-T1-weighted MR images, axial, sagittal, and coronal views, respectively) show?
- What pathological condition is affecting this child?
- What is the best way to manage this condition?

A 236

Figures 2, 3 show the tumor localized mainly in the right lower tegmentum of the pons. The tumor has a ring enhancement of irregular shape. The MR imaging study suggests a high-grade glioma with central necrosis (such as anaplastic astrocytoma and glioblastoma multiforme) firstly, and inflammation/infectious change secondarily.

In this case, the pontine tumor has damaged the abducens nerve fiber and/or its nucleus but not the facial nerve. The facial nerve fiber runs around the abducens nerve nucleus and could be damaged together. The combined symptoms of unilateral facial and abducens nerve palsy and contralateral hemiparesis due to the basal pontine lesion point to Millard-Gubler syndrome. This syndrome is usually caused by ischemia, but sometimes also by a tumor.

This tumor is located in the pontine base near the floor of the fourth ventricle. Therefore, surgical extirpation of the tumor is considered feasible.

The tumor was removed subtotally. Histology showed an anaplastic astrocytoma (WHO grade 3). The operation was performed without any complication. Figure 4 shows a postoperative T1-weighted image with Gd administration.

The girl underwent chemotherapy and radiation after the operation. Thereafter, she was transferred to a rehabilitation institution. At the time of writing, the hemiparesis and ataxia were improving.

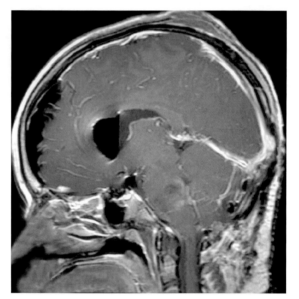

Fig. 4

Suggested Reading

1. Epstein FJ, Farmaer JP. Brain-stem glioma growth patterns. J Neurosurg 1993; 78:408–412
2. Kane AG, Robles HA, Smirniotopoulos JG, Heironimus JD, Fish MH. Radiologic-pathologic correlation. Diffuse pontine astrocytoma. AJNR Am J Neuroradiol 1993; 14:941–945
3. Kwon JW, Kim IO, Cheon JE, Kim WS, Moon SG, Kim TJ, Chi JG, Wang KC, Chung JK, Yeon KM. Pediatric brain-stem gliomas: MRI, FDG-PET and histological grading correlation. Pediatr Radiol 2006; 36:959–964
4. Tortosa A et al. Prognostic implication of clinical, radiologic, and pathologic features in patients with anaplastic gliomas. Cancer 2003; 97:1063–1071

Q 237

Masayuki Fujioka, Carl Muroi, Nadia Khan, and Yasuhiro Yonekawa

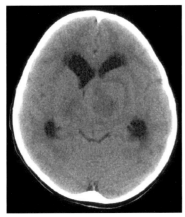
Fig. 1

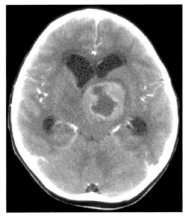
Fig. 2

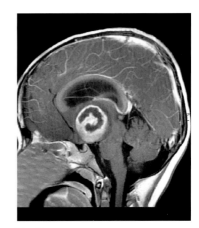
Fig. 3

A 5-year-old boy had started complaining of general fatigue and visual acuity disturbance 3 weeks earlier. The boy had been relatively lethargic for 1 week and had been suffering from vomiting for the last 3 days.

During the first medical examination, his consciousness level was 14 on the Glasgow Coma Scale. The general physician performed a CT study.

- What do Figs. 1 and 2 (pre- and postcontrast CT scans) show?

A T1-weighted MR imaging study showed that the cyst wall appeared isointense and that the content of the cyst exhibited hypointensity. T2-weighted MR imaging revealed a cystic lesion (the wall and the contents) and surrounding edema with hyperintensity.

- What does Fig. 3 (Gd-T1-weighted) show?
- What pathological condition is affecting this child?
- What is the best way to manage this condition?

A 237

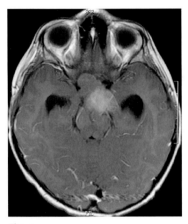

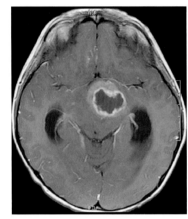

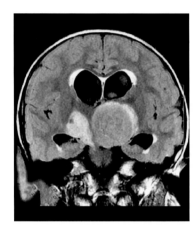

Fig. 4   **Fig. 5**   **Fig. 6**

Figures 1 and 2 show the cystic tumor with a solid component in the left prethalamic and hypothalamic areas. The tumor pushes the foramen of Monro toward the contralateral side. The precontrast CT scan shows an isodense wall with central low density. The postcontrast CT scan shows a cystic wall of irregular shape with moderate enhancement effect. The tumor has some surrounding edema. Dilatation of the anterior horns and the trigones of the lateral ventricles indicates obstructive hydrocephalus.

Figure 3 shows that the cystic tumor has a mural nodule enhanced on T1-weighted images. The tumor occupies the premesencephalic cistern and the third ventricle. The foramen of Monro is pressed toward the right. The midbrain is compressed and pushed away posteriorly.

Figure 4 indicates that the solid portion of the tumor is located mainly in the optic pathway. The enhancement effects of the solid component and the wall seem relatively heterogeneous on Figs. 4 and 5 (Gd-T1-weighted images). Figure 6 [fluid attenuated inversion recovery (FLAIR) MR imaging] shows that both the solid portion/cyst wall and the cyst contents appear isointense (partly hyperintense) to the gray matter. The FLAIR image shows the surrounding edema clearly as hyperintense change.

The differential diagnosis includes glioma (hypothalamus or optic pathway) and craniopharyngioma.

The boy underwent surgical removal of the tumor (subtotal expiration, supine position, left frontomedial craniotomy, interhemispheric approach). The tumor arose from the left optic tract. The histological diagnosis was pilocytic astrocytoma. A detailed study revealed no evidence of neurofibromatosis 1 (von Recklinghausen's neurofibromatosis). The boy had no additional deficits after the operation. At the 6-month follow-up, he was in good condition and was going to school.

Suggested Reading

1. Coakley KJ, Huston J, Scheithauer BW et al. Pilocytic astrocytomas: well-demarcated magnetic resonance appearance despite frequent infiltration histologically. Mayo Clin Proc 1995; 70:747–751

2. Fernandez C Figarella-Branger D, Girard N, Bouvier-Labit C, Gouvernet J, Paz Paredes A, Lena G. Pilocytic astrocytomas in children: prognostic factors—a retrospective study of 80 cases. Neurosurgery 2003; 53:544–553

3. Komotar RJ et al. Pilocytic and pilomyxoid hypothalamic/chiasmatic astrocytomas. Neurosurgery 2004; 54:72–80

4. Riccardi VM. von Recklinghausen neurofibromatosis. N Engl J Med 1981; 305:1617–1627

Q 238

Masayuki Fujioka, Carl Muroi, Nadia Khan, and Yasuhiro Yonekawa

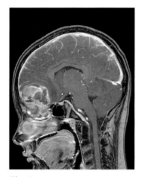
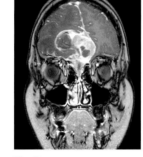
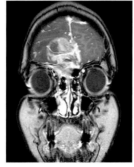
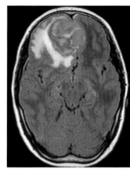

Fig. 1   **Fig. 2**   **Fig. 3**   **Fig. 4**

An 11-year-old boy had intermittent frontal headaches for 5 months. The headache had become more severe in the last 6 days. The boy had also been suffering from vomiting for 3 days.

The precontrast head CT scans showed a space-occupying lesion of isodensity to moderate hyperdensity with the surrounding edema in the right frontal lobe (frontal base). The CT study also showed bone destruction (osteolysis) in the frontal skull base and the ethmoid.

- What do Figs. 1–3 (Gd-T1-weighted images) and 4 (FLAIR MR imaging) show?
- What pathological condition is affecting this child?
- What is the best way to manage this condition?

A 238

The MR images (Figs. 1–4) show a mass lesion in the frontal cranial base (involving the bilateral olfactory groove and the right sphenoidal plane) with surrounding edema in the right frontal lobe. The Gd-T1-weighted images demonstrate a heterogeneously enhanced tumor. The tumor margin is irregular and the tumor seems lobulated. The extending portion of the tumor interdigitates with the brain. The tumor has an extracranial portion extending into the frontal sinus and the ethmoid sinus. The FLAIR image (Fig. 4) shows a tumor of mixed intensities and marked peritumoral edema. The cerebral falx is also strongly enhanced on the Gd-T1-weighted images (dural tail sign). This is an intra- and extracranial tumor associated with bone destruction. This tumor appears as a dural-based enhancing mass partially associated with a peritumoral CSF band. The differential diagnosis for such a tumor includes atypical (WHO grade 2) or malignant (WHO grade 3) meningioma, dural metastatic tumor, and sarcoma (ex. osteosarcoma and meningeal sarcoma).

The patient underwent surgical removal of the tumor (macroscopical total removal, supine position, frontomedial craniotomy). The histopathological study showed an atypical meningioma (WHO grade 2). The postoperative Gd-T1-weighted MR images show that the tumor was removed by >95% (Figs. 5, 6). No postoperative additional neurological deficits developed. At the 3-month postoperative follow-up, the patient was doing well and going to school.

Suggested Reading

1. Alvernia JE et al. Preoperative neuroimaging findings as a predictor of the surgical plane of cleavage: prospective study of 100 consecutive cases of intracranial meningioma. J Neurosurg 2004; 100:422–430
2. Chen TC, Zee CS, Miller CA et al. Magnetic resonance imaging and pathological correlates of meningiomas. Neurosurgery 1992; 31:1015–1022
3. Takeguchi T et al. The dural tail of intracranial meningiomas on fluid-attenuated inversion-recovery images. Neuroradiol 2004; 46:130–135

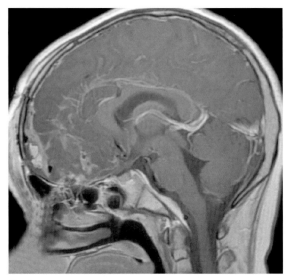

Fig. 5

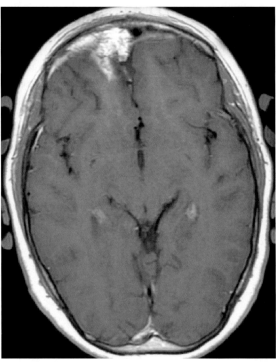

Fig. 6

Q 239

Jacob C. Langer and Priscilla Chiu

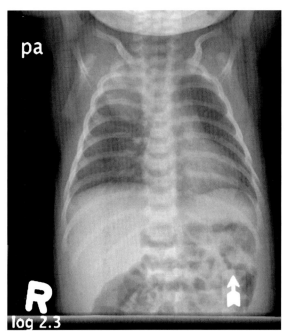

Fig. 1

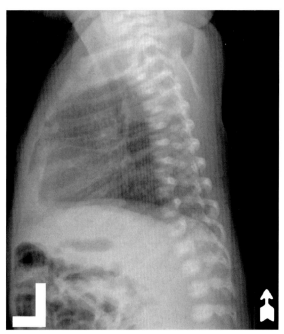

Fig. 2

A 3-week-old term female infant presented to the local emergency room with a history of increasing lethargy, fever, and poor oral intake. On physical examination, the infant was febrile at 39°C with normal vital signs and appeared well hydrated. She had normal breath sounds and no evidence of murmurs on auscultation. Her neurological examination was normal. Her birth history and family history were unremarkable.

She underwent a septic work-up which included a chest radiograph, as shown in Figs. 1 and 2.

- What do Figs. 1 and 2 show?
- What is the differential diagnosis?

The patient was transferred from the local hospital to the tertiary pediatric hospital. Intravenous antibiotics were started.

- What investigations would you order for this patient?

The patient's fever resolved and she was discharged home without any symptoms.

After 3 months, the patient was still symptom-free and doing well. She tolerated oral intake well and was growing.

- How would you manage this patient?
- What are the considerations in the surgical treatment of this lesion?

A 239

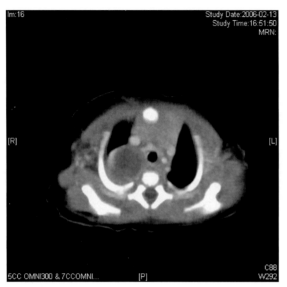

Fig. 3

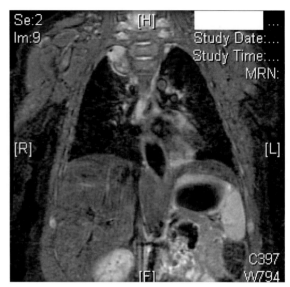

Fig. 4

This infant's chest radiograph showed a lesion in the apex of the right lung field. The lateral view showed the lesion to be in the posterior mediastinum.

The differential diagnosis for this lesion includes neurogenic tumor (most common), primitive neuroectodermal tumor, foregut duplication cyst (including neurenteric cyst), and anterior thoracic meningocele (extremely rare).

The radiological modality of choice is MR imaging, which provides excellent multiplanar imaging for neurogenic and spinal lesions, and is optimal for accurately detecting intraspinal extension. However, this procedure requires sedation or general anesthesia for optimal imaging resolution. Ultrasound is a less invasive study that can differentiate between solid and cystic lesions in the periphery of the chest. CT is also helpful in revealing the identity and extent of the lesion and is complementary to MR imaging in both aspects.

Neurogenic tumors (neuroblastoma and ganglioneuroma) arising from the thoracic sympathetic chain are the most common lesions of the posterior mediastinum in infants and children. The chest is the third most common site for neurogenic tumors after the adrenal gland and other retroperitoneal sites.

Neuroblastomas, arising from neural crest cells with immature neural elements, are the most common and lethal solid tumors of childhood. However, spontaneous regression may occur, especially in those identified early in infancy. In some cases, the neuroblastoma may mature into a benign ganglioneuroma.

Neuroblastomas produce vasoactive substances detectable in the serum and urine. Urinary metabolites of epinephrine, particularly vanillylmandelic acid (VMA) and homovanillic acid (HVA), are useful as diagnostic tests and for detection of recurrent disease. Elevated serum levels of neuron-specific enolase, lactate dehydrogenase, and ferritin correlate with the diagnosis of neuroblastoma and provide prognostic value.

Thoracic neurogenic tumors may infiltrate the spinal canal ("dumbbell" tumors) causing spinal cord compression and paraplegia, which may require emergency laminectomy to decompress the spinal cord.

This patient's urine tests showed elevated HVA and VMA. The lesion was subsequently imaged with CT (Fig. 3) and MR imaging (Fig. 4).

No other lesions were found, suggesting that this was an isolated thoracic neurogenic tumor with no metastases.

The definitive management of isolated thoracic neurogenic tumors is surgical resection via thoracoscopy or thoracotomy. At 3 months, the lesion was resected thoracoscopically without complication.

Q 240

Jacob C. Langer and Priscilla Chiu

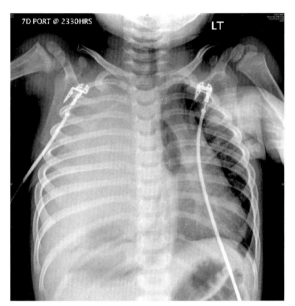

Fig. 1

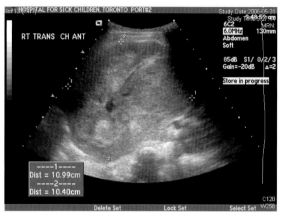

Fig. 2

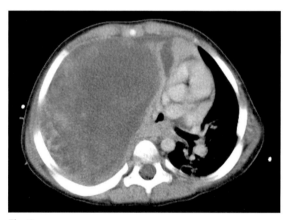

Fig. 3

A 5-year-old child presented to our emergency room with progressive cough and recent weight loss. He had no significant past medical history and no travel history.

The initial physical examination by the emergency physician revealed decreased breath sounds in the right chest.

The child was sent for a chest radiograph, shown in Fig. 1.

- What does Fig. 1 show?
- What is the differential diagnosis for the chest radiograph findings?

The emergency physician ordered the next investigation shown in Fig. 2.

- What does Fig. 2 show?

The patient was referred to the pediatric general surgeon after these investigations. He became progressively more dyspneic requiring supplemental oxygen and admission to the intensive care unit.

The multidisciplinary oncology team was consulted. The surgical team requested the investigation shown in Fig. 3.

- What does Fig. 3 show?
- What is the differential diagnosis now?
- How would you manage this patient?

A 240

This patient's chest radiograph showed loss of right lung volume (the "white-out"). The mediastinum was displaced into the left chest.

It was not clear on the radiograph whether fluid or solid tissue occupied the right chest. Lateral decubitus positioning may show air–fluid levels suggestive of an effusion, unless it is multiloculated or extremely large.

Ultrasound is a useful initial study to distinguish fluid and solid tissue in the chest. The patient's ultrasound (Fig. 2) showed a complex, solid mass with very little fluid.

The differential diagnosis includes benign and malignant tumors of the chest. Benign tumors include myxoma, hemangioma, teratoma, lipoma, and rhabdomyoma. Malignant tumors include Ewing's sarcoma, malignant teratoma, rhabdomyosarcoma, lymphoma, primitive neuroectodermal tumor, lipoblastoma, and pleuropulmonary blastoma.

CT scan can identify features of solid chest tumors and aid in their diagnosis. Vascular tumors will enhance with intravenous contrast medium. The presence of fat and calcification is typical of teratoma. Rib deformity may suggest Ewing's sarcoma. Disseminated lymphadenopathy would suggest lymphoma. Lung nodules in children should be investigated with CT imaging of the head, abdomen, and pelvis, as lung lesions may represent metastatic spread from other primary tumors.

The chest CT scan showed a large, nonhomogeneous mass with minimal intravenous contrast enhancement and a small effusion. No areas of fat or calcification within the tumor were seen and no lymphadenopathy or rib lesion was noted. The CT appearance suggested a primary mesenchymal tumor.

Definitive diagnosis of the lesion was obtained with a core biopsy showing malignant cells consistent with pleuropulmonary blastoma.

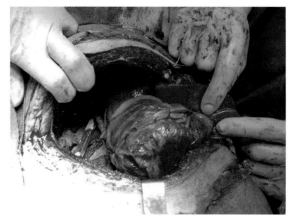

Fig. 4

Pleuropulmonary blastoma is a rare but aggressive tumor of the pleuropulmonary mesenchyme. There has been controversy over the association between congenital lung cysts and the risk of malignant degeneration in the cyst giving rise to this malignancy.

Following tissue diagnosis, this patient underwent surgical resection. The lesion involved the right middle and lower lobes and was adherent to the pericardium and chest wall. The lesion was completely resected through a "clam-shell" incision by complete pneumonectomy and partial resection of the pericardium. The pericardium was then reconstructed using Surgi-sis (Fig. 4).

The patient did well postoperatively and was discharged home. The role of postoperative chemotherapy for pleuropulmonary blastoma is unclear and subject to multidisciplinary oncology evaluation.

Suggested Reading

1. Dang NC, Siegel SE, Phillips JD. Malignant chest wall tumors in children and young adults. J Pediatr Surg 1999; 34:1773–8
2. Hill DA. USCAP specialty conference: case 1-type 1 pleuropulmonary blastoma. Pediatr Dev Pathol 2005; 8:77–84
3. Tagge EP, Mulvihill D, Chandler JC, Richardson M, Uflacker R, Othersen HD. Childhood pleuropulmonary blastoma: caution against nonoperative management of congenital lung cysts. J Pediatr Surg 1996; 31:187–9

Q 241

Frédéric Gauthier, Sophie Branchereau, and Chiara Grimaldi

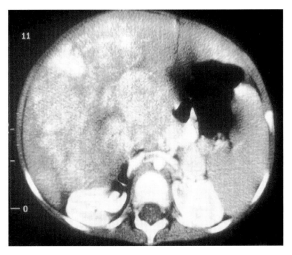

Fig. 1

A 2-year-old girl with no significant medical history presented to the pediatric emergency department with an abdominal mass. A US study and an abdominal CT scan were performed; the scan is shown in Fig. 1. A thoracic scan was normal.

- What is the initial diagnosis and how can you confirm it with blood tests?
- According to the different international protocols and the localization of the lesion, what are the treatment options?

At the end of preoperative chemotherapy, the alpha-fetoprotein levels had decreased to 632. The volume of the lesion also decreased on the CT scan and no extension to the fourth segment was detected.

- What type of resection would you plan?

A 241

A hepatic lesion is localized in the right hepatic lobe. The alpha-fetoprotein level is diagnostic measuring 61,200 (normal <15). The diagnosis is nonmetastatic hepatoblastoma.

We used the SIOP protocol SIOPEL 3 for this patient.

The localization of the lesion allows a right hemihepatectomy to be performed (Fig. 2).

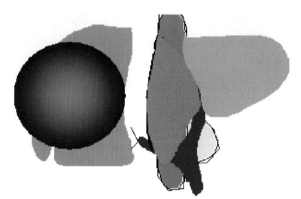

Fig. 2

Suggested Reading

1. Blouin P, Brugieres L, Tabone MD, Leverger G, Rubie H, Branchereau S. Carboplatin-epirubicin regimen for the treatment of hepatoblastoma. Pediatr Blood Cancer 2004; 42(2):149–54

2. Czauderna P, Otte JB, Aronson D, Gauthier F , Mackinlay G, Roebuck D, Plaschkes J, Perilongo G. Guidelines for surgical treatment of hepatoblastoma in the modern era—Recommendations from the Childhood Liver Tumour Strategy Group of the International Society of Paediatric Oncology (SIOPEL). European Journal of Cancer 2005; 41:1031–1036

Q 242

Amedeo Fiorillo

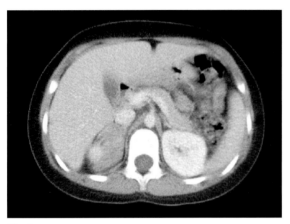

Fig. 1

A 6-year-old white girl was admitted to our department because of severe abdominal pain and fever. On admission, the child was febrile, and her general condition was compromised. Physical examination showed generalized lymphadenopathy and an extremely enlarged abdomen; a firm mass was palpable 10 cm below the right costal margin. Abnormal laboratory test results included: WBC, 15,460/μl with 74% neutrophils; platelets, 1,000,000/μl; erythrocyte sedimentation rate, 70 mm/h; and ferritin, 340 mg/dl. CT scan of the abdomen (Fig. 1) showed a huge retroperitoneal mass—5.2×3.2 cm in di-

ameter—closely connected to the superior vena cava, to the liver, and to the homolateral kidney; multiple fine calcifications and one large calcification were also evident.

- What is the diagnosis?
- What differential diagnosis do you take into consideration?
- Which other diagnostic tests do you perform to confirm the suspected diagnosis?
- What is the role of surgery in this condition?

A 242

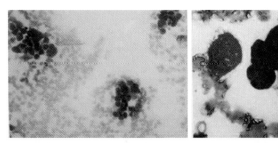

Fig. 2

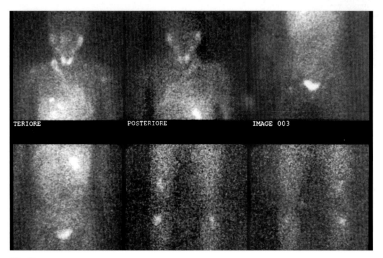

Fig. 3

This child was affected by neuroblastoma, arising from her right adrenal gland.

The primary tumor should be differentiated from a renal abnormality such as a multicystic kidney or a Wilms' tumor. Usually, as in this case, it is possible to demonstrate that the tumor is extrarenal, displacing rather than involving the kidney. Moreover, metastatic sites may be confused with other small, round, blue-cell tumors such as rhabdomyosarcoma, Ewing's sarcoma, or lymphoma.

Other tests useful in establishing the diagnosis are:

1. Measurement of urine catecholamines and metabolites such as homovanillic acid (HVA) and vanillylmandelic acid (VMA) (in our case the VMA level was 15 mg/24 h and the HVA level was 20 mg/24 h, both greater than 3.0 SD above the mean for age)
2. Bone marrow aspirate and trephine biopsy to search for unequivocal tumor cells (in this case bone marrow aspirate was positive; Fig. 2)
3. Metaiodobenzylguanidine scan, applicable to all sites of disease (Fig. 3)

4. Serum markers of predictive value such as neuron-specific enolase, ferritin, lactate dehydrogenase (LDH)
5. Definitive pathological diagnosis can be made from tumor tissue obtained by excisional biopsy (in this case it was neuroblastoma, schwannian stroma-poor)

The recommended minimum testing to define the clinical stage (from stage 1 that defines the localized tumor to stage 4 that defines any primary tumor with distant dissemination other than skin, liver or bone marrow, according to the International Neuroblastoma Staging System) also comprises bone radiographs and scintigraphy by technetium 99m scan, chest radiograph (AP and lateral), and chest CT or MR imaging if the chest radiograph is abnormal.

Surgery plays a pivotal role in the management of neuroblastoma in order to establish the diagnosis, to provide tissue for biologic studies, and to completely remove the tumor or the residual disease in delayed primary or second-look surgery.

Q 243

Amedeo Fiorillo

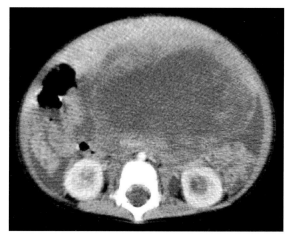

Fig. 1

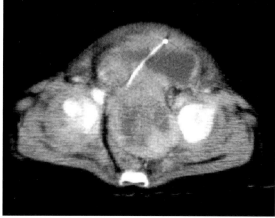

Fig. 2

A 1-year-old white boy presented with an enlarged, painless abdomen; no other sign or symptom was reported apart from occasional episodes of diarrhea. On admission his general condition was good; on physical examination a large abdominal mass was palpable and arterial hypertension was registered.

Pertinent laboratory test results were found to be in the normal range.

A CT scan of the abdomen (Fig. 1) showed a large, inhomogeneous, mainly solid mass extending from the second lumbar vertebra into the pelvis; the bladder was displaced to the left (Fig. 2). A radiographic skeletal survey, standard chest radiograph, CT of the chest, and a brain CT scan were all normal.

- How would you achieve the diagnosis?
- What is the differential diagnosis?
- What are the prognostic factors in this disease?
- What is the role of the surgeon?

A 243

The diagnosis, made on tumor tissue obtained by excisional biopsy, was "embryonal rhabdomyosarcoma" (RMS).

Traditionally, histologic classification includes embryonal, botryoid, alveolar, and pleomorphic variants; nearly two-thirds of cases, like our case, are of embryonal histology.

RMS belongs to the category of small, round, blue-cell tumors of childhood; therefore it must be differentiated from lymphoma, neuroblastoma, Ewing's sarcoma, and primitive neuroectodermal tumor.

The major prognosticators are:

a) Age (with a relatively poor outlook for infants with advanced disease)

b) Primary site (locations associated with little opportunity for spread, i.e., the orbit, share better prognosis compared with deep, poor confined areas, i.e., retroperitoneum)

d) Histologic type (the best prognosis is associated with embryonal, the poorest with alveolar variant)

e) Stage of disease (group I: localized disease is completely resected; group II: localized tumor, with or without spread to regional lymph nodes, is grossly resected with microscopic residual disease; group III: localized or locally extensive tumor shows gross residual disease after resection or biopsy only; group IV: distant metastases are present at onset)

RMS may spread by local extension, but metastases via the venous or lymphatic systems are rare at onset, diagnosed in no more than 20% of cases.

The goal of surgery should be to achieve complete resection of the primary tumor with an adequate margin of normal tissue; this will allow local control of the non-metastatic disease and possibly cure. Therefore, treatment should be individualized for each patient, based on clinical stage, site, and resectability of the primary tumor.

Suggested Reading

1. Lawrence W Jr et al. Pretreatment TNM staging of childhood rhabdomyosarcoma. A report of the Intergroup Rhabdomyosarcoma Study Group. Cancer 1997; 80:1165

2. Rodary C et al. An attempt to use common staging system in rhabdomyosarcoma: a report of an international workshop initiated by the International Society of Pediatric-Oncology (SIOP). Med Pediatr Oncol 1989; 17:210

Q 244

Amedeo Fiorillo

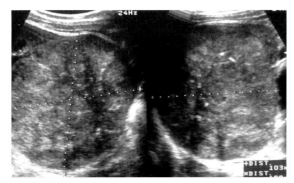

Fig. 1

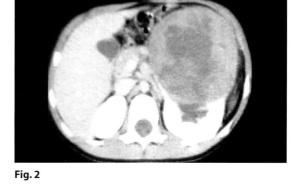

Fig. 2

A 5-year-old white girl was admitted to our department because of abdominal swelling first noticed 1 month earlier. On admission she was febrile and had severe abdominal pain. Physical examination showed a large left flank mass that did not move with respiration. The initial laboratory evaluation revealed elevation of the erythrocyte sedimentation rate (56 mm/h), lactate dehydrogenase (LDH) (1,967 IU/l), neuron-specific enolase (68.3 mg/ml), and ferritin (626 µg/l). However, a normal renal function, including urinalysis, was found and urinary vanillylmandelic and homovanillic acids were in the normal range for age. Moreover, an abdominal ultrasound examination (Fig. 1) showed a large (10×10 cm in diameter) mainly solid intrarenal mass. Contrast-enhanced CT of the abdomen (Fig. 2) confirmed the presence of a left dishomogeneous renal tumor and a CT of the chest (Fig. 3) revealed multiple pulmonary densities also evident on standard chest radiographs.

- What is the diagnosis?
- What is the differential diagnosis?
- Which other tests would you perform in this case?
- What is the role of surgery in this disease?

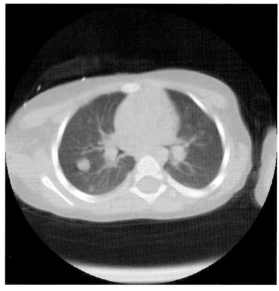

Fig. 3

A 244

In this case, the final diagnosis was three-phase Wilms' tumor without anaplasia, stage IV.

The chief differential diagnosis is neuroblastoma; however, the distinction is usually made on imaging studies because nephroblastoma is intrarenal, whereas most neuroblastomas arise from the adrenal gland and only displace the kidney. Other benign and malignant intrarenal neoplasms, such as mesoblastic nephroma, renal cyst, multicystic kidney, or renal rhabdomyosarcoma, require the benefit of biopsy to be properly diagnosed.

A radionuclide bone scan and radiographic skeletal survey should be obtained in children with pulmonary or hepatic metastases.

All pediatric renal tumors can be staged according to the National Wilms' Tumor Study Group (NWTSG) Criteria:

a. Stage I: the tumor, confined to the kidney, is completely resected
b. Stage II: there is penetration of the renal capsule or invasion of the renal sinus vessels, or biopsy of the tumor before removal or spillage of the tumor during removal, but the tumor is completely resected
c. Stage III: gross or microscopic residual tumor remains postoperatively
d. Stage IV: distant metastases, more commonly to the lung (80% of cases) and to the liver (15% of cases).
e. Stage V: bilateral renal tumors

The single most important prognostic factor is the histologic finding of anaplasia. However, lymph node involvement and, of course, stage of disease retain their importance as predictors of outcome.

Immediate and complete removal of the primary tumor, if feasible, is mandatory even in the presence of lung metastases. However, NWTSG recommends delayed surgery and preoperative chemotherapy for patients with tumor extension into the inferior vena cava above the hepatic veins, for lesions judged to be unresectable, and for patients with bilateral tumors.

Suggested Reading

1. Beckwith JB. National Wilms' Tumor Study: an update for pathologists. Pediatr Dev Pathol 1998; 1:79
2. Breslow NE et al. Clinicopathologic features and prognosis for Wilms' tumor patients with metastases at diagnosis. Cancer 1986; 58: 2501
3. Ritchey ML et al. Management and outcome of inoperable Wilms' tumor. A report of National Wilms' Tumor Study-3. Ann Surg 1994; 220:683

Q 245

Amedeo Fiorillo

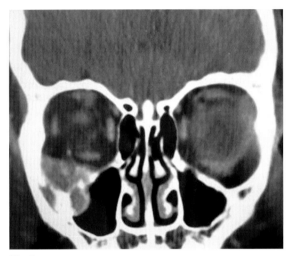

Fig. 1

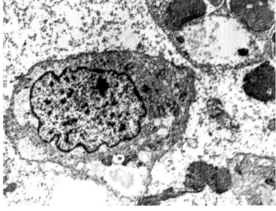

Fig. 2

A 7-year-old boy was admitted to our department with a 4-month history of a painless swelling of the lower orbital region. On admission, his general condition was good. Physical examination showed a painless swelling involving the lower right eyelid and the corresponding malar region; mild proptosis was also evident, but ocular motility was preserved. Pertinent laboratory test results were normal. A CT scan of the head showed a destructive lesion extensively involving the right maxillary bone (Fig. 1), without evidence of surrounding soft tissue involvement.

The initial diagnostic imaging evaluation included a CT scan of the neck region, chest, and abdomen, a skeletal radiographic survey, a radionuclide 99mTc bone scan, and a bone marrow biopsy; all were normal.

Histologic examination of tumor tissue, obtained by an excisional biopsy, revealed a small cell tumor. Special staining revealed the presence of a large amount of periodic acid-Schiff-positive material, consistent with intracellular glycogen. Electron microscopy showed undifferentiated neoplastic cells of a round shape, the predominant feature being abundant glycogen deposition corresponding to the vacuolated cytoplasmic areas (Fig. 2).

- What is the diagnosis?
- What evaluation should be performed?
- What is the prognosis?
- What is the treatment strategy?

A 245

The clinical and histologic features of this case are all consistent with a diagnosis of Ewing's sarcoma. More commonly, it is an undifferentiated tumor of the bone, but it may also arise from soft tissues. A more differentiated form of this disease, known as peripheral primitive neuroectodermal tumor (PPNET), also occurs. It is now widely accepted that all these entities represent a spectrum of a single disease.

Ewing's sarcoma must be differentiated from other small round-cell tumors such as neuroblastoma, rhabdomyosarcoma, lymphoma, and from inflammatory disease, especially if the patient is febrile and an elevated erythrocyte sedimentation rate is found. Neither a blood test nor a urine test provides specific markers of Ewing's sarcoma; however, immunocytochemistry is of value. Typical undifferentiated Ewing's sarcoma is defined as a neoplasm that has immunoreactivity only for vimentin and is negative for neuron-specific enolase (NSE); in contrast, PPNET reacts with vimentin and with a number of neural markers (NSE, beta2-microglobulin). Rhabdomyosarcoma shows positivity to desmin, myoglobin, and actin. Neuroblastoma may be differentiated by using monoclonal antibody NCL-NB84, which is expressed in more than 90% neuroblastomas but not in Ewing's sarcoma.

Major prognosticators are the localization of the primary tumor (axial localization implies a very poor prognosis) and presence of overt metastases at diagnosis. However, evaluation of chemotherapy-induced necrosis is also of prognostic value.

According to the histologic response grading method, based on the four-tiered semiquantitative grading system for osteosarcoma treatment effect, grade I is tumor necrosis of less than 50% of the tumor, grade II is tumor necrosis of more than 50% to less than 90%, grade III is tumor necrosis of 90% to 99%, and grade IV is tumor necrosis of 100%. Event-free survival at 5 years was 0% for grade I, 37.5% for grade II, and 84% for grade III and IV.

It is widely accepted that prompt chemotherapy is necessary to treat occult micrometastases, present in over 80% of cases at diagnosis. However, it is also mandatory, for definitive cure of these patients, to achieve and maintain local control of the primary tumor. This could be obtained by radical surgery for accessible sites and when the patient would not be exposed to the risk of unacceptable mutilations. Alternatively, as in the present case, radiation therapy can be used, provided that it is optimally delivered in terms of total dose and planning of treatment.

Suggested Reading

1. Dunst J and Schuck A. Role of radiotherapy in Ewing tumors. Pediatr Blood Cancer 2004; 42:465
2. Ginsberg JP et al (2002) Ewing's sarcoma family of tumors: Ewing's sarcoma of bone and soft tissue and the peripheral primitive neuroectodermal tumors. In: Pizzo PA, Poplack DG (eds) Principles and Practice of Pediatric Oncology. Lippincott, Philadelphia, pp 973–1016
3. Wunder JS et al. The histological response to chemotherapy as a predictor of oncological outcome of operative treatment of Ewing sarcoma. J Bone Joint Surg Am 1998; 80:1020

Q 246

Amedeo Fiorillo

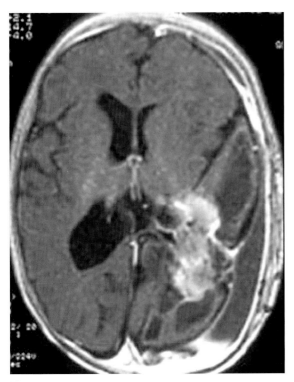

Fig. 1

A 3-month-old white boy presented with signs of increased intracranial pressure. MR imaging of the head showed a contrast-enhanced intraventricular mass and subdural fluid collection (Fig. 1). Following partial surgical removal of the tumor, microscopic examination revealed a papillary lesion with columnar epithelium (Fig. 2); neoplastic cells showed cytologic atypia and increased mitotic activity (Fig. 3).

- What is the diagnosis?
- What is the prognosis of this disease?
- What is the best therapeutic strategy?

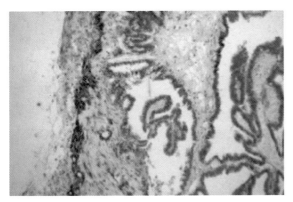

Fig. 2

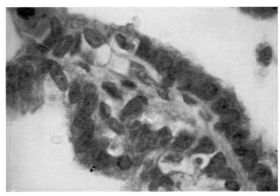

Fig. 3

A 246

The intraventricular location together with the histological features point to the diagnosis of choroids plexus carcinoma; this condition is to be differentiated from embryonal tumors, malignant ependymoma, and germ cell tumors. However, immunohistochemistry is highly useful for differential diagnosis. In choroid tumors, neoplastic cells usually show immunoreactivity for cytokeratins and staining for S-100 protein and vimentin, whereas glial fibrillary acidic protein (GFAP), carcinoembryonic antigen (CEA), and placental alkaline phosphatase (PLAP) are negative.

The disease accounts for less than 1% of childhood brain tumors and is characterized by a very dismal prognosis with few patients surviving more than 6 months after a partial surgical resection.

The most favorable prognosticator is represented by the gross total resection of the tumor, usually hampered by its high degree of vascularity and friability.

Systemic chemotherapy has been used, with some success, before surgical intervention in order to reduce the tumor volume, to diminish its vascular response, and in turn to facilitate its surgical removal. Furthermore, there is recent evidence that systemic chemotherapy can be of value, as adjuvant therapy, even in patients with partially resected tumors; alkylating agents, etoposide, vincristine, and platinum compounds have been mainly used. More recently, excellent results have been obtained by the association of doxorubicin and methotrexate with carboplatin and cyclophosphamide.

Suggested Reading

1. Fiorillo A et al. Efficacy of sequential chemotherapy including methotrexate and doxorubicin in an infant with partially resected choroid plexus carcinoma. Pediatr Neurosurg 2003; 38:21
2. McEvoy AW et al. Management of choroid plexus tumors in children: 20 years experience at a single neuro-surgical centre. Pediatr Neurosurg 2000; 32:192
3. Souweidane MM et al. Volumetric reduction of a choroids plexus carcinoma using preoperative chemotherapy. J Neurooncol 1999; 43:167

Q 247

Christophe Chardot and Sylviane Hanquinet

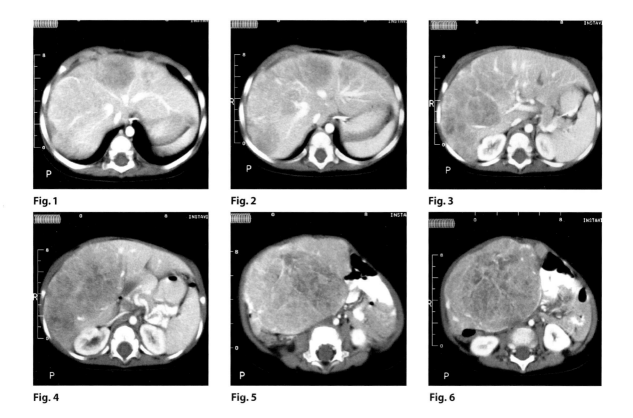

Fig. 1   Fig. 2   Fig. 3

Fig. 4   Fig. 5   Fig. 6

A 13-month-old boy presented with increasing abdominal distension, which had been recently noticed by his parents. His general condition was good. Clinical examination revealed a large mass of the right upper quadrant of the abdomen.

- Which diagnosis can be suspected?

Abdominal US revealed a multinodular liver tumor.

- What biological test is likely to confirm the diagnosis of hepatoblastoma?

Figures 1–6 represent the CT scan at diagnosis.

- How would you define the extension of the tumor?
- How would you stage this tumor according to the SIOPEL PRETEXT classification?

The diagnosis of hepatoblastoma was confirmed by needle biopsy.

- What are the main rules for the treatment of such a tumor?

This child was treated with initial chemotherapy, according to the SIOPEL 3 protocol. Chemotherapy was well tolerated, and the oncological response was good, with significant tumor shrinkage and a decrease of the alphafetoprotein (AFP) level to 242 UI/l. Preoperative imaging showed residual tumor in the right liver (segments 4 to 8), and two small nodules in segments 2 and 4, without extrahepatic disease.

- What is the preoperative stage of the tumor?
- What are the surgical options?

A 247

The abdominal mass in the right upper abdominal quadrant is likely to be a tumor. The most common abdominal tumors in this age group are nephroblastoma, neuroblastoma, and hepatoblastoma; choledochal cyst, benign hepatic tumors (cystic mesenchymal hamartoma), duodenal duplication, pancreatic tumor, and lymphoma are also possible.

The serum alpha-fetoprotein level is 15,00,000 UI/l (normal value <5 UI/l): the diagnosis of hepatoblastoma is almost certain. Another rare cause of multiple liver nodules and elevated AFP is tyrosinemia. Normal AFP levels do not exclude malignant liver tumors: mainly nonsecreting hepatoblastomas or hepatocarcinomas and sarcomas.

When describing the extension of the tumor, the following questions should be addressed:
- Uni- or multifocal tumor?
- Confined to the liver or extrahepatic extension?
  - Intra-abdominal fluid (ruptured tumor?)
  - Perihepatic extension: diaphragm, liver hilum, other intra-abdominal organs
  - Pulmonary metastasis
  - Extra-abdominal and extrathoracic involvement (brain, bone, etc.): imaging according to clinical findings
- The intrahepatic extension is defined by localization of the tumor as compared to the main vessels, portal bifurcation and hepatic veins:
  - Portal bifurcation delimits
    • Couinaud's segment 1 behind the portal bifurcation
    • The rest of the liver (Couinaud's segments 2 to 8) anterior to the portal bifurcation
  - Hepatic veins define four hepatic sectors:
    • Right lateral sector (Couinaud's segments 6 and 7) on the right of the right hepatic vein
    • Right medial sector (Couinaud's segments 5 and 8) between the right and the median hepatic veins
    • Left medial sector (Couinaud's segment 4) between the median hepatic vein and the umbilical scissure
    • Left lateral sector (Couinaud's segments 2 and 3) on the left of the umbilical scissure
- Patency or invasion/thrombosis of the hepatic veins and portal vein

In this case, the tumor is multinodular, without extrahepatic extension. The main tumor invades segments 5 to 8 (Figs. 2–4), with intra-abdominal protrusion of the tumor (Figs. 5, 6). There are also nodules in segments 2 and 4 (Figs.1, 2). The right portal vein is compressed by the tumor, but there is no radiological evidence of vascular invasion.

SIOPEL (Liver Tumors Study Group of the International Society of Paediatric Oncology) has created the PRETEXT (Pre-Therapeutic Extension) classification, which reflects the intrahepatic extension of the disease, and allows stratification of the patients into several therapeutic and prognostic subgroups. The PRETEXT categories are based on the number of hepatic sectors (cf. supra) free of tumor:
- PRETEXT 1: three adjacent hepatic sectors free of tumor
- PRETEXT 2: two adjacent hepatic sectors free of tumor
- PRETEXT 3: one hepatic sector, or two nonadjacent sectors, free of tumor
- PRETEXT 4: all four hepatic sectors invaded
- Extrahepatic growth is indicated by adding one ore more of the following characters: V (main hepatic veins or vena cava invaded), P (portal vein or large portal branches invaded), E (intra-abdominal extrahepatic invasion), M (distant metastases: mostly lungs)

In the case described here, all hepatic sectors are invaded, without apparent vascular or extrahepatic involvement: PRETEXT 4 tumor, V-, P-, E-, M- (Fig. 7).

The main rules for the treatment of hepatoblastomas are:
- The patient must be treated according to one of the current international protocols, using a multidisciplinary approach.
- Complete excision of the primary liver tumor is necessary: this can often be achieved by partial hepatectomy, but may necessitate total hepatectomy (and liver transplantation) in some cases. All modern techniques and expertise in liver surgery are required. If total hepatectomy and liver transplantation are necessary (PRETEXT 3 and 4 tumors), the child should be referred early on to a pediatric liver transplantation center for assessment, planning of the treatment

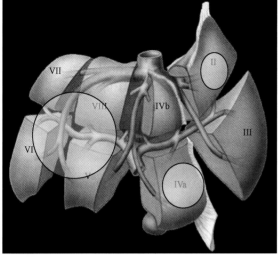

Fig. 7

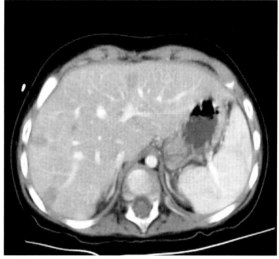

Fig. 8

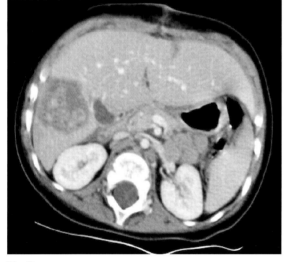

Fig. 9

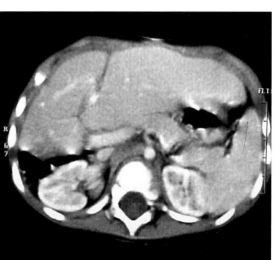

Fig. 10

(including possible living related liver donation), and family information.

– Hepatoblastomas usually have a good response to chemotherapy. Preoperative chemotherapy is therefore recommended in most protocols in order to induce tumor shrinkage; it allows safer surgery with lower risk of incomplete resection and/or tumor spillage.

The preoperative stage of the tumor is a multinodular nonmetastatic PRETEXT 4 hepatoblastoma. In order to completely remove all residual intrahepatic tumor, total hepatectomy and liver transplantation are currently (2008) recommended in such a case. Due to the risk of prolonged waiting times for a cadaveric liver graft, and subsequent tumor regrowth while waiting for transplantation, living related donation is proposed to the family in order for surgery to be performed at the optimal time after the initial chemotherapy.

Nevertheless, when this child was treated in 2001, conservative surgery was preferred. Since right hepatectomy and tumorectomies of the nodules in the left liver may have exposed the child to postoperative liver insufficiency (due to potential shortage of remaining liver parenchyma), a two-stage surgery was chosen: first tumorectomy of the nodules in segments 2 and 4, and right portal vein ligation; then 1 month later, after growth of the remaining left liver, right hepatectomy. The child underwent uneventful surgery and postoperative chemotherapy. Histology revealed viable hepatoblastoma in all three resected tumors, with surgical margins free of disease. Figure 8 shows tumor shrinkage after initial chemotherapy. Figure 9 shows the liver 4 weeks after the first operation: the left liver has grown, and the right portal branches are not opacified. Figure 10 shows the liver 6 months after the second operation: the remaining left liver is hypertrophied without tumor recurrence. The child was alive and well 7 years after surgery.

Acknowledgements: To Prof. Claude Le Coultre and Gilles Mentha, who operated on this child.

Suggested Reading

1. Aronson DC, Schnater JM, Staalman CR, Weverling GJ, Plaschkes J, Perilongo G et al. Predictive value of the pretreatment extent of disease system in hepatoblastoma: results from the International Society of Pediatric Oncology Liver Tumor Study Group SIOPEL-1 study. J Clin Oncol 2005; 23(6):1245–52
2. Brown J, Perilongo G, Shafford E, Keeling J, Pritchard J, Brock P et al. Pretreatment prognostic factors for children with hepatoblastoma—results from the International Society of Paediatric Oncology (SIOP) study SIOPEL 1. Eur J Cancer 2000; 36(11):1418–25
3. Czauderna P, Otte JB, Aronson DC, Gauthier F, Mackinlay G, Roebuck D et al. Guidelines for surgical treatment of hepatoblastoma in the modern era—recommendations from the Childhood Liver Tumour Strategy Group of the International Society of Paediatric Oncology (SIOPEL). Eur J Cancer 2005; 41(7):1031–6

Q 248

Yves Aigrain and Pascale Philippe-Chomette

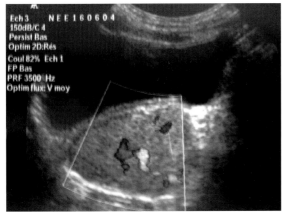

Fig. 1

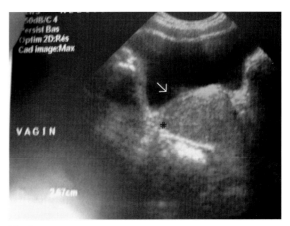

Fig. 2

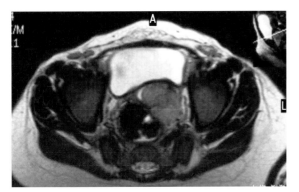

Fig. 3

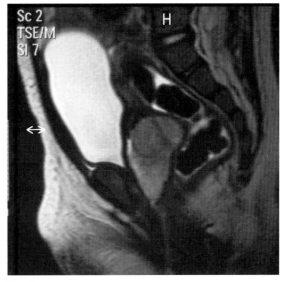

Fig. 4

A healthy 20-month-old girl presented with vaginal bleeding.

Clinical examination revealed active vaginal bleeding. A solid anterior pelvic mass was found at digital rectal examination prolapsing from the vaginal area, without any sign of precocious pseudopuberty.

A US examination was performed (Figs. 1, 2).

- Can you describe the US findings?
- What other radiological examinations would you ask for?
- Can you describe the examination shown in Figs. 3 and 4? What are your hypotheses?

Biological tests were performed, yielding the following results: alpha-fetoprotein (AFP), 6,500 UI; beta human chorionic gonadotropin hormone, 0.

- What is your diagnosis?
- What is your strategy?
- What other explorations could be proposed in this case?

A 248

There is a solid vaginal mass with bleeding as the principal symptom.

The US examination confirms the vaginal site and the vascularized character of the tumor. In this age group, there is the possibility of vaginal rhabdomyosarcoma or vaginal germ-cell tumor.

A chest radiograph and an abdominal and pelvic MR imaging examination should be requested.

The pelvic MR imaging examination shows a vaginal tumor with tissular component and blood inside.

With a high AFP level, the diagnosis is yolk sac tumor, also called endodermal sinus tumor. This is a malignant germ cell tumor. The elevation of AFP serves as a diagnostic tumor marker and a method with which to evaluate response to treatment and monitor postoperative recurrence.

Primary chemotherapy should be started to reduce the tumoral volume; endoscopy with biopsy could be useful simply to localize the origin of the tumor before chemotherapy, but not imperative. The diagnosis is established with the high level of AFP (Fig. 5).

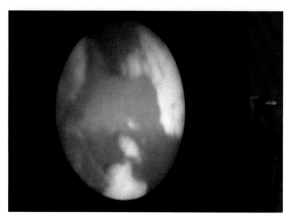

Fig. 5

Suggested Reading

1. Handel LN, Scott SM, Giller RH, Greffe BS, Lovell MA, Koyle MA. New perspectives on therapy for vaginal endodermal sinus tumors. J Urol 2002 Aug; 168(2):687–90

2. Lacy J, Capra M, Allen L. Endodermal sinus tumor of the infant vagina treated exclusively with chemotherapy. J Pediatr Hematol Oncol 2006 Nov; 28(11):768–71

3. Terenziani M, Spreafico F, Collini P, Meazza C, Massimino M, Piva L. Endodermal sinus tumor of the vagina. Pediatr Blood Cancer 2005 Sep 30

Q 249

Craig T. Albanese

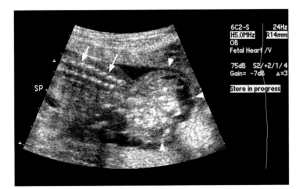

Fig. 1

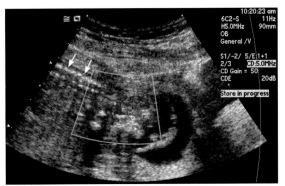

Fig. 2

An 18-week prenatal ultrasound (Fig. 1) of the lower fetal spine revealed a large caudal mass (*arrowheads*; spine, *arrows*). A color Doppler sonogram (Fig. 2) demonstrates blood supply to the mass, which is derived from enlarged branches of the middle sacral artery and internal iliac arteries (spine, *arrows*). A fetal MR imaging study (Fig. 3) with a fluid-sensitive sequence demonstrates that the mass (*arrowheads*) is largely fluid-containing with a small solid (*asterisk*) component.

- What are the findings and what is your diagnosis?

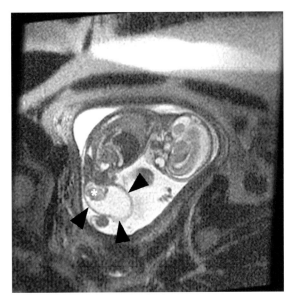

Fig. 3

A 249

This is a sacrococcygeal teratoma. This lesion is complex (cystic and solid). Predominantly solid lesions have a very rich blood supply that can cause fetal hydrops due to high output cardiac failure. Note the bright calcifications (Fig. 1) in the mass. They are rarely malignant.

Suggested Reading

1. Bittmann S, Bittmann V. Surgical experience and cosmetic outcomes in children with sacrococcygeal teratoma. Curr Surg 2006 Jan–Feb; 63(1):51–4

2. Makin EC, Hyett J, Ade-Ajayi N, Patel S, Nicolaides K, Davenport M. Outcome of antenatally diagnosed sacrococcygeal teratomas: single-center experience (1993–2004). J Pediatr Surg 2006 Feb; 41(2):388–93

3. Schmidt B, Haberlik A, Uray E, Ratschek M, Lackner H, Hollwarth ME. Sacrococcygeal teratoma: clinical course and prognosis with a special view to long-term functional results. Pediatr Surg Int 1999; 15(8):573–6

Index

Contents Page by Page

4 Genitourinary Disorders 255

5 Cardiovascular Disorders 319

Subject Index